Behavioral Methods in Social Welfare

Behavioral Methods in Social Welfare

Helping Children, Adults, and Families in Community Settings

Edited
by Steven Paul Schinke

Foreword by James Whittaker and Scott Briar

AldineTransaction
A Division of Transaction Publishers
New Brunswick (U.S.A.) and London (U.K.)

Second paperback printing 2009

This book is printed on acid-free paper that meets the American National Standard for Permanence of Paper for Printed Library Materials.

Library of Congress Catalog Number: 2008002648
ISBN: 978-0-202-36214-4
Printed in the United States of America

Library of Congress Cataloging-in-Publication Data

Behavioral methods in social welfare : helping children, adults, and families in community settings / edited by Steven Paul Schinke.
p. ; cm.—(Modern applications of social work)
Originally published: New York: Aldine Pub. Co., 1981.
Includes bibliographical references and indexes.
ISBN 978-0-202-36214-4 (alk. paper)
1. Social service. 2. Behavior modification. 3. Social psychology. I. Schinke, Steven Paul. II. Series.
[DNLM: 1. Behavior Therapy. 2. Social Work. 3. Community Mental Health Services. 4. Psychology, Social. WM 425 B41995 1981a]

HV37.B43 2008
361.3'2—dc22 2008002648

Table of Contents

Acknowledgments

Most of the people deserving credit for this book are acknowledged in the Table of Contents. Thus, my mentors, Sheldon Rose and Bill Butterfield, continue contributing to my education. I am indebted to both. My University of Wisconsin chums, Rob Schilling, Rick Grinnell, Stan Witkin, Jeff Edelson, and Ray Berger, further helped me along the way. Representing a recent stage in my development, Seattle colleagues Lew Gilchrist, Betty Blythe, Sharon Berlin, and Cheryl Richey show their influence. Also represented are a pair of conspirators who earn my respect and gratitude. In an insidiously effective effort, Scott Briar and Jim Whittaker ply continuous reinforcement to shape my interests and habits.

Owning much of my prosperity are special people at two places where I pass many happy hours. The University of Washington Child Development and Mental Retardation Center sustains my clinical and research foci through the beneficence of its Director, Irvin Emanuel, its Administrator, Henry Schulte, and its harmonious crew, embodying Lois Winters, Dick McDonald, Kyum Ha Lee, Greg Owen, Ed Lowe, Jeanne Scott, Marion Johnson, Jim Sackett, Sharon Landesman-Dwyer, Jerry Sells, Helen Hoffman, Mary Pierce, and Mary Richardson. Fellow social workers Peggy West, Judi LeConte, Jan Garretson, and Jim Hall keep me in line too. University of Washington School of Social Work accomplices in part responsible for my behavior are Associate Deans Naomi Gottlieb and Ted Teather, Administrator Elissa Dyson, and stalwarts Elsie Faires, Vern Bryant, Henry Maier, Jim Anderson, Gail Mathieson, Gail Nyman, Rino Patti, Guela Johnson, Mike Austin, Stephanie Prince, Dave Snyder, Rona Levy, and Tony Ishisaka.

The geography separating us does not hamper four Easterners from markedly advancing my career. Virginia Insley and Juanita Evans from Maternal and Child Health in Rockville, freely give me their counsel, sagacity, and succor in good times and bad. I feel privileged to have these social workers as professional associates and, more important, as dear friends. Ted Tjossem and Mike Begab from the National Institute of Child Health and Human Development in Bethesda kindly sponsor my more recondite research. I look forward to lots of future collaborations with each of these gentleman.

Over the years, tangible aid at least indirectly touching this volume was given by Maternal and Child Health Training Project No. 913 from the Bureau of Community Health Services (Health Services Administration), by Mental Retardation and Development Disabilities Branch Grant HD 02274, and Center for Population Research Grant HD 11095 from the National Institute of Child Health and Human Development (National Institutes of Health), all administered through the United States Public Health Service, Department of Health and Human Services, and awarded to the University of Washington Child Development and Mental Retardation Center.

Collegiate and concrete support are necessary to start any book. No matter how brilliant, felicitous, and rich, however, ideas produce fruit only when nurtured by those committed to myriad, intermediate tasks. Contributors to the present product are fortunate to have a small cohort of highly competent professionals willing to take on and follow through on such commitments. I, and my co-authors, humbly thank a sextet of ghost writers: Anna Bolstad, Joan Hiltner, Lois Holt, Lesley Link, John Wander, and Edith Watson.

Authors

Raymond M. Berger, Ph.D.
Assistant Professor
School of Social Work
University of Illinois at Urbana-Champaign
Urbana, Illinois 61801

Sharon B. Berlin, Ph.D.
Assistant Professor
School of Social Work
University of Wisconsin
Madison, Wisconsin 53706

Betty J. Blythe, M.S.W.
Associate
School of Social Work
University of Washington
Seattle, Washington 98195

Scott Briar, D.S.W.
Professor and Dean
School of Social Work
University of Washington
Seattle, Washington 98195

William H. Butterfield, Ph.D.
Associate Professor, and Chair of the Doctoral Program
George Warren Brown School of Social Work
Washington University
St. Louis, Missouri 63130

Edmond T. Dimock, M.S.W.
Manager, Group Home Program
Children's Home Society of California, Northern District
Chico, California 95926

Wayne D. Duehn, Ph.D
Professor
Graduate School of Social Work
University of Texas at Arlington
Arlington, Texas 76019

Jeffrey L. Edleson, Ph.D.
Assistant Professor
School of Social Welfare
State University of New York at Albany
Albany, New York 12222

Benjamin S. Friedman, Ph.D.
Health Care Consultant
Community Health Management Corporation/
Community Health Foundation
Evanston, Illinois 60201

Eileen D. Gambrill, Ph.D.
Professor
School of Social Welfare
University of California, Berkeley
Berkeley, California 94720

Lewayne D. Gilchrist, M.S.W.
Doctoral Candidate
School of Social Work
University of Washington
Seattle, Washington 98195

Richard L. Gorsuch, Ph.D.
Professor of Psychology and Director of Research
Graduate School of Psychology
Fuller Theological Seminary
Pasadena, California 91101

Richard M. Grinnell, Jr., Ph.D.
Associate Professor
Graduate School of Social Work
University of Texas at Arlington
Arlington, Texas 76019

Alice Lieberman, M.S.W.
Doctoral Student
School of Social Work
University of Washington
Madison, Wisconsin 53706

Mary Ann Lynch, M.A.
Program Evaluator
Dallas County Mental Health and Mental Retardation Center
Dallas, Texas 75206

Nazneen Sada Mayadas, D.S.W.
Professor
Graduate School of Social Work
University of Texas at Arlington
Arlington, Texas 76019

Elsie M. Pinkston, Ph.D.
Associate Professor
School of Social
Service Administration
University of Chicago
Chicago, Illinois 60637

Richard A. Polster, Ph.D.
Assistant Professor
Graduate School of Social Work
University of Texas at Arlington
Arlington, Texas 76019

Cheryl A. Richey, D.S.W.
Associate Professor
School of Social Work
University of Washington
Seattle, Washington 98195

Sheldon, D. Rose, Ph.D.
Professor
School of Social Work
University of Wisconsin
Madison, Wisconsin 53706

Robert F. Schilling, II, M.S.W.
Clinical Instructor
Child Development and Mental Retardation Center
University of Washington
Seattle, Washington 98195

Steven Paul Schinke, Ph.D.
Associate Professor, School of Social Work, and
Director of Social Services, Child Development and
Mental Retardation Center
University of Washington
Seattle, Washington 98195

Theodore J. Stein, D.S.W.
Associate Professor
Jane Addams School of Social Work
University of Illinois at Chicago Circle
Chicago, Illinois 60680

Judith Werking, M.S.W.
Private Practice
16 Phillip Road
Oxford, Mississippi 38655

James K. Whittaker, Ph.D.
Professor
School of Social Work
University of Washington
Seattle, Washington 98195

Stanley Witkin, Ph.D.
Assistant Professor
School of Social Work
Florida State University
Tallahassee, Florida 32306

John S. Wodarski, Ph.D.
Professor, and Director of the Research Institute
School of Social Work
University of Georgia
Athens, Georgia 30602

Foreword

This book offers proof positive that behaviorism has come of age in social work. Steven Schinke and his contributors are social work practitioners/teachers who document their attempts to extend the basic tenets of behavioral psychology from the laboratory, clinic and classroom to the full range of client groups and social problems that make up the present practice scene.

It has not always been so. Even today, in many agency settings, the acceptance of behavioral methods remains tentative. Take, for example, the frustration evident in the statement recently made by a British social work colleague attempting to implement a behavioral approach in a child guidance clinic: "My colleagues say, you deal with the encopresis, bedwetting and fire-setting, we'll handle the core problems in psychotherapy!"

In social work education, things were often not much better in terms of behavioral content, which, to the extent it appeared in the curriculum at all, appeared in electives or in courses not focused on practice. It is a true measure of progress, amply evidenced by the selections in this volume, that behavioral methods are now a more visible, integral component of both social work education and practice.

With this new visibility has come an explosion of some of the myths and clichés surrounding behavioral practice in general:

—— *It is mechanistic and de-humanizing.* Read Richey's sensitive account of how women become help-mates to each other in acquiring assertiveness skills.

—— *It ignores cognitive process.* Read Berlin's, Duehn's and Mayadas's accounts of how cognitive and behavioral approaches can be combined to deal with sensitive interpersonal problems.

——*It can't work with the kind of complex problems faced by social workers.* Read Dimock and Stein and Gambrill on multi-problem family interventions.

Taken as a whole, these contributors show how far we have come in developing an empirically based approach to social work practice—and how much work remains to be done.

Behavioral methods offer no panacea to social work and, despite the impressive documentation contained in the present volume, no conclusive evidence as yet. What behavioral methods *do* offer, however, is a systematic format for both problem intervention and evaluation that, over time, will produce a more empirically based practice. One promising sign, well documented in the present effort, is the facility with which Schinke and his contributors have subjected their practice procedures to the rigor of research and evaluation.

Though this beginning attempt to blend clinical practice and research is not without its own set of special problems, as we are well aware from our own experience here at the University of Washington, it offers many benefits as well, notably the sense of competence that student-practitioners acquire in understanding and controlling both the art and science of their clinical practice. For example, behaviorists have rediscovered the importance of "relationships" in the casework process—and have given new and specific meaning to that term. Thoughts and feelings along with concrete operant behavior now figure prominently in the behavioral perspective.

Whether all of this will end in a new conceptualization of the casework process is not entirely clear. Steven Schinke and his colleagues do not offer a definitive model for practice, but a series of "snapshots" of important work in process. Their collective effort provides a fresh perspective and new stimulus for all social work practice, as well as an affirmation that disciplined, responsive and sensitive social work intervention can and does make a difference in the lives of people.

James K. Whittaker
Scott Briar
University of Washington School of Social Work

Introduction

Social work attempts to understand and to solve human problems. The practice of social work translates abstract theory into concrete methods for analyzing and alleviating personal and societal stresses. Within a range of settings, organizations, and roles, social workers address the complete life-cycle. Hospital nurseries, daycare centers, public schools, public welfare agencies, residential treatment and correctional facilities, and nursing homes for older persons alike are organizational structures for social work. Social workers serve in these agencies as therapists, supervisors, consultants, educators, adminstrators, researchers, and policy analysts.

Despite this diversity, common goals unify social work practice. Social workers help people. In the seventeenth edition of the *Encyclopedia of Social Work,* spokesman Scott Briar concludes that taken together the many goals of the profession "express a desire to enhance the quality of life and opportunities for maximum self-development and well-being for all persons" (1977a, p. 1530). Subsumed under our help-giving mission are interpersonal practice functions of individual counseling, group therapy, client advocacy, and resource coordination. Professional objectives are met through one or more of these functions.

Help is given in a myriad of ways, most guided by underlying theory. Whittaker (1974) outlines twenty-one social work methods including activity-group therapy, behavior modification, conjoint family treatment, existential psychotherapy, guided group interaction, milieu treatment, play therapy, self-help groups, and transactional analysis. Each offers a perspective from which to understand, assess, or change human behavior. Choice of a particular helping method rests on multiple factors. Factors relevant for social work practice span agency setting, client population, presenting problem, worker training, prevailing attitudes and biases, and logistical arrangements of time, physical space, and caseload. The theme of the present chapter—indeed of the entire volume—is that regardless of the relative weights assigned these factors, prepotent social work occurs when help is given via behavioral methods.

Thus, the thesis advanced here is that behavioral social work presages considerable profit for professional practice. Behavioral methods have come of age in social work. They must now become vital, integral components of our practice wisdom. This introduction gives a rationale for assigning importance to behavioral methods and suggests why social workers are hesitant to embrace behavior modification. Reviewed is the evolution of behavioral technology from research in controlled settings to social programs conducted in the natural environment. Adumbrated and detailed are advantages of applied behavioral programs, pitfalls encountered in such programs, and guidelines for avoiding these pitfalls. Moral and ethical issues of behavioral social work are specified. A prologue to the remainder of the book devotes special attention to the clinical-research approach for teaching the practice of behavioral social work.

RATIONALE AND RESISTANCE

Behavior modification has clear relevance for social work. Behavioral methods center on the client by focusing practice on overt action and change. Examining overt behavior brings to light the client's strengths, weaknesses, and goals. The behavioral approach unifies assessment, intervention, and evaluation so client and worker jointly share diagnosis and treatment. Principles and techniques of behavior modification are applicable to direct practice, case consultation, large social programs, and policy formulation and implementation. Further, its positive, preventive nature makes behavior modification germane to any social work setting. And, the ease of empirically validating behavioral intervention makes the methodology useful for process and outcome research, demonstrations of professional accountability, and data-based feedback.

Still, behavioral practice is eschewed by many social workers. Some may disdain behavior modification because of its origins in experimental psychology. Others may suspect that the heritage in laboratory research render behavioral methods incompatible with field practice. A good number of workers, especially those entering the profession prior to the upsurge of applied behavior modification, seem misinformed about the modality. Another explanation of our colleagues' reluctance to adopt behavior modification is its somewhat tarnished reputation. indisputably, negative stereotypes have been assigned to the paradigm.

Associations with such undistinguished things as cattle prods, psychosurgery, the unwarranted withholding of food and money, rigid adherence to immutable rules, and Machiavellian control of body and mind all give the critic plenty of grist (Hilts, 1974; Hollis, 1968; LeShan & LeShan, 1968). Just the label "behavior modification" conjures up less than objective judgments from lay persons and professionals (Turkat & Feuerstein, 1978; Woolfolk, & Woolfolk, 1979; Woolfolk, Woolfolk, & Wilson 1977).

Slow acceptance of behavior modification does not mean social workers seldom use this intervention in their professional and personal lives. Quite the contrary. Possibly no intervention methods are employed more than those taken from social-learning theory. For example, we routinely apply the Premack Principle (Premack, 1965) by making attractive activities contingent on less attractive ones: "First I have to finish this doggone report, then I can have lunch." Or, "Billy, you can watch TV after you clear the table and load the diswasher." Completing tasks and engaging in social interactions nearly always involves conditional payoffs. Parents give children privileges for doing chores around the house. Employees get smiles, pleasant words, and salary raises for jobs well done. During therapy, nonbehavioral Rogerians reward their clients with verbal contingencies of "Um-hm," "I see," and so forth (Truax, 1966).

Nonethless, unscientific and inconsistent use of behavioral techniques negates and abuses this technology. Reinforcement given at the wrong time strengthens maladaptive behavior. Removal of clients from social stimulation, as happens with the technique of time-out, and implementation of aversion techniques will have untoward effects if not done properly. Certainly, negative procedures must be offset by copious reinforcement of clients' positive responses. Poorly planned behavioral methods delivered within large-scale programs will compound bad side effects and outcomes. Even though they are rare, shocking reports on misuses of these methods (Buckholdt & Gubrium, 1980; Risley, 1975) mandate a good grasp of behavior modification theory and practice before any clinical application.

EVOLUTION OF BEHAVIORAL TECHNOLOGY

Contemporary behavioral methods spring from research on respondent and operant conditioning. Respondent or classical conditioning embodies principles that explain how behavior increases or decreases when paired with some stimulus. A child may remain seated in the car because her parents sharply say "No!" whenever she stands. The child has learned new behavior by responding to the environment. Operant conditioning begets learning when behavior is followed with rewarding or punishing events. As an instance, the author patronizes a local saloon that serves complimentary hors d'oeuvres; he avoids the bar next door that has a loud juke box. Such discrimination was acquired by operating on the environment and experiencing pleasant or unpleasant consequences.

Research on the two social-learning approaches started with analogue investigations of infrahuman behavior. Dogs, cats, pigeons, monkeys, rats, and rabbits are subjects for respondent and operant conditioning studies (Adams & Hughes, 1976; Pavlov, 1928; Whaley & Malott, 1973). To a large part, initial investigation of human behavior stays with analogue responses like memorizing nonsense syllables, engaging in rote motoric tasks, or learning to avoid mild electric shock (Kazdin, 1978a). Heuristic findings from analogue research, may however, direct behaviorists to areas with clinical relevance. The bulk of these new directions are into situations of tightly controlled investigations with clients in fairly restricted environments.

Research in Controlled Settings

Accordingly, problems are approached in places affording vigorous research control. Children are studied in university child development centers, experimental preschools, and institutions for retarded persons. Early investigations remedy children's fear (Jones, 1924), enuresis (Mowrer & Mowrer, 1938), temper tantrums (Williams, 1959), thumbsucking (Baer, 1962), crying (Hart, Allen, Buell, Harris, & Wolf, 1964), poor reading (Staats & Butterfield, 1965), face-scratching (Allen & Harris, 1966), inadequate verbalization (Baer, Peterson, & Sherman, 1967), antisocial play (Hart, Reynolds, Baer, Brawley, & Harris, 1968), and hyperactivity (Patterson, Ray, & Shaw, 1968). Controlled behavior modification research with adults occurs in psychiatric hospitals, outpatient clinics, and college counseling centers. Research in these settings modifies alcohol abuse (Voegtlin, 1940), sexual deviancies (Raymond, 1956), negative reactions to marital sex (Brady, 1966), phobias (Davison, 1968), nondating (Martinson & Zerface, 1970), anxiety (DiLoreto, 1971), poor study skills (Beneke & Harris, 1972), marital disharmony (Azrin, Naster, & Jones, 1973), lack of assertiveness (Hersen, Eisler, & Miller, 1973), hypertension (Elder, Ruiz, Deabler, & Dillenkoffer, 1973), and depression (Hersen, Eisler, Alford, & Agras, 1973).

Laboratory and other experimental sites permit control of key variables that affect results and thereby provide the opportunity to establish cause and effect relationships. Researchers arrange and manipulate the physical surroundings. They precisely define intervention (the independent variable) and accurately measure the outcome of interest (the dependent variable). Experimenters direct therapists and research assistants. Study participants are usually committed and compliant. Self-referred participants portray their motivation by independently seeking help. Psychiatric inpatients and college students receive recompense for study involvement—special privileges, money, quiz points.

Work in the Natural Environment

Clinical research practitioners in social agencies and in the community work outside of an experimental structure. The various settings, of the home, public welfare office, school, family service agency, and substitute-care facility, inhibit control of program design, intervention delivery, and outcome evaluation. On the positive side and overwhelmingly in favor of these sites are chances to validate behavior modification procedures with problems, persons, and real-life situations not seen by researchers in controlled environments.

A pioneer demonstration of behavioral intervention in the community was produced by Schwitzgebel and Kolb (1964) who describe work with delinquent youths. Overall program goals were reduced delinquency and more involvement in school, vocational training, employment, or military service. Approaching these goals, Schwitzgebel and Kolb concentrated on building rapport to foster positive change. The street-level researchers gave tangibles—money, cigarettes, and food—when youths visited a neighborhood office "just to talk." Youths later received rewards when active in recreational and vocational programs. Thenceforward, the former delinquents discovered new opportunities and became able to secure trade-school training and jobs. This gradual process of behavior change is evident in the way community workers engage one wary youth. A worker first meets the young man in a pool hall; next, at a subway entrance near the pool hall; then in front of the subway tollgate; then inside the tollgate; and finally, at a subway exit. Contingent on meeting the worker at a designated spot, the young man gets social and tangible rewards. The investigators compared the outcomes of youths in their program with a group of young delinquents having parallel backgrounds and police records. Three-year follow-up data show youths in Schwitzgebel and Kolb's program with fewer arrests and less months of criminal incarceration than youths in the comparison group.

Another example of community-based behavioral intervention is Achievement Place, a group-home program for delinquent and predelinquent adolescents. Elery Phillips (1968), one of the founders of Achievement Place, tells of a token economy system that enables young residents to earn points for completing home chores and schoolwork; points are lost if youths disobey or lash out physically. Achievement Place residents and staff negotiate individual behavior-change projects, subsequently evaluated through research designs and objective measures. The scores of reports made by Phillips and colleagues portray Achievement Place as a community-based intervention that keeps predelinquency in adolescence from potentially turning into a criminal behavior in adulthood (Phillips, Phillips, Fixsen, & Wolf, 1971; Phillips, Phillips, Wolf, & Fixsen, 1973; Wolf, Phillips, Fixsen, Braukmann, Kirigin, Williner, & Schumaker, 1976).

Child-management training for families in their own homes has obvious ramifications for behavioral social work. According to parent-training expert, Gerald Patterson:

> It seems likely that some families...will find that training in an interview, laboratory or group situation will be ineffective, simply because the procedures are not systematic enough to control their behavior or because the relevant reinforcing contingencies (for parent and child) cannot be properly presented. The necessity for additional precision in training for such families is provided by having the behavior modifier go into the home and carry out the training program in that setting. (1971, p. 756)

A legacy of home-based family training confirms Patterson's statement. Representative work by Hawkins, Peterson, Schweid, and Bijou (1966) takes place in the natural home and helps a mother use operant techniques to reduce her child's temper tantrums, self-injurious behavior, and aggression. Summaries from Graziano (1975), O'Leary, O'Leary and Becker (1967), and Wahler, Winkel, Peterson, and Morrison (1965) establish the predictable success of child-management training in the home. Due to these and other equally committed researchers, community workers have within arm's reach comprehensive instructional materials for home intervention and evaluation (Christophersen 1977; Patterson, 1975; Patterson, Reid, Jones, & Conger, 1975; Reid, 1978).

This review and any similar effort would be incomplete without coverage of the community-based Behavior Research Project. Detailed by Tharp and Wetzel (1969), the Project served behaviorally disordered and predelinquent children and their families across a three-state region. Nonprofessional behavior analysts took care of case planning and evaluation, and parents, teachers, and social caseworkers were in charge of intervention. Field notes from one behavior analyst express processes of assessment, intervention, and evaluation that typify this ambitious endeavor.

> Case #79. David had been picked up for stealing hubcaps and for entering an apartment and dismantling a phone. He was also under suspicion of setting a fire and stealing a large check from a nearby home. David had been getting

> professional help from child guidance agencies, counselors, and probation officers since the first grade, when he began stealing....David was the family scapegoat: the father resented him, felt no responsibility for him, and was physically abusive....For several months we made fruitless attempts to shape the father's mediating behavior. Realizing the necessity of a male reinforcer we introduced an external mediator—a male college student volunteer—who took David out on Saturdays if he met the criterion of not bullying his sibs for a specific length of time. David bullied his sibs on 94% of the baseline days. The 89 days following intervention he engaged in this behavior on 62% of the days. After the introduction of the external mediator, this behavior decreased to 20% of the following 75 days. (Tharp & Wetzel, 1969, pp. 93-94).

Results of the Behavior Research Project are drawn from single-case designs, behavioral ratings, and institutional records of police contracts, school, attendance, and vocational achievement. Based on these data, Tharp and Wetzel posit:

> We believe that the case for behavior modification in the natural environment has now been established in the following areas: contingencies can be managed in the natural environment; behavioral changes can be recorded and assessed; for the behaviorally disordered child, desirable changes can be effected, and, last, it is possible to work in and with the natural environment, according to an operational model derived from nonmedical learning theories. (1969, p. 185)

Like-minded behavioral programs occur in daycare centers (Hall & Holmberg, 1974); Head Start facilities (Madsen, Madsen, & Thompson, 1974): public schools (Filipczak, Archer & Friedman, in press); community mental health agencies (Johnson & Geller, 1980); residential treatment settings (Cuvo, 1973; Libb, House, & Green, 1973); group homes for mentally retarded persons (Schinke, 1979a; Schinke & Wong, 1977(b)); youth detention institutions (Jesness, 1976); youth clubs (Wodarski, Feldman, & Pedi, 1976); campus housing cooperatives (Miller & Feallock, 1975); and industrial sites (Hermann, de Montes, Dominguez, Montes, & Hopkins, 1973). Clinical research in these places has grappled with job finding; (Azrin, Flores, & Kaplan, 1975); employment interviewing (Schinke, Gilchrist, Smith, & Wong, 1978); job placement (Mills & Walter, 1979); work performance (Pierce & Risley, 1974); cigarette smoking (Schinke, Blythe, & Doueck, 1978, 1979); juvenile delinquency (Filipczak, Archer, Neale, & Winett, 1979): shoplifting (McNees, Egli, Marshall, Schnelle, & Risley, 1976); crime prevention (Schnelle, Kirchner, Galbaugh, Domash, Carr, & Larson, 1979): litter dropped by people (Clark, Burgess, & Hendee, 1972) and that left by dogs (Jason, McCoy, Blanco, & Zolik, 1980); waste reduction (Geller, 1980); energy consumption (Winett & Neitzel, 1975); and use of public transportation (Everett, 1980).

ADVANTAGES OF APPLIED BEHAVIORAL PROGRAMS

Behavioral programs conducted in the field have distinct advantages over laboratory research. Extant literature (Davids & Berenson, 1977; Gambrill, Thomas, & Carter, 1971; Jason, 1977, 1978; Meyers & Schleser, in press; Thomas and Walter, 1973) and this author's experiences point to at least seven advantages. Elucidated below, these include focus in situ, indigenous reinforcement, tailored intervention, problem solving, treatment packaging, social validation, and carry-over of change.

Focus In Situ

A focus on problems where they happen is a clear advantage of behavioral social work in applied settings. Contrasted with work having a community locale are traditional programs in which clients are removed from everyday milieus and given group and individual counseling within a specific treatment setting. A community program running counter to formal treatment is that of Schwitzgebel and Kolb (1964) where delinquent youths are met on street corners and in pool halls, and thus engaged in neighborhood recreation and habilitation.

Indigenous Reinforcement

Clients in the natural environment have opportunities to choose from an array of meaningful reinforcers. Schwitzgebel and Kolb find their youths selecting cigarettes, candy, and money as preferred rewards. Our group at the University of Washington plies young people who participate in skills-training programs with bus tokens, tokens for pinball machines, pizza, cold cash and soda pop, and the infamous Twinky—always popular with the younger crowd. More traditional programs infrequently proffer these attractive incentives. Also, use of the already mentioned Premack Principle is significantly aided by programs designed and implemented where clients live and work. In the home, family members literally survey their immediate environment to discover tangible and social reinforcers. These could take into account watching the goldfish, listening the to the stereo, playing with the cat, giving or receiving a backrub, raiding the refrigerator, working on the car, going for a walk, and simply doing nothing at all.

Tailored Intervention

Adapting behavioral techniques and procedures to fit individual clients will create efficient and effective intervention. Even formidable impediments to case planning and service delivery can be skirted when intervention is not bound by a predetermined structure. Tharp and Wetzel (1969) relate how their work tailors intervention to the natural environment:

> When Carl asked for an increase in his allowance the Behavior Analyst suggested to the mother that this was an opportunity to work on his use of obscene language which had been annoying her. The mother began giving Carl an extra quarter with his Saturday morning allowance, but required that a nickel be forfeited in a ceramic pig each time she heard Carl use an obscenity. The necessity of "pigging" Carl rapidly decreased (p. 110).

Such tailoring makes optimal use of natural systems to bring the presenting problem under control and to then positively change behavior.

Problem Solving

Behavioral social work in the community draws from techniques of general problem solving. In no way limited to narrow prescriptions for treatment, fundamentals of recognizing and specifying problems, coming up with various ways to solve problems, and evaluating these potential solutions will give clients tools to deal with personal and social struggles on their own. With Carl and his mother in the case above, the behavior analyst so modeled the problem-solving procedure of negotiation as well as the principle of response cost—or "pigging." Systematic models of problem solving (D'Zurilla & Goldfried, 1971; Mahoney, 1974, Schinke, Gilchrist, & Blythe, 1980) mesh well with the natural environment since each conceptual, step is operationalized through daily trials and experiences.

Treatment Packaging

Community-based behavioral programs demonstrate that combinations of techniques have greater clout than one or two techniques used alone (Azrin, 1977; Schinke & Wong, 1978). Emphasis on treatment technique packaging is attractive to caseworkers, parents, teachers, and clients who react negatively to some behavior-change techniques but not to others. Parents relying on discipline through punishment might be convinced to manage their child's whining and temper tantrums by counterbalancing punishment with neutral or positive procedures. Toward this end, they could ignore whining, reinforce the child for not whining and for interacting pleasantly, and resort to punishment only when the obstreperous behavior got out of hand.

Social Validation

Serving to strengthen behavioral social work in the natural environment are the many opportunities to validate behavior change. An area of growing interest in behavioral science (Kazdin, 1977a; Whittaker, 1975, 1979; Wolf, 1978), social validation requires the client and significant persons in the client's life to subjectively judge improvements that follow intervention. Subjective measures are on equal par with objective ones and allow social workers to quantify levels of consumer satisfaction with clinical outcomes. Tharp and Wetzel (1969) initiate telephone follow-up to learn patients' subjective happiness with their children's postintervention behavior. Achievement Place researchers query group home residents about how well they like staff members who received special training (Willner, Braukmann, Kirigin, Fixsen, Phillips, & Wolf, 1977). This author and his associates incorporate one or more measures of consumer satisfaction in every study. We have asked consumers to judge the intervention process (Blythe, Gilchrist, & Schinke, 1980), outcome (Schinke, Gilchrist, & Blythe, 1980), value (Schinke, Smith, Myers, & Altman, 1979), and overall impact (Schinke, Gilchrist, Smith, & Wong, 1978).

Carry-over of Change

The likelihood of generalization and future maintenance of change is a clear advantage to behavioral social work in extraclinical environments. When important persons in the client's life are included in program planning and implementation, when intervention is conducted in situ, and when natural rewards, treatment packages, and problem-solving are tailored to client needs, all persons involved are more likely to stick to some form of the treatment approach. This gratifying carry-over is denoted by Tharp and Wetzel (1969) who ascertain that most of their clients are employing behavioral techniques up to two years after treatment ends.

PITFALLS AND HOW TO AVOID THEM

Behavioral programs in the natural environment betoken an exciting future for social work practice. As with any frontier, however, workers must temper their explorations of behavioral methods with caution and skepticism. Well organized, succinct reports cause some programs to appear deceptively easy. Not often do investigators exhibit candor like Tharp and Wetzel when holding forth on data from the Behavior Research Project. "These results are encouraging and frustrating: the land has bees as well as milk and honey" (1969, p. vii). To continue this metaphor, behavioral social workers who advance too hastily or too cavalierly will get stung.

Conservative clinical researchers stay cognizant of common pitfalls during the implementation of behavioral social work in the community.

Continuing awareness of them prepares workers, clients, and colleagues for the inevitable exigencies of real-life practice, that may, nonetheless be anticipated and by applied strategies minimized in terms of deleterious effects. We must remain cognizant of organizational and political constraints, accountability, resource limitations, research control, intervention programming, flexibility, and collaboration. Neither exclusive nor exhaustive, consideration of each should stimulate careful analyses of this volume's subsequent chapters and of any current or proposed behavioral social work.

Organizational and Political Constraints

Community social programs occur within organizational systems. Organizations are physically distinct: a residential treatment center, group home, social service agency, daycare center. Or, they are some abstract entity: a family, street gang, or the Greater Seattle Consortium of Social Agencies Serving Needy, Lost, and Shipwrecked Life-Voyagers. Regardless of structure, no community program operates independently. Every organization has written and unwritten regulations and never written but potent political rules. Before planning any behavioral program in the community, social workers must be familiar with the constraints that attend these rules and regulations.

Organizational and political constraints are best understood by assessing communication patterns and decision processes, learning who controls the reinforcers (incentives, raises, promotions), and identifying mechanisms through which reinforcers are dispensed (cf. Wodarski, 1976). Sometimes this information is easily obtained; more often it is not. Because every family, agency, cottage, or institution has a process for determining day-to-day operations, shrewd workers examine all relevant processes through contacts with members of the organization. Workers interview key persons in the vertical hierarchy—director, operations manager, financial secretary, supervisor, line worker, client. Interviewing several people who represent each rung on the hierarchical ladder helps ensure reliable and accurate data. What should interviews cover? Any discussion, no matter how informal, yields rich information. Just as important, face-to-face contact enhances personal relationships and cements a base for the worker's credibility. Topics to cultivate during interviews are the proposed program and how it may affect operations in the short run and longitudinally, a history of similar programs, a rundown on who works for whom, candid appraisals of job satisfaction, and individuals' feelings about life in the organization.

The problems caused by organizational and political constraints have been borne out by Reppucci and Saunders' account (1974) of one community behavioral program. Recounting experiences with the reorganization of a residential center for delinquents, the investigators relate attempts to convert a work-for-pay system to a token economy:

> Institutional restraints have been largely responsible for our inability to change the work-for-pay program. At the top level of administration, the commissioner of the state department responsible for the training school was agreeable to our plan of theory, but he pointed out that, in practice, any changes in the allocation of work-for-pay money would require approval by the state legislature—a task outside the realm of political possibility. At the middle level of administration, the head of the business office seemed interested, but insisted that the business office could not become involved in exchanging points for money. At the bottom level, various staff who normally supervised youngsters in the work-for-pay program pointed out that they were responsible for doing work the right way and that teaching skills at the same time would impair their effectiveness and might even be dangerous. Thus, at every level there were institutional constraints that blocked any changes in the work-for-pay program (p. 651).

The present social worker's experiences with client families, group homes, public welfare agencies, daycare centers, and other community settings corroborates organizational and political bumps at every turn in the road.

Accountability

The behavorial approach necessitates the collection of objective data on program progress and outcome. Collecting data implies performance evaluation and challenges extant *modus operandi* (Hersen & Bellack, 1977; Schinke 1979b). Program plans, therefore, will reduce these challenges by the sharing of collection procedures and intended data uses before assessment and evaluation start. If data collection threatens staff or clients, the procedures are renegotiated until acceptable. Throughout the program, workers communicate changes in procedures for data collection. All data are directed back to clients, families, and colleagues. If plans go astray, workers should immediately inform all who may be affected. Bad tidings are better presented by someone with an explanation and possible solution than by another party not privy to the facts.

When the project is completed, behavioral social workers bear the burden of reporting to anyone whose life was or will be touched by the program. They should be apprised of outcome results and the imputed reasons for success or failure. Workers suggest directions for congeneric programs with the target group and problem. Clients and people interested in the client's welfare are given opportunities to relate their feelings about the behavior-change endeavor. What were the first-hand benefits and adverse effects they felt? How can future efforts be improved? This reciprocity of feedback and inquiry will remove many of the stigmata from social program evaluations. A fortiori, such care signifies high ethical standards and effective professional practice.

Resource Limitations

Allocations of time, personnel, and money resources may moderate the scope and magnitude of behavioral programs. Intervention that involves expensive reinforcers, equipment, and facilities is especially vulnerable to resource limitations. Realistic cost estimates in advance of program implementation will obviate the embarrassment of not being able to make good on what may prove to have been precocious commitments. During and after the program, workers should keep exact records of all time and resources expended. Contrasting these data with later outcomes will give some notion—even if only a crude one—of the cost effectiveness of behavioral intervention (Kirchner, Schnelle, Domash, Larson, Carr, & McNees, 1980; Masters, Garfinkel, & Bishop, 1978; Romans, 1979). This parameter is receiving considerable emphasis as social welfare programs undergo budget cutbacks (Shepard & Thompson, 1979; Schinke, 1979b; Yates, 1979).

Research Control

Insufficient research control is perhaps the greatest restriction to evaluation of community behavioral programs (Cowen, 1978). By and large, community practitioners are dissuaded from conventional research designs to evaluate social programs. Professional ethics go against relegating needy clients to no-treatment control conditions. Instead of placing members of their cohort in no-contact control groups, for example, Schwitzgebel and Kolb (1964) study a comparison group of youths from outside their catchment area. Some single-case research can be contraindicated in social program evaluations. Requisite preintervention baselines are not amenable to serious antisocial, delinquent, highly noxious, or health-damaging behavior. On this limitation Tharp and Wetzel report:

> In the Behavior Research Project the establishment and recording of baseline rates for behaviors occurring in the natural environment proved difficult, at least as a standard procedure. There was much pressure from the environment to intervene rather than take baseline recordings. School personnel and parents would not easily tolerate observations over long periods of time if the behavior was a disturbance to them. Behavior analysts usually stated that these initial observations were valuable and intervention was difficult to assess without them. Most often this helped mediators tolerate delay in intervention, though not always. (1969, p. 151)

Even so, as outlined in my later chapter and in the one by Gorsuch, a modicum of research control may be garnered through an acquaintance with the literature and the use of a bit of imagination.

Intervention Programming

Precisely defined techniques developed in the psychology laboratory research often deliquesce into ambiguous jargon in social work practice. Meticulously detailed procedures aside, intervention techniques will be given different connotations by everyone involved. An example is provided by Reppucci and Saunders.

> At the Connecticut School for Boys the term *time-out* (short for "time out from positive reinforcement") was readily adopted and its meaning clearly understood (i.e. twenty minutes of sitting quietly with no stimulation of any kind). Within six months, however, *time-out* had many meanings, not only across cottages but within the same cottage. To some it had its original meaning, but to others it meant an undesignated time period of sitting quietly, a quiet period plus time-off weekend visits home; one hour of sitting and doing nothing; or calming down and then talking about the reason for the *time-out* (1974, p. 653, italics in original).

Ill-defined target behaviors can also eventuate in the case of unsystematic programming. A plan to "increase Anna's social approach responses with authority figures" will probably be misinterpreted. Does "social approach" mean sitting and smiling? or, walking within three feet of another individual? or, grabbing someone's hand and saying: "Hi, the name is Anna, what's your handle?" Are authority figures older siblings? Police officers? Social workers? Given this ambiguity, Anna's social approaches may go unrewarded; at best her behavior will be reinforced inconsistently. Avoiding such problems demands propaedeutics. Prior to intervention delivery, workers should write out specific outcomes and behavior-change techniques. These are iterated, discussed, role played, and practiced with anyone expected to use them.

Flexibility

Behavioral social work has to be flexible. Allegedly powerful techniques are less impressive in natural settings. Behavioral methods validated with analogue populations can be quite weak when applied clinically (Kazdin, 1978a). For these reasons, expectations for change remain open to negotiation and renegotiation. Since intervention goals are generally developed from assessment data not accessible until the beginning of the program, absolute or unchangeable goals can never be abolute. Rather, flexible objectives mirror the vagaries of real-world interactions: "Joan and her mother will have demonstrated their new learning when Joan complies with her mother's requests 20% over the baseline rate." The novelty of behavioral methods and the negative feelings many people have about behavior modification indicate methodological rigor balanced by flexibility. Contingency plans and modest goals facilitate this balance.

Collaboration

Social work has a tradition of delivering intervention though the interpersonal dyad of worker and client. With its long and respected history as a primary vehicle of therapeutic change, the dyadic relationship will remain important in professional practice. Nevertheless, workers in community settings cannot practice exclusively within a dyadic framework. Most community-based professionals—certainly those using behavioral methods—depend on a triadic model of service delivery. Here, social work practice involves consultants, mediators, and targets. Social worker consultants give direction, support, and encouragement to mediators, who are likely to be parents, teachers, peers, and substitute-care paraprofessionals. Mediators in turn act as reinforcing agents, provide feedback, and instruct the targets of behavior change.

Uncomplex conceptually, operations of the triadic model have ramifications for community programming. Smooth entry into a social system, agency, or institution requires more than the approval of people at the top—administrators, superintendents, principals, directors, department heads. Although no program should be launched without administrative support, success ultimately rests with line-staff mediators. The crucial period of initial program development, termed the port-of-entry phase (Reppucci, 1977), is wisely marked by contacts with all potential mediators. As with organizational and political networks, workers will be hard pressed to find an alternative as good as the one-to-one interview.

Programmatic and individual case planning further involves mediators. Soliciting mediators' input shows concern for their ideas and generates means for reaching program ends. Who should be engaged? Whittaker (1970) suggests that plans for child-care training encircle any staff who will have contact with targets, from custodians to administrators. Furthermore, program planning should early on involve staff in order to vitiate subsequent sabotage of behavior—change efforts, whether intentional or unintentional. This involvement should not neglect labor union representatives. Virtually critical in private industry, union endorsement may determine the success of programs within social organizations. (Dean, 1971; Reppucci, 1977).

Programs may be implemented solely by mediators. Of premier concern is that mediators harmoniously interpret and carry out the intervention. After mediators are given time to comment on them, intervention specifics are modeled and rehearsed. Noted before, lack of clarity leads to inconsistency which may mean failure for the most admirable project. For instance, a program aimed at reducing some negative action by extinction procedures will not succeed if just one person attends to the maladaptive target response. Misunderstandings among those delivering intervention are easily thwarted through group practice sessions. In these pratice sessions social work consultants provide instructions, feedback, reinforcement, and coaching to individual mediators while others watch and learn vicariously (Schinke & Wong, 1978).

Collaboration with mediators does not end when intervention commences. Feedback and reinforcement are ongoing. Since initial and continued successes are very rewarding, such are expressly designed into the program. Posting graphed performance records or data that describe positive progress will engender esprit de corps and motivation (Barnard, Christophersen, & Wolf, 1972; Panyan, Boozer, & Morris, 1970). By monitoring mediator and client advancements, workers establish their interest and gather feedback on weaknesses of the program. These data can guide ways to strengthen the program before it is too late to make changes. When movement toward goals cannot be monitored or is not progressing, the goals are ill-specified or unreachable. These must be quickly dropped or renegotiated. Program failure does not imply mediator failure; rather, it indicts poor incentives for mediator success.

Mediators sometimes disagree with an intervention goal, plan, or technique. Tharp and Wetzel (1969) illustrate:

> Benny was a low achieving ninth grader who felt he was getting an unfair deal from his home environment as well as his school environment. He had struggled through two very inconsistent stepfathers and a number of nonmotivated teachers. The only thing that kept him in school and out of the grasp of the police was his devotion to his mother.
>
> After overcoming a number of crises at the school, and establishing a concrete reinforcer at home, we intervened into Benny's intermittent work habits in the classroom. He began to work quite diligently in all his classes except math, where he had the greatest teacher friction. The math teacher had been opposed to Benny and to the intervention all along. Two weeks after the intervention plan was started, Benny was suspended from math, on the slim pretext that on that day he didn't bring his book to class. The teacher accused him of stealing the book and told him the homework he had been turning in was not up to par. He was called a "no-good bum" and told he would be better off out of school, and certainly out of math class. For Benny this was the last straw. He feared that the same thing would eventually happen in all his classes. He stopped coming to school. His mother, whom we had almost convinced that the school was finally giving her son a new opportunity, sympathized with Benny, and did not demand that he return. She allowed Benny to get a job. Benny was a drop-out (or "push-out"); the case was terminated (pp. 132-133).

Instances as this can be checked when the social worker carefully explains the rationale, goals, and procedures of behavioral intervention. Nonetheless, particularly difficult goals should be abandoned—at least temporarily. Flexibility, treatment packages, involvement of all mediators, and early program successes together minimize problems in program implementation.

PROFESSIONAL ETHICS

Behavioral social workers face moral and ethical issues. As helping professionals, social workers wrestle with human problems, social deviancies, and interpersonal dilemmas. Professional encounters with such suffering predictably brings up controversy. In a clinical research capacity, social workers put forth values relative to data collection, protection of client rights and privacy, and assurance of fair treatment for research participants (Schinke, in press-a).

Social workers who adopt behavioral methods must live with additional values-related principles, many of which were noted above in my mention of the negative stereotypes ascribed to behavior modification. Hereupon, attention can be turned to the ethical issues social workers must address in the design and orchestration of behavior-modification programs, transfering the discussion from global ethical issues to discrete procedural ones.

Professional prerogatives to specify clinical outcomes and values in order to direct behavior change are inherent in every intervention program. Few will argue with the principle that behavior modification, like all psychotherapies, is founded on much subjectivity and precious little objectivity. When behavior therapy was in its infancy, theoretician Perry London (1964) stated that this methodology and "every aspect of psychotherapy presupposes some implicit moral doctrine" (p. 6). Sixteen years later Allen Bergin (1980a) amplifies the treatise: "As an applied field, psychotherapy is directed toward practical goals that are selected in vague terms. It is even necessary when establishing criteria for measuring therapeutic change to decide, on a value basis, what changes are desirable. This necessarily requires a philosophy of human nature that guides the selection of measurements and the setting of priorities regarding change" (p. 97). Recognizing the impossibility of a value-free climate, ethical social workers should make their value judgments as explicit as possible, in order to permit clients, mediators, colleagues, and the lay public to scrutinize, substantiate, or refute behavior-change goals and means.

An obvious ethical issue is the control professionals have over their clients' lives. Therapeutic control is neither unintended nor undesired. Any psychosocial intervention zeroes in on goals such as improved thoughts, responses, and interpersonal behavior (Strupp, 1978, 1979). Human service professionals facilitate such improvement by exerting control. In regard to this issue in nonbehavioral counseling, Carl Rogers says: "In client-centered therapy, we are deeply engaged in the prediction and influencing of behavior, or even the control of behavior. As therapists, we institute certain attitudinal conditions, and the client has relatively little voice in the establishment of these conditions. We predict that if these conditions are instituted, certain behavioral consequences will ensue in the client" (Rogers & Skinner, 1956, p. 1063)[1].

Behavioral social workers translate control into helping clients shed light on who and what governs their behavior. Clients can then decide if they want to maintain or to alter relationships with reinforcing persons and activities. In this fashion, behavioral social work lets clients identify their reinforcers, see which ones they control, and act according to their best interests.

Accordingly, the ethics germane to the procedures of behavioral programs center on the definition and use of reinforcers. Besides being a strategy for responsive intervention, giving clients free choice of their reinforcers operationalizes the implicit value that clients must eventually assume control of their treatment. Though before they have full reign over their behavior-change programs, concerns may be voiced about the giving out of reinforcers as bribes (O'Leary, Poulos, & Devine, 1972).

Such concern is often posed by mediators reluctant to reward behavior that is expected of clients. Children, students, spouses, patients, and intmates may be viewed as having the "moral" duty to engage in a prescribed manner because they want to or are supposed to, not because they will receive some added payoff. Apart from the fact that the definition of a bribe is "Anything, esp. money, given or promised to induce a person to do something illegal or wrong" (Webster's New World Dictionary, 1974, p. 176), workers must deal with the issue. One strategy is to observe how everyone is contingently rewarded by salaries, kisses, letters of commendation, educational degrees, professional certification and licensure, promotions, compensatory time off, and so forth. Workers should note that ultimately clients have full reign of their behavior-change program when they know about external controls on their actions. Should conditional rewards remain distasteful, behavior modification may not represent treatment of choice for client or mediator.

[1]He considers control to be a matter of attitude and therapeutic situation.

Ethical issues can arise around selection of the locus of intervention. Obviously, social workers must choose and exclude those people who will participate in program planning. Workers and included collaborators then set outcome goals and select means to achieve them. It is basic to deciding whether to increase or to decrease the behavior in question. Selecting among positive and negative behavior-change techniques will logically follow.

Sequent ethical issues include choosing when to begin transfer of change and termination phases of intervention. As previously noted, subjective value judgments come into play during program evaluation, use of data, and follow-up. Open struggling with these ethical issues is difficult and not generally mirrored in the majority of professional public welfare practice (Bowie, 1979). But, as Bergin wrote recently:

> Although there is widespread aversion to (a) taking overt value positions and (b) justifying them, both of these must be done for the sake of clarity and honesty. It will not do for therapists to hide their prejudices behind a screen of scientific jargon. Not only do ethical clarity and honesty demand a change, but consumerism is also pressing all of us to be explicit about what we are inviting clients into, why, and with what consequences. (1980b, pp. 11-12)

Regardless of client group, presenting problem, agency setting, or practice role, social workers must scrutinize the values underlying professional judgments and straightforwardly address personal values that differ from those held by clients. Such continuous self-evaluation will allow behavioral social workers to implement client-centered ethics in every phase of professional practice.

PROLOGUE OF COMING CHAPTERS

The next eighteen chapters review behavioral social work that represents the vanguard of effective, efficient, rigorous, and humane client service. Documentation comes from social work with children, families, and adults, and from material on professional competence and accountability. The authors who contribute this evidence span our field in terms of geographic setting, institutional affiliation, and areas of interest. Each contributor has a record of professional practice, empirical research, classroom teaching, in-service training, and scholarly writing. These workers' behavioral credentials are displayed in the programs and procedures they detail.

The chapters put their respective contents into an applied clinical research framework. This common frame organizes behavioral methods across the panoply of social work practice. The transformation of behavior modification theory into practice thus focuses on actual clients, presenting problems, and social work settings, so that these clinical applications move abstract concepts into the realities of client service.

Real too, however, are the flaws in the behavioral methods presented. The contributors are mindful of disparities and disappointments when theory meets with practice. None masks these lacunae. None suggests that the described application completes the bridge between textbook and real world. Instead, each attempt to apply behavioral methods is meant as a penultimate validation. Final trials will happen after readers replicate the methods, achieve success, realize shortcomings, and refine the procedure to match unique client conditions.

Replication is the objective of every chapter. It is hoped that the level of specificity and attention to routine, the crucial issues of actual implementation woven into these contributions will help foster increased practice of behavioral social work. To be sure, fruitful uses of all methods will have to consider differences among client groups, their difficulties, and agency sites and resources. Polster's work with underachieving students in public schools, for instance, requires adaptation to be responsive to special education children in the learning disabled classroom. Necessary modifications to the various practice models will profit from this chapter's discussion of pitfalls and guidelines for behavioral programs in the natural environment.

Because the contributions are intended to complement each other, readers should review all related chapters before formalizing their plans. Practice with marital problems will benefit from procedures outlined by Pinkston, Friedman and Polster; Berlin, Richey, Duehn and Mayadas, and Witkin. Practice-level evaluation will be easier if my chapter and Gorsuch's are read preparatory to assessment and intervention.

In closing, an analytic reading of the coming chapters should be coupled with the goal of deductively using the outlined procedures. Readers must transfer these methods from clinical application to conceptual understanding, and go on to apply the concepts to their own practice. When this cycle is completed, the reader can rightfully take credit for advancing the practice and understanding of behavioral social work.

I

Methods for Children and Families

Social work is much occupied by the wants of children and families. The profession's commitment to economic and social services for young people and their parents is evidenced by our roots in settlement homes and orphanages, our advocacy for humane child-labor laws and for the health and safety of children in their own homes, and our preeminence in child welfare institutions and agencies. Over the years our concern for the well-being of children and families continues and expands. Public and private social work assists young clients and their adult caretakers by zeroing in on poverty, mental health, education, corrections, child and family policy, and the law. Current moves in child welfare portend its relevance for future social services planning and delivery.

Contemporary issues and problems faced by the American family are articulated in the next seven chapters. The chapters cover topics of predelinquency, parenting, school performance, youths' social competence, substitute care, crisis intervention, and child abuse. Each of these areas is reviewed, put in the perspective of our professional mission, and analyzed within a practice framework. The authors go on to describe behavioral methods appropriate for social work with the client constituency and their difficulties. All chapters are thus bonded by an interest in services for children and families, a social work orientation to child welfare, and the application of behavior modification.

Without question, it is the bond of behavioral social work that sets this text apart from other references on social work with children and families. The following contributions, for instance, commonly recognize the merits of social work emphasizing and increasing positive behavior. John Wodarski encourages the reinforcement of positive responses and discourages the punishment of antisocial interactions in his work with aggressive and disruptive boys. Elsie Pinkston and her colleagues require parents to choose and increase a positive response to offset the negative behavior that stimulated referral for family counseling. Rick Polster and associates show school underachievement as reversible via tangible and social rewards.

With adolescents, Lew Gilchrist argues for social skills training as a way to thwart deleterious health habits, promiscuous sexuality, criminal delinquency, unemployment, and conflicts with parents. Ted Stein and Eileen Gambrill depict written contracts as a means for alleviating painful processes that attend foster care placement, restoration of children into their homes, and termination of parental rights. Also addressing the out-of-home placement, Ed Dimock supports positive methods for social work with young people in group homes and those engaged in family crises. In the last chapter of this section Rob Schilling brings a refreshing approach to our ability to understand and remediate child abuse. Schilling's closure is most fitting since he demonstrates how child welfare workers who adopt behavioral methods optimally help their clients, themselves and the field.

1

Groups for Anti-Social Children

John S. Wodarski

Behavioral therapeutic approaches with pre-delinquent, delinquent, and antisocial children have had a successful history (Braukmann and Fixsen 1975; Graziano 1975; O'Leary and Wilson 1975;). Although most of these approaches deliver services through a one-to-one intervention mode, social work practice with delinquent children has utilized the group as a major vehicle for service delivery. This chapter documents the application of behavioral group techniques in the treatment of the antisocial child. Based upon the author's experiences with two research projects funded by the National Institute of Mental Health, Center for Studies of Crime and Delinquency, this chapter provides a general introduction to the target area, a review of supporting literature, a description of the intervention paradigm, program consequences, and implications for practice.

The first project involved implementing and evaluating a community-based treatment program for antisocial children (Group Intergration and Behavioral Change: The St. Louis Project); the second involved developing follow-up procedures for Preparation Through Responsive Education Program (PREP), a community-based program founded on behavioral principles. The majority of issues discussed stem from the St. Louis Project. Where relevant, items from the PREP project are included to elaborate issues originating with the St. Louis study.

INTRODUCTION

Setting

The study site was a community agency providing recreational, leisure time, and educational services for 16,000 enrolled members and for the community at large. Agency funding included membership dues, the United Way, The Jewish Federation, and various federal grants. The agency's physical plant included two modern buildings, a 100-acre site with day camp facilities, and a 400-acre site with residential camping facilities. Each year the professional group work staff, consisting of eighteen M.S.W.s with specializations in group work, organizes approximately 200 clubs and classes for children ranging in age from six to eighteen years. M.S.W. service roles include planning and organizing the agency program for children and youth and supervising the graduate and undergraduate college students who lead the groups. The majority of graduate students are enrolled in accredited graduate schools of social work; the majority of undergraduates are majoring in one of the social sciences. Usually the M.S.W. supervisors have provided supervision for at least two years. As part of its regular service the agency has admitted physically handicapped and mentally retarded children to its program. Similarly, it has sponsored discussion groups for parents of children with socio-behavioral difficulties. Historically, the agency's research endeavors have been in the field of aging (Goodman 1972), mental retardation (Pumphrey, Goodman, and Flax 1969), and community action.

Participants were antisocial boys ranging in age from eight to sixteen years. During the three years of the program 750 antisocial children were referred to the community center from various agencies, including a special school district, mental health centers, juvenile courts, and children's homes. Participants were defined as antisocial according to various diagnostic measures utilized by members of the professional therapeutic community: teachers, counselors, psychologists, and social workers. The rationale for referral to this program was to provide a new service for adolescent males not served by other means in the metropolitan area and to provide children the opportunity to interact with peers who had no official records of delinquency.

To help professionals determine which children should be considered for referral, the investigators devised a checklist illustrating the types of behaviors that a child should exhibit at home, school, or at their agencies. Professionals were asked to estimate the average incidence of antisocial, non-social, and pro-social behavior a child would exhibit in a week. Children with the highest scores were accepted into the program and were stratified according to age and placed randomly into groups. Behaviors denoted on the checklist were analogous to those listed on an

Table 1

Number of antisocial children referred, number accepted, and number of groups according to year of study.

Year of Study	Number of Children Referred	Number of Children Accepted	Number of Groups
I	157	47	7
II	338	114	14
III	255	90	11
Total	750	251	32

observational scale used for the research and to those reported on a self-inventory completed by the children, referral agency personnel, parents, behavioral observers, and their group workers. Table one illustrates the number of children referred, the number accepted and the number of groups formed each year. Approximately 20% of the children dropped out of the program each year during the baseline period (i.e. during the first eight weeks preceding the application of treatment) due to factors such as vacations, illnesses, and unwillingness to attend. Statistical analyses executed on selected variables such as age, percentage of antisocial behavior exhibited, race, and socio-economic status indicated no signficant differences between participants in the study as compared with dropouts. Furthermore, the dropout rate was distributed evenly among the groups.

Attendance averaged five members per meeting at antisocial groups ranging from four to twelve members. Groups met at the Center for the two-hour period once weekly to engage in various physical activities such as basketball, hockey, swimming, or nature hikes, and to discuss topics of mutual interest, such as difficulties at school, with parents, drugs, and sex. The groups met for an average of twenty two times, ranging from fourteen to twenty-eight meetings. Every precaution was taken to avoid undue stigmatization of the referred children: they were treated as regular agency members, given regular membership cards, and were encouraged to participate in other activities offered at the Center. In addition, efforts were made to assure that relatively similar expectations would be held for all children in the program, including the referred children. Therapists were assigned randomly to groups and to a particular treatment method.

Presenting Problem Characteristics

In order to select children for the program it was necessary to systematically assess the frequency of antisocial behavior exhibited by each child during a uniform time period. Consequently, personnel from the referral agencies were asked to estimate the number of times that each referred child exhibited one of five categories of antisocial behaviors during the preceding one-week period. Additionally, referrers estimated the incidence of pro-social and non-social behaviors. The antisocial behavioral categories were: 1) interpersonal aggression of a physical nature (hitting, kicking, shoving, biting, pinching, slapping, hair pulling, and sticking or poking with a held or thrown object): 2) interpersonal aggression of a verbal nature (aggressive statements such as "I'll kill you"); 3) object aggression (damaging or destroying the property of others); 4) disruptive behavior towards peers (temper tantrums, restlessness, climbing out of windows, poor concentration on tasks, and purposeful tapping, whistling, making loud noise, throwing objects such as paper, candy, erasers, chairs, or other diversions) and 5) disruptive behavior toward adults (temper tantrums, running away, and refusal to carry out reasonable requests).

THEORETICAL FRAMEWORK

Every treatment program should be established on the best theoretical rationale existing. We have discussed elsewhere the reasons for the consistent negative findings of classic studies involving the treatment of antisocial children through traditional methods and means (Feldman, Wodarski, Flax and Goodman 1972, 1973). Those literature reviews led to the isolation of two theoretical frameworks with substantial empirical support providing a rationale for conceptualizing our program. These frameworks are labeling theory and behavior modification.

Labeling Theory

From the review of the literature it was evident that there is a pronounced tendency in our society for the helping professions to group clients together in the same context for treatment purposes. We place mentally ill persons in mental hospitals, adult criminals in prisons, and mentally handicapped children in schools for the retarded. This process, in many instances, is supported through legal sanctions. Two reasons probably account for the segregation of exceptional individuals from interactions with so-called "normal" individuals. They are based on economic and theoretical factors, often inter-related. For economic reasons, helping institutions treat individuals in the same context because it is easier, more efficient, and less costly to deliver services to homogeneous clients. For theoretical reasons, it is believed that homogeneous groups may lead to greater empathy among clients and increased understanding of common social problems, in turn leading to therapeutic improvement. In addition, if successfully treated, clients provide adequate role models for others from the same homogeneous group. Data are lacking, however, indicating that these benefits actually accrue.

Client grouping is used extensively in the treatment of antisocial children despite little success with this process (Bednar and Lawlis 1971; Radzinowicz and Wolfgang 1971; and Warren 1970). Our observation has been that the following consequences result from the grouping process:

1. As antisocial children go through the many institutional procedures to secure services they become labeled, resulting in stigmatization.
2. Antisocial children are not provided opportunities to experience adequate role models since interaction with normal peers is discouraged and role

models provided in segregated treatment settings may be more deviant than the ones provided in other settings. Thus, antisocial children have a reduced likelihood of positive reinforcement from peers for pro-social behavior.

3. Homogeneous groupings prevent interactions between antisocial children and others with "regular" self concepts which may lead to antisocial children developing self concepts of deviancy.

4. The ability of antisocial children to learn pro-social behaviors is limited in segregated contexts; when pro-social behaviors are learned, the ability to generalize these behaviors to the open environment is minimal.

If treatment took place in the open community, it is feasible to assume that more generalizability of behavior would occur. Hence, it was our belief that it is more desirable to locate treatment endeavors for antisocial children within agencies serving primarily pro-social clientele, such as community centers, YMCA's, and neighborhood settlement houses (Feldman, et al. 1972). This would alleviate many of the dysfunctional consequences discussed above.

Behavior Modification

On the basis of the information available at the time of the conceptualization of our treatment paradigm, a group level behavioral program was well supported by prior research (Burchard and Harig 1976; Fixsen, Phillips, and Wolf 1973; Heaton, Safer, Allen, Spinnato, Prumo 1971). The model we used is outlined below.

BASIC PRINCIPLES OF GROUP LEVEL BEHAVIOR MODIFICATION

Basic Assumptions

1. The majority of behavior is learned.
2. Behavior must be observable and countable.
3. Behavior can be changed by altering the antecedent events and/or the consequences occurring after the behavior.
4. Antisocial children exhibit antisocial behavior primarily because their environments reinforce this behavior.

General Techniques for Working with Children

1. Positive consequences increasing behavior are called reinforcers (candy, smiling, positive physical contact, for example).

2. Three means of eliminating antisocial behaviors are to ignore the behaviors, to increase the reinforcement for exhibition of pro-social behavior and/or to

reinforce children who exhibit desired behavior to facilitate the other group members modeling the behavior. Children most readily model behavior exhibited by physically attractive children similar to them in relevant characteristics such as age, sex, race, and social class. Thus, group workers should reinforce children who can serve as models.

Types of Contingencies

1. A contingency is a statement specifying conditions of reinforcement. Contingencies can be structured at individual or group levels. An example of an individual contingency would be to provide a child who has generally engaged in withdrawn behaviors with candy, sufficient praise, or positive physical contact when he participates in a group activity.
2. Group contingencies can be structured for the whole group or for selected members. When the group contingency is structured for one or two members, reinforcement for the whole group depends on these members exhibiting a behavior at a certain level, such as decreased fighting, decreased disruptive verbalizations, or increased participation in group activities. Such a contingency exerts considerable pressure to conform. Group contingencies can be structured to decrease disruptive and withdrawn behaviors and to increase planning behavior to desired criterion levels. Under the group contingency, everybody shares equal amounts of reinforcement. Group contingencies are particularly potent for working with antisocial children since they provide the necessary tools to modify the peer reinforcement structure which in many instances is maintaining the behavior.

Use of Punishment

On the whole the use of punishment and contingencies that imply threats are discouraged. It is best to phrase a contingency in the positive. Thus, state that if the group or particular individuals exhibit certain behaviors, a certain type of reinforcement will be available to the group. An example of negative contingency structuring is to indicate that if a particular group does not exhibit a certain type of behavior, members will not receive reinforcement. To structure a positive contingency, one can indicate that if the group accomplishes a criterion behavior, reinforcement will be provided. Reinforcers that can be utilized are praise, money, food, having a party with a group of the opposite sex, sports tickets, and so forth.

Shaping

It is often desirable to utilize the concept of shaping—reinforcing closer and closer approximations to the desired behavior. An example of a behavior lending itself to shaping is group attentiveness. The group leader might state; "If we can discuss a topic for ten minutes, then we will all have an extra treat at the break." At the next meeting the span could be increased to fifteen minutes, then to twenty minutes, and so forth. Thus the concept of shaping rests on stating an initial goal easy for the group to obtain.

Decreasing Dropout Rates

A crucial element affecting the ability to alter an antisocial child's behavior is the client's decision to remain in therapy. Dropout rates are extremely high for all professions concerned with helping antisocial children. To assure that antisocial children evaluate the treatment contexts positively, workers should choose program activities high in reward value, enhance initial behavioral exchanges by concurrently presenting members with positive reinforcers, and use minimal punishment.

Behavioral Group Work Approach

Group work with antisocial children is based on a number of rationales. First, the presence of other children in the group setting can provide an arena for the observation of appropriate behavior through the models group members present, and for the acquisition and practice of socially relevant behavior.

Moreover, groups provide a context where new behavior can be tested in a realistic atmosphere; that is, group contexts provide feedback necessary to acquire social behavior. Additionally, when behavior is learned in a group context, it is likely to come under the control of a greater number of discriminative stimuli; therefore, greater generalization of the behavior can occur for a broader variety of contexts.

Group interaction frequently typifies many kinds of daily interactions. Services facilitating the development of behavior enabling antisocial children to interact in groups are likely to better prepare children for participation in society—i.e., with social skills necessary to secure "natural" reinforcement (Feldman and Wodarski 1975).

Groups provide a valid locus for accurate diagnosis and a potent means for changing client behavior (Meyer and Smith 1977; Rose 1974, 1977). Lastly, the provision of services through groups greatly increases the number of clients served by an effective treatment program. All these factors provide the rationale for the larger use of groups for social group work practice with antisocial children (Meyer and Smith 1977; Wodarski and Feldman 1975).

DESCRIPTION OF INTERVENTION PARADIGM

For the present projects, children were selected on the basis of referred incidence of estimated antisocial behavior. They were stratified according to age, then randomly assigned to a treatment group. Their worker was also assigned randomly. Each group was in a baseline condition for eight weeks preceding treatment.

During baseline the group leaders seldom structured group behavioral contingencies, activities, friendship relationships, or task relationships. The leader permitted members to select their own activities from a list of fifty activities and to develop their own friendships, tasks, and interpersonal relationships with one another. The leader planned no systematic series of interventions to change members' behaviors. His interactions with the group tended to be spontaneous, leaders were instructed not to consciously plan any intervention that would increase or decrease a child's or group of children's behavior. Only when the psychological or physical safety of a member was in significant jeopardy were workers to intervene.

Thus during baseline, workers did not plan systematic interventions likely to influence the display of pro-social, non-social, or antisocial behavior within the group. This is analogous to a traditional group work diagnostic technique postulated by Churchhill (1965). In this phase practitioners refrain from intervention so they can assess client needs without contamination from intervention efforts. After the children's observed incidence of antisocial behavior reaches a stabilized, or "natural" level, treatment is introduced and members' behavior is monitored.

After a six to eight week baseline period was completed, workers filled out the Social Learning Evaluation Form for Individuals and the Social Learning Evaluation Form for Groups. Following an adequate diagnostic baseline period, implementation can be faciliated through the use of schematic aids such as these to help identify treatment objectives. As noted on the Individual form under the heading of "Problem Behavior," workers should describe in detail the key observable behaviors exhibited by a child, especially those interfering with group functioning. Examples are hitting, slapping and whistling loudly. One should list only observable and quantifiable behavior. After describing disruptive behavior, workers place the name of the target child in the next column. Under "Preceding Events" (antecedent stimuli), workers list those behaviors the child and/or the worker exhibited immediately before the child displayed the behaviors. For instance, if a target was: "Johnny fought after the others teased him," under "Following Events" (consequences), we might find: "Three other children clapped." Under "Duration," workers estimate how long the child exhibited the requisite behaviors, in terms of minutes and seconds each time that they occurred. "Frequency" simply requires a count of the occurrence of behavior. Next, workers note the type of individual or group contingency likely to increase targeted pro-social behaviors and/or decrease antisocial or non-

Social Learning Evaluation Form for Individuals

Worker's Name ______________________________ Date ______________

Name of Child	Problem Behavior	Preceding Events	Following Events	Duration	Frequency	Type of Individual or Group Consequence Structured	Reward

Social Learning Evaluation Form for Individuals

Worker's Name ____________________ Date __________

Problem Behavior	Exhibited By How Many Children	Names of Children	Preceding Events	Following Events	Duration	Frequency	Type of Group Consequences Structured	Reward

FIGURE 1b

social behaviors. It is important to remember that a group contingency can be used to increase or to decrease the behavior of one child, or several children, or of the entire group. Whether an individual or group contingency is chosen depends on the situation and the behavior to be modified. Finally, under "Reward" workers indicate reinforcement to be provided for the child or children. The group evaluation form is similar to the individual social learning evaluation. Under "Problem Behavior," one lists behavior two or more individuals exhibit simultaneously, especially if they disrupt the group. Workers indicate how many children exhibited the behavior, and their names. Preceding events, following events, duration, frequency, type of group contingency, and reward are completed in the same fashion as specified in the instructions for the individual evaluation. It should be noted that the individual and group evaluation forms may be completed after each group meeting, thus resulting in the accumulation of schematic process recordings through the duration of treatment.

Examples of Modified Behavior

Table two presents typical behavior and contingencies structured by the The table includes a majority of behavior modified for the duration of the five-year project.

Intervention Methods: Case Illustration I

The following two case records exemplify some of the points discussed, especially regarding formulation of behavior modification plans.

Fred, sixteen years old, was referred by a residential treatment center for antisocial children. He exhibited the following problematic behavior: 1) not staying with the treatment group; 2) not participating in group activities; 3) doing things to distract other members from planning activities (making bird calls and whistling); and 4) physically threatening group members if they did not go along with him. The worker decided to work on all four behaviors by structuring the following contingencies. To help Fred stay with the group, stimulus control would be employed. The worker would meet with the children away from the agency to not enable the child to leave the group meeting: most meetings were held at a member's house or at the leader's house. At the same time, it was agreed that group members would try to structure activities appealing to Fred to help make the group more attractive to him and to exert influence on his behavior. To deal with his fighting it was decided to structure a group contingency. If no fights occurred during the meeting, all members could buy ice cream, go bowling, or go out for a pizza. Finally, as treatment progressed, as Fred could stay with the group for increasingly longer

Table 2

Behaviors and Contingencies

Behavior	Contingencies
A. Withdrawn	
1. Non-participation (physical and verbal) in group activities exhibited by one or more members.	Group contingency Develop project that needs total group cooperation for its *completion* such as planning a party. Upon completion every member secures the reinforcer.
	Individual contingencies Attention for participating, including praise, eye contact, and physical reinforcement such as a pat on the back. Likewise, candy, fruit, and other material reinforcers can be utilized.
2. Sitting in corner, withdrawn.	Group contingency Make statement to the effect that if everyone can participate in the group activity then everyone will have treats.

Problem	Contingencies
B. Lack of togetherness	Group contingencies
1. Group members do not stay together, e.g. if group activity is playing in the gym, some members go to the snack bar, others run in the halls.	Make statement to the effect that if *all* members can stay together for activities, then after the activities they will all have a coke together. Other reinforcers to be utilized—trips, food, having a party with another group, utilization of various facilities in the center, and tickets for sporting events.
C. Inadequate role behaviors	Individual contingencies
1. Improper role behaviors exhibited by child.	1. Reinforce proper role actions through verbal and physical reinforcement.
2. Unsuccessful attempts at constructive leadership.	2. Give attention to attempts at leadership such as give reinforcement for adequate suggestions, completion of requisite task for the group, and so forth.
3. Very selfish.	3. Make statement to the effect that when the group engages in any type of project they will all receive sodas if they work together.
D. Resistance to group activity	Individual contingencies
1. Doesn't follow directions.	1. Make reinforcer contingent upon following directions.

2. Won't cooperate with the group.	2. Make reinforcer contingent upon cooperation with the group.
E. Inability to make decisions	Group contingencies—Make verbal statements such as the following:
1. Inadequate attention span. Members don't listen to each other.	1. "If we have a good planning session for X minutes then we will go to the hockey game next week."
2. Lack of creativeness for activities.	2. "Think of something new and exciting, then we can have a treat."
3. Talking about inappropriate subjects, for example, about cars when the group activity is to plan for an outing.	3. "If we can finish with this topic first then we will talk about cars."
4. Inability to make decision concerning future activities.	4. "If group can decide on the activity for the next two weeks, then we will go bowling."
F. Descriptive	Group contingencies
1. Verbalization not directed at the group discussion. The child talks to another child and thus disrupts the other child's participation in the group activity; the child speaks without directing the conversation toward anyone; the child engages in name calling, crying, screaming, laughing loudly, coughing loudly, disruptive singing, and whistling.	1. Ignore outbursts. Indicate to the group that if this behavior continues the members will not receive reinforcers. Leaders should reinforce individual behaviors such as attention to task and co-operation. Also each child should be required to return one reinforcer to leader if individuals continue to yell and scream.

2. Gross motor behaviors: If the children are seated around the table, a child is out of his seat without the group worker's permission, running, jumping, skipping, standing up, hopping, moving a chair, or walking around which disrupts the group activities.	2. "If these behaviors continue, you and the others cannot participate in the next group activity. If you can participate in painting without any running, jumping, skipping, standing up on your chair, then we can participate in any activity you like."
3. Physical aggression: Contact is initiated by one child toward another who is participating in the group activity. This contact disrupts the latter child's participation. The contact may include hitting, kicking, shoving, punching, slapping, striking with an object, throwing an object which hits another person, poking with an object, biting, pulling hair, touching, patting, or disturbing another child's property.	3. "If this continues then we will not have our game of football." Reinforce group and individuals with verbal praise when they exhibit pro-social behavior.
4. Object interference: A child plays with some object that interferes with another child's participation in the group; taps a pencil or other objects, claps, taps feet, rattles or tears paper, throws book on table, or slams things on furniture.	4. "If you do not throw chairs then you can go for a walk through the woods, take a treasure hunt, or tell stories."
5. Distracting behaviors: A child engages in physical movement that attracts another child's attention and stops participation in the group activity. The former child may rock in a chair, sit out of position, clean or rummage in furniture.	5. Suggest a party with another group if they improve social behavior.

6. Children ostracize and pick on one child.	6. “If you get along with each other, especially Ron, then the group will go skating in two weeks.”

* All of the reinforcers mentioned here can be used interchangeably on a group or individual contingency basis to modify behaviors contained in A through F. The particular contingency structured would depend on the children and context.

sessions, meetings were returned to the agency. At the same time, the worker reinforced Fred's participation in planning activities through physical reinforcement, such as pats on the back, praise, and attention.

Interventive Methods: Case Illustration II

Stan is a nine-year-old boy in the fourth grade of one of the most progressive schools within the metropolitan area. His parents are affluent. Stan is of normal height, weight, intelligence, and health for his age. Stan's behavior during the baseline period included pushing and throwing furniture at people, running in the halls, disrupting other groups by name-calling, making loud noises, and withdrawing from group activities. Diagnosis suggested that his antisocial behavior was maintained by positive reinforcement through peer attention, particularly from his buddy Tom, who laughed, joined with him, and physically reinforced him for such behavior by pats on the back and smiling. Additionally, it was apparent that the group worker's reprimands to Stan tended to reinforce such behavior, rather than diminish it, particularly by reaffirming Stan's behavioral problems among his peers.

Contingencies of behavioral change were implemented after baseline. The worker began by engaging the group in an interesting activity. However, as in previous instances, Stan and Tom attempted to disrupt the activity. Because the majority of members wished to engage in the activity, the group worker reinforced them for their participation with smiling and praise. At the same time, he ignored Stan's and Tom's behavior. In a short time, disruptions by Stan and Tom ceased; they began to participate increasingly in the group's activities. As they did, the worker reinforced them with smiles and verbal praise.

In order to enhance member's efforts to build cooperative relationships, and to plan and complete increasingly demanding tasks, the group worker paired the children with one another in subsequent sessions and structured further contingencies. Specifically, members were told that each person would earn twenty cents if the group could plan an activity in which everyone would participate. Likewise, members were informed that all would receive an additional twenty cents if *everyone* participated in the chosen activity. These contingencies helped Stan and Tom participate more effectively and more consistently in group activities. Additionally, as they earned social reinforcement from the worker and from their peers, they were more readily accepted by others and felt more comfortable in the group. To avoid satiation with monetary reinforcements, other group contingencies and other reinforcers were introduced at periodic intervals. For example, the group was asked to engage in an activity without anyone disrupting the others, after which members could have a party, go swimming, and have refreshments.

Near the termination of the group, the monetary contingency was given less frequently to ensure maintenance of the behavior. If everyone participated in planning and performing an activity without disruptive behavior such as fighting and throwing objects, each member received thirty cents; for each disruption the group was penalized five cents per person. Throughout, the leader's reinforcers of praise, smiling, head, eye contact, and physical touch fostered Stan's and Tom's pro-social behavior.

Evaluation Criteria and Outcome

In the last decade, much research has focused on antisocial children (Davidson and Seidman 1974; Empey and Erickson 1972; Lundman, McFarlane, and Scarpitti 1976). This research is characterized by few efforts measuring therapist behavior or evaluating change on multiple criterion measures, i.e. rating scales completed by children and therapists and behavioral data secured by trained observers. In view of the multidimensional nature of human behavior, it seems necessary to evaluate more than a single behavioral dimension. Thus, we employed multicriterion measures to execute a comprehensive evaluation of our program.

Self-Inventories

A checklist measuring perceived incidence of antisocial behavior for one week was filled out on each child at the beginning of the program and at its conclusion by referral agencies, parents, children, group leaders and behavioral observers. Behaviors noted on the checklist were analogous to those listed on the observational scale used for the research. (Copies of these instruments are available from the author.) In addition, children also completed a subclass of the Jesness Inventory (1969) designed to measure self-reported tendencies toward aggression. This scale consists of thirty-one items Jesness contends reflects awareness of unpleasant feelings, especially of anger and frustration, tendency to react readily with these emotions, and other discomforts concerning the presence and control of such feelings.

Behavior Observation of Children and Therapist

An observation technique was devised to measure frequencies of pro-social, non-social, and antisocial behavior exhibited by children and frequencies of worker therapeutic behavior. This procedure had seldom been implemented in open settings such as community centers. An observer in each group was instructed to remain as unobtrusive as possible and to avoid social interaction with the group. Upon introduction, children were informed that observers would not interfere in any way with the group, that all information obtained would be confidential—reviewed only by the research team—and that they could help observers do their work by ignoring them.

Child Behavioral Categories

Pro-social behavior was defined as any behavior directed toward completion of group tasks or toward participation in group activities. Non-social behavior was defined as behavior not directed toward the completion of group tasks or activities. Antisocial behavior was defined as behavior preventing members from participating in group tasks or activities. Specific behaviors used in the definitions are available from the author; for an extended discussion see Wodarski (1978).

Therapist Behavior Categories

Observers rated therapist behavior according to the general category of whether therapists intervened on an individual level, i.e. individual intervention with one child, or on a group level, i.e. group intervention with two or more children. Observers then specified therapist behavior with respect to the following categories: directions, physical contact, praise, positive attention, holding, criticism, threats, negative attention, and time-out. To conserve space these categories are not elaborated. For an extended discussion, see Wodarski, Feldman, and Pedi: (1976).

Observational Protocol and Rater Agreement

A cohort of forty-two trained raters, assigned to the various intervention groups, collected observational data on all children and therapists according to a predetermined protocol. Every ten seconds, raters recorded a group member's behavior. Rotating around the group, raters observed all children and therapists numerous times each session. Agreement among raters was quantified by having different raters observe identical videotaped group sessions. Using data collected for each ten second interval, rater scores were compared through dividing instances raters agreed on an observational code by instances they agreed and disagreed. For 257 such agreements checks, raters showed a mean of .91, with a range of .82 to .99, across all child and therapist behavior code recordings.

Subjective Evaluation

Subjective evaluation included assessment by agency and research staff, parents, group leaders, observers, children, and referral source workers.

Subjective evaluations by agency staff and the behavioral observers were both positive and negative. Overall, it appeared that staff and observer general reaction was neutral. This could be due to their use of less specific outcome criteria, their concern not for method effectiveness but for how treatment helped each individual child, and their concern with how much time and energy was involved in adequately implementing the method.

Research staff learned how difficult it was to implement and evaluate an intervention in terms of outcome criteria, ensuring quality of instruction and supervision, ensuring the consistency of implementation, and in terms of the complexity of developing methods measuring the relationship between intervention and change.

Criteria employed by parents, children, group workers and referral agency personnel did not reflect criteria employed by agency or research staff. Most evaluated the project positively, indicating through verbal reports and questionnaires that it helped them or their children, and was a good and enjoyable experience. Such assessments, however, were not collaborated by other data. These data suggest that consumers use different criteria for evaluation than do researchers. Consumer assessment of benefits is a difficult issue to resolve, especially when consumer criteria differ from researcher criteria.

How Evaluation Addressed our Needs

Most behavioral researchers have isolated highly specific variables for study—group vs. individual contingencies, for example. However, when working with large, evaluative studies, which might be designated as process studies, data are less clear cut. Such ambiguity usually results because the implementation of the independent variable, such as method of therapy, is not consistently conceptualized and monitored.

Thus, a first requirement for systematic study is adequate conceptualization and operationalization of intervention and of the dimensions indicating its implementation. These steps provide the basis for adequate evaluation and a more precise analysis of intervention effect. Our data may have shown no observed behavioral differences between group therapies because the observational categories were too broad or because they did not include relevant behavior. If we assume the categories were valid and should yield different behavior rates between methods, a next step involves developing mechanisms assuring that different group therapies were implemented. This may involve providing mechanisms through which therapists can gain feedback on how they are implementing methods. Such channels would incorporate data from observers on therapists and children behavior, data from self-inventories, and a periodic review of videotapes on therapy implementation. These procedures would increase the probability that intervention was being implemented, which in turn increases the probability of adequately testing the intervention.

Thus, lack of intervention differences may lie in the observation system—broad coding categories not conceptually consonant with intervention—in deficiencies in the implementation, such as too global conceptualizations of intervention, or in poor therapist training and supervision. Hence, therapist data facilitate evaluating whether methods were implemented correctly.

Moreover, our experiences indicate that securing adequate referrals is essential for a proper test of community-based intervention. We believe that only through behavioral measurement in the natural and intervention environment can various interventions be validated and compared. Since financial and administrative constraints on the present effort did not permit such procedures, we had to depend on professional opinions as to whether children would exhibit antisocial behavior at the intervention site with the same frequency this behavior was manifested in the natural environment.

INTENDED PROGRAM CONSEQUENCES

Adequate evaluation of intervention did occur through behavioral observation and self inventories completed by children, referral sources, group leaders, parents, and observers. Evaluation was facilitated by detailed conceptualization of behavioral group work with antisocial children and development of a reliable scale for measuring child and therapist behavior. Researchers learned much about requisites for the establishment, implementation, and evaluation of community-based intervention.

Cost-effectiveness

Successfully applying behavioral group work can be costly. Behavioral group work is a complex approach in terms of choosing appropriate intervention to achieve desired change. Likewise, adequate supervision is an absolute necessity. Videotaping, another costly investment, should provide data indicating how behavioral methods are being applied. Data derived from tapes are then used to alter application of the techniques.

Initial training for the St. Louis project consisted of a five-hour seminar in which behavioral techniques were applied. Thereafter, supervision was provided twice weekly. Prior to the seminar, practitioners acquired a general knowledge of behavioral principles through selected readings from Feldman and Wodarski (1975) and others. Next, professional group workers role-played various aspects of group meetings, illustrating specific concepts, and hence serving as therapist models.

After practitioners had occasion to observe professionals, they were afforded an opportunity to lead groups. Immediate feedback from practitioners and colleagues enhanced learning. Videotapes were another feedback mechanism. Tapes provided a medium where various facets of practice could be replayed and examined immediately and repetitively. Beginning practitioners reviewed tapes, made behavioral diagnoses, and designed corresponding intervention plans. Performance on such tasks met the following criteria: 1) clear explication of behavior to be modified, especially in terms of observable referents; and 2) clear explication of intervention selected to achieve requisite change. Practitioners also were trained to collect systematic behavioral data. This necessitated that they become skilled in observational techniques.

The requisites of behavioral group work are substantial. Developing behavioral goals for each child and for the group is costly in terms of supervisor time. Likewise, provision of data to workers through videotaping or behavioral observation is expensive both in time and money. Costly data analyses are necessary to evaluate the effectiveness of behavioral group work. If traditional control group designs are employed, expenditures of money, energy, and administration can be substantial. Such considerations should be examined carefully before a decision is made to implement behavioral group work.

Continuance of Initial Work

Various social service agencies dealing with antisocial children have adopted the described behavioral group work model with antisocial children. Unfortunately, the model is not currently being subjected to as extensive an empirical testing as occurred during the St. Louis project. This investigator and others have executed additional work attesting to the efficacy of group contingencies as viable means of behavior change (Slavin and Wodarski 1978).

UNINTENDED PROGRAM CONSEQUENCES

Organizational Barriers

Staff resistances mentioned previously by other researchers were encountered in the present work. Concerns centered on additional supervisor paperwork controlling the quality of intervention and supervision, additional in-service staff training, fears of evaluation, and uneasiness regarding behavioral observers and videotaping.

All procedures were readily accepted when rationales were provided for their inclusion. It should be stressed, however, that adoption was facilitated through agency executive sanctions and through care on the part of the researchers to address the concerns of practitioners. Had these procedures not been followed and had the staff become anti-program, the project most assuredly would have failed (cf. Wodarski and Feldman 1974; Feldman and Wodarski 1975).

Stereotypes

Most stereotypes concerning behavior modification were encountered and dealt with. Since words hold different connotations to practitioners and researchers, successful execution of a project sometimes depends on the choice of terms. When such labels as "control group," "randomness," "antisocial child," and "behavior modification" are introduced researchers should be certain that there is a clear understanding of terms so workers do not assign incorrect or unintended meanings. The same procedures should be utilized in the interpretation of a behavioral project to lay boards and citizens of the general community. A misinterpretation occurred, for example, when intervention was labeled "behavior modification" during a presentation to community center staff. Some staff responded that they viewed such treatment to include "shocking" children and similar punitive measures. Clear explication of the method was necessary for staff to understand its goals and implementation. Thus, it was explained that group leaders using behavior modification were taught to avoid punitive measures and, instead, to set rewards for behavior and to decrease behavior by not attending to it. The same procedure had to be used to illustrate the rationale of baseline, how symptom substitution would not occur, and so forth.

Serendipitous Findings

Based on our experience, the need to increase accuracy of the referral procedures is evident. The self-inventory used in the referral procedure was a satisfactory initial step in operationalizing the referral process. But, a more accurate selection of children who could have benefited from the intervention may have occurred if more measurements of antisocial behavior were carried out in the natural environment. Administrative obstacles, noted earlier, precluded this procedure.

This project could have benefited from better worker preparation, despite extensive training with videotapes, role plays, and practice. More comprehensive and systematic training involving additional practice in making behavioral diagnosis, designing and implementing intervention, and evaluating change would facilitate program implementation. Finally, the reliability of the self-inventories was low. Had they been available, inventories that more accurately measure antisocial behavior may have yielded better data.

IMPLICATIONS FOR THE FUTURE

Practice

More accurate referral procedures should be developed. Revised referral procedures of self-inventories and behavioral data might ensure that children will exhibit antisocial behavior in the intervention context. Second, clinicians must maintain realistic expectations of what can be done for a child. The behavior repertoire of a child considered antisocial cannot be altered significantly through a one- or two-hour intervention program once weekly. More comprehensive services are needed to combine family therapy, group work, and vocational therapy, for example.

As behavioral group work becomes more adequately conceptualized, agencies must be equipped to help workers become proficient in applying behavioral methods, i.e. developing feedback mechanisms assessing how well methods are being implemented.

Further, no one attempting to do behavioral group work should initiate such complex intervention without professional supervision; and supervisors must be willing to spend necessary time and energy in program development and implementation.

Research to be Done

We need to establish better measurement of antisocial behavior—i.e. improve correlations among behavioral methods, self-inventories and other modes of data collection. Future research should establish "non-deviant" behavior rates to provide guidelines for decisions to offer services. Moreover, future research should center on the delineation of variables influencing the referral process such as clients' race, socio-economic factors, and age to facilitate connecting children with appropriate services.

Any behavioral intervention program should include procedures for the maintenance and generalization of change. Programs should also include follow-up. Follow-up would enable researchers to ascertain whether gains were maintained and how antisocial behavior changes over time. Since such steps require developing means to collect data outside of the intervention context, methodological and administrative costs will be substantial. Finally, conceptualization of behavioral group work should continue to be advanced through research and practice endeavors such as those described in this chapter.

2

Parents as Agents for Behavior Change

Elsie M. Pinkston
Benjamin S. Friedman
and
Richard A. Polster

Changing dysfunctional interactions between parents and their children should be the highest priority in family mental health. Although therapists may disagree regarding etiological and treatment factors in emotional disturbance of children, it is generally agreed that negative interactions help maintain angry and aggressive child behavior (Patterson, Reid, Jones, and Conger 1975). Without major changes it is unlikely that improvement can be achieved with severely disturbed children. Accordingly, parents, teachers, and even siblings are taught to encourage prosocial behaviors of targeted children. From the behavioral clinician's perspective this process is one of education in social learning techniques, teaching parents reinforcement techniques and contingency management procedures to enhance and maintain improved social interaction between them and their children (Berkowitz and Graziano 1972; Hall, Christler, Cranston, and Tucker 1970; Johnson and Katz 1973; O'Dell 1974).

This move toward using family members and other nonprofessionals as part of the intervention team is part of the evolution from intervention with individuals in institutions and other therapeutic settings toward a more community-oriented approach. The technology for studying human behavior, originally developed in institutions for retarded and emotionally disturbed children, provides the base for research in naturalistic settings.

The Parent Education Program (PEP) is designed for parents of aggressive children between five and twelve years old, referred by school and community outreach social workers. Founded on social reinforcement theory, the program regards interpersonal breakdown in families as the result of infrequent reciprocal reinforcement of positive behaviors between parents and children and teaches family members to increase rates of positive reinforcement for appropriate interpersonal task-oriented behavior. This chapter outlines fundamental steps in the PEP intervention and assessment process. Data from individual children and families illustrate these steps. Assessment includes questionnaires and direct observation during baseline and intervention of parent and child behavior, and evaluation of tape recordings of family conversations during baseline and intervention to assess generalization of effects. A consumer questionnaire is administered to the parents by mail following termination and follow-up interviews are conducted by telephone 2 years beyond termination.

Intervention focuses on establishing positive interactional patterns via modeling, rehearsal and contracting. During parent training, behavioral contingencies are modeled by the therapist and are rehearsed with parents and children. Contracting procedures are practiced and subsequently instituted in each home.

Intervention

After referral to PEP, social workers contact the family by telephone to explore the possibility of program participation. Initial agreement to collaborate is then followed by mailed out questionnaires and an invitation to come to an orientation session at the PEP lab.

At the beginning of this face-to-face interview, workers explain that parents will be taught skills that will help them with current problems, and be useful in handling future ones. Emphasis is on discriminating and modifying problems early so parents can begin to work independently.

The Parent Education Program is presented as a vehicle for helping families learn to interact appropriately through more positive means. Social workers' responsibilities are defined as teaching parents data collection and procedures for independent intervention with future child-interaction problems, helping implement school intervention programs if necessary, and being available for consultation by telephone or home visit. Parental responsibilities include attending two clinical sessions, collecting data on their child's behavior, reading *Parents Are Teachers* (Becker, 1971), and carrying out negotiated intervention programs.

Baseline Data Collection

Using information from telephone contact, paper and pencil checklists, and the clinical interview, parents specify troublesome behaviors or those needing improvement. Specific descriptions of behaviors are written on an observation form, preserving much of the parent's language. Typically, a positive and a negative behavior are selected for baselining.

Once behaviors and chores are defined, instructions are provided specifying use of data collection forms. A frequency count of targeted behaviors is recorded by the parents during a one- to two-week period in which the problems were most likely to occur. These data are telephoned to answering service for daily monitoring by the worker. Also, each family is visited in the home during the baseline period. Purposes of this visit are to collect additional data on parents and children, to determine whether or not relevant targets had been defined, to compare independent observer data with that recorded by parents, to answer any questions regarding the data collection or the program, and to pick up any paper and pencil data.

Teaching Behavioral Principles

Baseline data accumulation is then followed by the first parent training session. Workers start by teaching operant principles through relevant examples. Discussing reinforcement, workers remind parents how they contributed to their child's early walking and talking by praising the child. The training session further addresses family communication in terms of its relationship to parent/child interaction. Workers emphasize the importance of parents in presenting a united front. Workers suggest that disagreements frequently result in children receiving different and confusing messages from parents. Parents are also told that analysis of family communications often reveal that children pit parents against each other to avoid negative consequences.

Parents are next introduced to a set of contracting rules. These include: setting aside a block of time to talk with the child, selecting one behavior and defining it in observable terms, describing all important aspects of the behavior (e.g. how often it should be done, when it should be done, and who will demonstrate and teach it), agreeing on a reinforcer for performing the behavior, deciding who will determine whether the behavior was completed, and noting all of the above information in a written and signed contract. Because program success relies heavily on reinforcement, parents and workers devote considerable time to identifying immediate and backup reinforcers. This process begins when parents are asked to list reinforcers already existing in their environment—television, free time, trips, and movies for example. Whenever possible, workers suggest that parents engage in a positive activity with the child to reward appropriate behavior.

Major child management techniques discussed with the parents are differential attention, shaping, time out, and overcorrection. Techniques are again described by examples, usually drawn from parents' own experience. Workers stress that the two latter procedures should only be used with predefined seriously negative behavior, such as hurting another person, and that punishment is most likely to be successful when combined with differential attention and the shaping of positive behavior.

Decisions regarding the selection of target behavior for home intervention are based on baseline data. In most cases, highly visible behavior and actions that occur frequently are selected. Occasionally, a behavior is dropped because parents no longer consider it to be a problem or because it occurs at such a low rate that it provides limited opportunity for parents to learn to treat it. Home point systems are jointly negotiated with parents and children until agreement among all involved family members is obtained with the most difficult behavior receiving the most points. Point systems are developed for siblings of the target child when desired by parents or requested by the children.

During the final segment of the first training interview, workers model differential use of parent attention, monitoring of point systems, time out, and overcorrection procedures. After modeling, parents are asked to rehearse each procedure with their child, with the trainers providing reinforcement and feedback. Parents unable to carry out a procedure are given positive feedback on some aspect of their performance and provided additional instructions and repeated modeling until the parent has performed each step. The many items that must be covered in this interview have resulted in an outline for PEP workers to complete at the first training session. Presented in Table one, the outline helps remind workers of their agenda and serves as a feedback source for later evaluation.

Subsequent Home Visits

Practical application is facilitated by visits to the home where workers record independent data on targeted behavior, make necessary revisions in the data collection procedures, discuss difficulties with the point system with the children, assist the parents in rehearsing praise, ignoring, awarding points, contracting, and using punishment procedures, while reviewing all intervention procedures; in most cases, only one visit is necessary.

Termination and Follow-up

Termination for PEP families occurs when they have achieved stable behavior changes for three weeks, and when children have been removed from the home point system. At this time, parents are provided data collection materials for the development of another home point system

Table 1. First Training Session Outline

Date: ______________________________
Worker: ______________________________
Parent: ______________________________

I. Present behavioral principles and examples.
____A. Reinforcement ______________ Example ______________
____B. Extinction ______________ Example ______________
____C. Punishment ______________ Example ______________
____D. Target Behaviors ______________ Example ______________

II. Communication.
____A. Reciprocal: parents teach children and children teach parents.
____B. Directions and requests should be explicit; no please or okay? at the end of a direction if compliance is expected.
____C. Parents must present a united front to the children.

III. Responsibilities of worker.
____A. Train skills.
____B. Organize program at home.
____C. Only work on parent specified behaviors.

IV. Responsibilities of Parent.
____A. Record data.
____B. Practice skill as trained and advise or discuss alternatives.
____C. Gain independence from PEP.
____D. Be specific and explicit in expectations.
____E. Follow through on behavioral assignments.

V. Contracting rules.
____A. Sit down with child.
____B. Select one behavior and define it in observable terms.
____C. Describe all the important aspects of the behavior, such as:
  ____1. how often should it be done
  ____2. when (the specific time) it should be done
  ____3. where it should be done
  ____4. who will demonstrate and teach the behavior to the child
____D. Agree on a reward which will be given for performing the behavior.
____E. Decide who will determine whether the behavior was completed according to the definition.
____F. Write down all of the above information in a contract format similar to the contract written in the training session.
____G. Both parents and child should agree and sign the contract.

VI. Time out and overcorrection.
____A. Specify behavior and procedure.
____B. Time out ______________ Example ______________
____C. Overcorrection ______________ Example ______________

VII. Decision on target behaviors at home.
____A. Initial information on questionnaire is used to determine target behaviors.
____B. Determine reasonable rewards, privileges, and bonuses.

VIII. Point system.
____A. Earning and spending of points.
____B. Specificity of expectations is facilitated.
____C. Bonus rewards are possible and helpful.
____D. Determine value of behaviors on point system form.
____E. Contract point system with child.

IX. Modeling.
____A. Praise ______________ Example ______________
____B. Ignoring ______________ Example ______________
____C. Points ______________ Example ______________
____D. Punishment ______________ Example ______________

X. Review program.

should other problems occur, and are asked to complete an evaluation form. Parents are also told to call workers if their child has further problems they feel need assistance.

Two to three months following termination, workers call parents to ascertain if they are still keeping data. If so, parents are asked to describe the behavior and any intervention. Parents are further asked to evaluate the program and describe its effectiveness in remediating their children's problems. Similar follow-up calls are repeated every six months for two years.

ASSESSMENT AND EVALUATION

The parent training program, as detailed in this chapter, is aided by the collection and use of a number of data sources, the most important being collection by the parent during the baseline and treatment phase of the program, when they tally the occurrence of targeted behaviors in a specified time frame, usually one to two hours, each day. These data are then reported daily by phone to enable the worker to monitor progress and continued parental participation.

An additional data source is an observer in the home during probes and reliability checks. This home visit, scheduled when the parents record data, establishes the reliability or accuracy of the parents' data. The observer's data, compared before and after treatment, demonstrates whether or not it reflects behavioral changes similar to those found in the parent-recorded data.

More subjective data regarding the program is provided through a consumer evaluation form mailed to the parent one or two months following termination to determine their opinon of the program's effectiveness, and supplemented by periodic telephone interviews soliciting parents' perception of the program's long-term value and of the behavioral procedures.

FINDINGS

Of sixteen families evaluated to date, thirteen have completed the intervention phase. Eleven families indicated program success, defined as a substantial decrease in inappropriate behavior and agreement between workers and parents that the program had helped improve the child's behavior. Two families completed the training program but did not implement the program in such a way as to gain a positive effect; three families were terminated following the initial interview because of unwillingness or inability to collect baseline data. As illustrations, three case studies are presented here as representative of program successes.

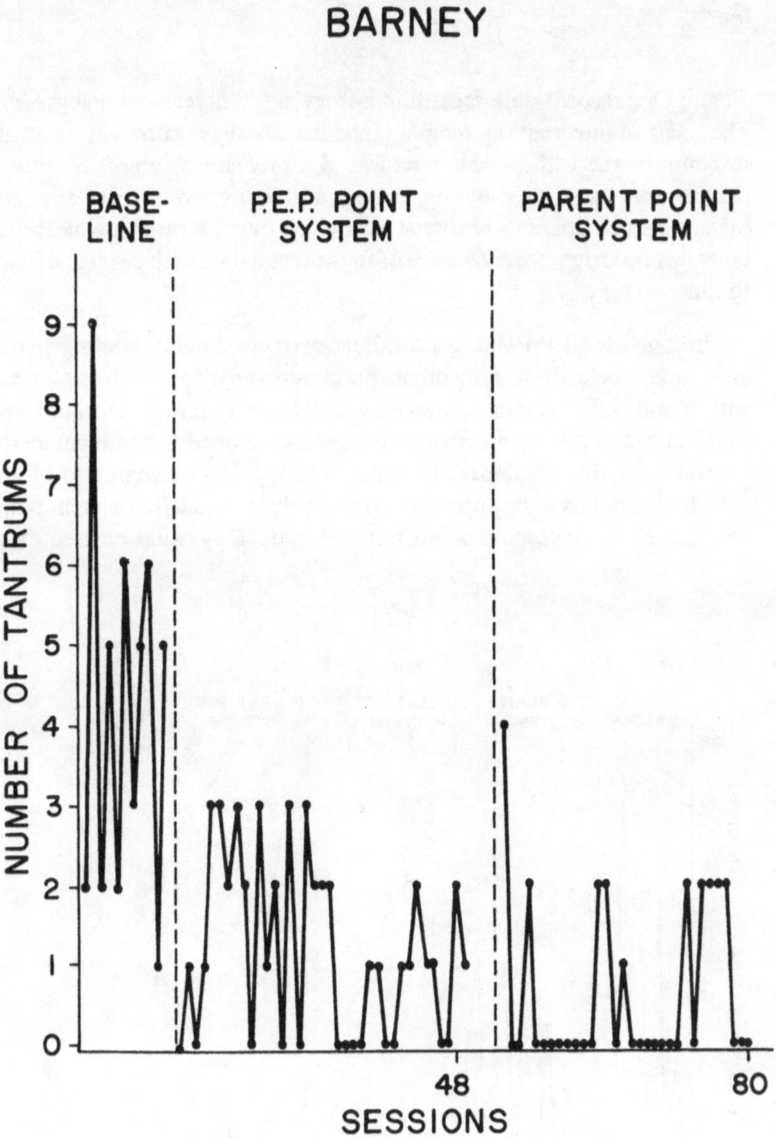

FIGURE 1. Number of Temper Tantrums by Barney During Daily 1-Hour Observation Session.

Barney

Figure One records data regarding Barney, a seven-year-old first grader. The focus of intervention, temper tantrums, usually occurred at home in response to the withdrawal or refusal of a privilege or object by either parent, and included shouting, crying, and aggressive threats directed toward Barney's parents or three-year-old brother. During baseline, brief tantrums occurred on an average of four times a day, with a range of one to nine.

Through the PEP Point System, Barney received points contingent on appropriate behaviors, daily points purchasing privileges such as playing with friends after school or watching television. Failure to earn at least fourteen out of twenty possible points per day resulted in confinement to his room for the remainder of the day. Daily points exceeding fourteen were bonus points to be applied to special privileges, such as a fishing trip with father. Once specific points were set aside, they could be used only

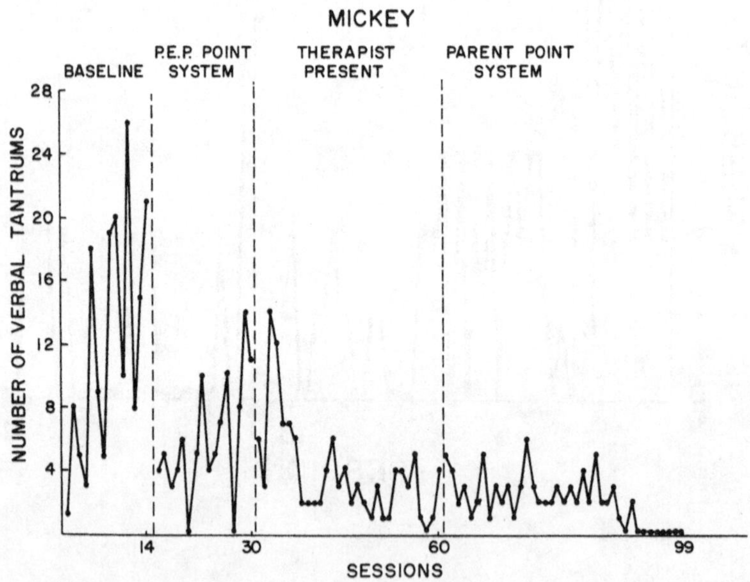

FIGURE 2. Number of Verbal Tantrums by Mickey During Daily 2-Hour Observation Session.

for that event. During this phase temper tantrums decreased to approximately one per day, with a range of zero to three.

In the second phase, Parent Point System, the number of behaviors included was reduced to eight. Instituted by parents, the new point system streamlined record keeping and allowed concentration on a few target responses—appropriate play and talking in a soft voice—rather than working on wider variety of household duties. Under this second point system, the daily number of tantrums decreased to an average of less than one per day, ranging from one to four over thirty two days.

Mickey

Data for Mickey, a seven-year-old first grader exhibiting high rates of verbal tantrums, are shown in Figure Two. Verbal tantrums included nagging, whining, and screaming. Since parents reported difficulty in teaching Mickey to comply with their requests in the face of such verbal barrages, they saw decreasing verbal tantrums as a step toward increasing positive interactions in the home. During the fourteen-day baseline period, Mickey's verbal tantrums averaged twelve times per day.

A point system instituted for sixteen days allowed Mickey to receive daily points contingent on engaging in appropriate household behavior—such as cleaning his room—as well as on behavior incompatible with verbal tantrums—compliance with parental requests and not yelling. By earning thirty out of a possible forty two points, Mickey could purchase daily privileges of television or play time. Points earned in excess of thirty were saved and exchanged for weekly bonuses. Failure to earn minimum points needed to purchase daily privileges resulted in the child staying in his room for the evening. Under the PEP Point System, verbal tantrums decreased to an average of six daily with an upward trend the final three days of the condition.

For the next thirty days, intervention was implemented with the social worker present five nights the first week, fading to four, three, two, one nights during subsequent weeks, and finally to an on-call advisory status. During this phase the worker modeled procedures and instructed parents in intervention with Mickey and with his younger sister. Verbal tantrums decreased to four per day, with a range of one to fourteen.

The third and final interventive phase, the Parent Point System, involved a chart constructed by Mickey and his parents with pictorial examples of point-earning behavior; Mickey was no longer reminded to engage in appropriate behavior, and daily report cards from school also permitted him to earn points for schoolwork. Quite successful, this thirty nine day phase saw verbal tantrums decreasing to less than two per day.

Jim

Jim, whose data are presented in Figure Three, was a six-year-old kindergarten student. Jim's parents expressed their extreme difficulty in teaching their child to comply with requests. Specifically, the parents were frequently unable to get Jim to follow instructions without nagging him into a "battle of the wills." Noncompliance, operationally defined as the third occasion on which either parent told Jim to engage in a task, frequently occurred around picking up toys and bath and bedtime routines. During baseline, noncompliance averaged six episodes per day, with a range of zero to fourteen for twenty eight days.

During intervention Jim earned points for behaviors that his parents were interested in adding to his repertoire of skills—e.g. making his bed and keeping toys in specific storage areas—as well as responses incompatible with noncompliance, such as complying with parental requests the first time they were made. Daily points, within a range of eighteen to twenty-eight, were redeemed for playing with toys, watching television, playing on the porch, and similiar activities. Bonus points,

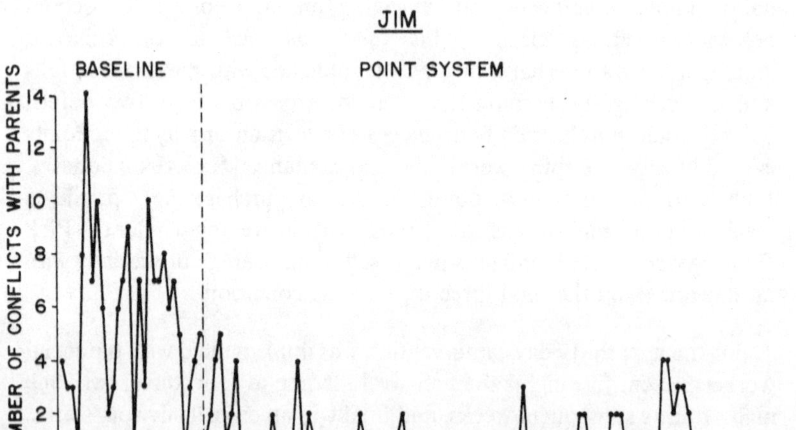

FIGURE 3. Number of Noncompliances With Parental Requests by Jim During Daily 2-Hour Observation Session.

earned over the minimum amount needed to purchase daily activities, were spent weekly for special treats, a movie, building and flying model airplanes with father, or going on a shopping trip, for example. Jim also earned a daily allowance contingent on earning minimum daily points.

Points for positive behavior at school were also added to the home point-system. Each day, Jim's teacher filled out a report card in which he could earn a total of eight points contingent on no time-outs, staying in his work area, raising his hand, and bringing papers home. To emphasize the importance of appropriate school behavior following decreased conflicts at home, first four points and later six school points were required for Jim to earn his daily privileges. Subsequently, noncompliance decreased to an average of less than one daily instance over 101 days.

CONCLUSION

Findings from other parent training programs (Berkowitz and Graziano 1972; Johnson and Katz 1973) and our research experiences indicate that parents can be taught to alter their children's inappropriate behavior through a combination of techniques including instructions, contracting, modeling, rehearsal, and feedback. In the case studies described, child behavior was positively altered by helping parents change their interactional approach. Objective data gathered on short-term improvements and long-range maintenance of learning support the Parent Education Program as a means for helping families in the community before their children's problems need costly professional and institutional services.

The program is designed to require a minimum number of in-clinic contacts between the social worker and the family and to focus attention on family interaction in the home. Because intervention is implemented in the home, it decreases the necessity of programming generalization of behavioral change from the clinic to home. It also reduces the difficulty parents encounter in making office appointments—i.e. obtaining babysitters, finding transportation, and getting time off from work—possibly an important variable in reducing discontinuance. Moreover, behavioral procedures, providing a positive alternative to the aversive control frequently encountered, can be modified to fit families with a variety of needs. Single parents, low-income groups, and intact families with adequate resources can equally prosper from this approach.

Unfortunately, few systematic attempts are made to teach people how to be good parents. We hope our efforts can help other social workers redress this serious neglect in preparing children to in turn become resonsible adults and better parents to their offspring.

3

Reaching Underachievers

Richard Polster
Mary Ann Lynch
and
Elsie M. Pinkston

SCHOOL SOCIAL WORK

The service responsibilities of school social workers are numerous, addressing many client groups, including students, families, teachers, and the community. Areas of involvement for school social workers encompass befriending lonely students, helping troubled families contact community agencies, helping students with academic decisions, and developing curricula and school policy. Regardless of service focus, school social workers influence and aid students in acquiring basic skills for the future. Ideally, such influence and aid results in improved opportunities for students to lead productive and successful lives. Social work participation in schools is not a new phenomenon; involvement in academic issues and one-to-one intervention are recent additions to school social workers' roles.

School social work in the United States dates to the early 1900's when social services were delivered through private agencies and civic organizations. Social work services were most often made available in
University students significantly improved mathematics performance

response to social legislation such as compulsory school attendance laws (Costin 1977). As social work participation in schools developed, the nature and direction of intervention changed. In 1922, Richmond emphasized important links between school and home, recommending social workers look to homes when dealing with school problems of inadequate scholarship, tardiness, and poor attendance. For example, Richmond described an early case in which a social worker helped a student organize his time to raise his grades (Richmond, 1922).

Despite an early emphasis on social social work, Costin concluded that in the 1960's neither educators nor social workers expressed appropriate concern about students' learning problems. She criticized social workers for failing to develop intervention programs for students not doing well academically and suggested the primary task of school social work was to help students acquire needed skills for adulthood (Costin, 1969). In 1972, Costin again addressed the issue, stating that although social workers had assumed new roles in schools, changes were neither "dramatic nor sufficient" (Costin, 1972(a); 348). She suggested changes in school social work approaches and that "the focus of work with pupils be shifted from an emphasis on emotion, motivation, and personality toward learning, thinking, and problem solving" (Costin 1972(a): 350). Radin also stressed social work involvement in academically related areas, not limiting services to "emotion" problems. One of Radin's goals was "to promote the maximum development of all children in school, particularly those whose potential has been grossly unrealized" (Radin 1975:605). Consequently, the scope and responsibility of social work involvement in schools has grown.

In light of issues raised by Costin and Radin and increasing caseloads, efficient programs for school-based intervention are essential. One example of a successful intervention program is Epstein's Task-Centered Project. Epstein found the Task-Centered approach particularly effective in helping children operationalize problems and work toward solutions (Epstein, 1977). Other examples of effective school-based intervention strategies come from applied behavior analysis. Unique properties of behavior analysis including operational problem definitions, consistent data recording, and outcome evaluation make possible efficient, problem-focused interventions. For these reasons, this chapter presents the use of behavioral procedures in the design, implementation, and evaluation of a social work intervention program for seventh and eight-grade underachievers.

Additionally, this chapter reviews the current literature on underachievement, focusing on behavioral research and procedures successful in related areas. We present a detailed explanation of the underachievement intervention program along with a discussion of the program's effectiveness and a consideration of implementation issues.

UNDERACHIEVEMENT

Research has correlated low interest in early schooling to termination of education prior to high school graduation (Savage, 1976). Moreover, a recent article cited poor academic performance as a major cause of dropping out of school (*U.S. News and World Report,* 1976). This phenomenon is not new: a survey conducted over twenty five years ago revealed underachievement as a prevalent social problem. Reviewing records of 1,162 suburban junior and senior high school students, Alter (1954) found that of the 7% having scores of 130 and above on the California Test of Mental Maturity 42% were classified as underachievers because grade-point averages were below their tested IQ's. Investigating two high school graduating classes, Ritler and Thome (1954) discovered only 35% had grade point averages as high as IQ scores. Such statistics are compelling evidence that underachievers may also be less likely to complete high school than average or high achievers.

What are the consequences of early termination of schooling? One appears to be a high likelihood of chronic unemployment. Recent labor statistics showed 25.3% of youths aged sixteen to nineteen with one to three years of high school unemployed; youths with four years of high school had an unemployment rate of 16.1% (Hedges, 1976).

Efforts to identify family types associated with underachievement have not revealed consistent patterns of interpersonal relations (Chance, 1965; Morrow and Wilson 1965; and Wellington and Wellington, 1968). Some studies described underachievers as being pushed and engineered; others see these students no more pressured than average or high achieving students. Thus, it may not be safe to assume that underachievers have unique family backgrounds.

Traditionally, those attempting to help underachievers have considered emotional problems primarily responsible for poor academic performance. Intervention through individual, group, and parent counseling produced mixed results in changing students' attitudes about achievement (Brodel, Ohlsen, Proff, & Southard 1965; Carr, 1971; Hummel, 1966; Walsh and Steggs 1972). No study reported counseling alone as being effective in improving students' grades. These failures may result from focusing on emotional problems rather than directly on underachievement. Other attempts to alleviate the problem have identified underachievement as lack of motivation. Studies following this orientation have used a variety of verbal and motivational incentives. Lowe (1973), for example, reported that verbal praise was insufficient in improving academic performance. Klein, Quarter, and Laxer (1969) determined that verbally rewarding in-class risk taking (e.g. raising one's hand when not completely sure of the answer) did not help raise students' grades; material rewards produced a more potent effect on grades.

when paid for improvement, but changes did not generalize to other academic areas, e.g. history or science (Kipnis & Resnick, 1971).

Programs focusing on study behavior have modified underachievement. In one program, Karnes, McCoy, Zehrbach, Wollersheim, and Clarizio (1965) improved the grades of adolescent underachievers by placing them in a class with high achievers. Exposure to contingencies emphasizing achievement may have been a key factor. An eight-week study skills training program, combined with using desired activities as rewards for studying, improved college students' grade-point averages (Foreman 1969). Positive results of these studies indicate that reinforcing academic performance and emphasizing the expectation for high achievement are essential program components.

By definition, underachievers are capable of doing their work. Indeed, a major reason for receiving poor grades appears to be noncompletion of homework assignments. To document this relationship, Wilson and Morrow (1965) surveyed teachers on the amount of student homework handed in and found 91% of high achievers turned in homework compared to 9% of the underachievers. Lack of work produced outside of school may underlie most underachievement. Incomplete homework assignments generally mean poor class preparation, often resulting in poor classroom performance. Below standard classroom performance precludes the possibility of positive attention for work effort. When students do not prepare for class, teachers may lower future expectations. A cycle of underachievement develops when students continue to perform below ever decreasing standards.

SELF-CONTROL

Programs stressing self-control and increased study time have generally had a positive effect on underachievement. Self-regulation programs have four distinct advantages: (1) Students have personal control and choice of target behaviors and reinforcers (Ballard and Glynn, 1975; Flowers, 1972; Klein and Schuler, 1974); (2) Students are the best agents for changing their own behavior; (3) Self-control programs teach technical and analytical skills useful in future attempts at self-change (Jeffrey, 1974; Phillips, Phillips, Wolf, & Fixsen, 1973); and (4) Self-monitoring gives immediate performance feedback and serves as reinforcement (Kazdin, 1974c).

Researchers have successfully implemented self-control procedures for problems of anxiety (Rehm and Marston, 1968), smoking (Keutzer, Lichtenstein, & Mees, 1968; McFall, 1970; Roberts, 1969), obesity (Goldiamond, 1965; Stuart and Davis, 1972; and Stunkard, 1972), and classroom disruptions (Bolstad and Johnson, 1972; Glynn, 1970; Lovitt and Curtiss, 1969). Broden, Hall, and Mitts (1971) and Johnson and White (1971) found self-monitoring sufficient to increase the total time pupils spent studying. Knapczyk and Livingston (1973) showed a combination of self-recording and tokens produced substantial reading improvement. Klein and Schuler (1974) implemented a self-monitoring program improving accuracy of math solutions.

Empirical research indicates that students can change their study behavior, monitor their own progress, and increase homework completion. Such research, combined with the action-oriented direction of school social work, was used to design and implement a program for ameliorating underachievement with seventh and eighth grade students in a public elementary school by addressing three questions: Do grades improve more for program participants than for nonparticipants? Can students be taught to manage programs without initial parent control? Can the program be implemented within the time constraints of school social workers' schedules?

THE METHOD

Students

Students in the seventh and eight grades of a large urban school with a difference of not less than 0.75 points between their average score on the Iowa Test of Basic Skills and their grade-point averages for the first and second grading periods of the 1975-1976 school year were categorized as underachievers and comprise the study sample. Of 180 seventh and eight graders, forty-four met the criteria.

Doubtless, there are potential problems using the IQ score grade-points average discrepancy for identifying underachievers. Some have suggested that performance on a one or two day test may not be comparable with long-term success (Allen, 1971). Extraneous variables—illiness, good guessing—can hinder or help short-term performance. Use of standardized scores, however, appears preferable to merely asking teachers' opinions or defining underachievement through other subjective measures.

Five of the forty-four underachieving students evidenced classroom behavior problems (e.g. physical or verbal aggression) requiring more intensive intervention, and hence were excluded from the present study. The thirty-nine remaining students were assigned numbers randomly. In order of number assignment, students' parents were contacted in groups of three until twelve families agreed to participate. In all, nineteen families were contacted; students from three families declining participation were assigned to the comparison group; four students were excluded from experimental and comparison groups when they declined participation.

Study Design

A multiple-baseline design (Baer, Wolf & Risley, 1968; Hersen & Barlow, 1976; Howe, 1974) evaluated differences in study behavior between self-control procedures alone and parent-control procedures followed by self-control procedures. To make program implementation more manageable, the twelve subjects were assigned to one of four groups: A, B, C, or D. Because each group began recording baseline data after the preceding group began intervention, participant interest was not diminished by long periods of baseline recording. Students began intervention after fulfilling two requirements: First, the social worker had to achieve at least 80% reliability agreement with the parents' observational recording of study behavior; second, a minimum of five days' baseline data were recorded.

Self-control procedures were implemented by all experimental group students. Groups B and D controlled their own programs at the beginning of the intervention phase; Groups A and C did not start self-control procedures until they had performed appropriately under parent-control conditions. The decision to allow students to progress to the self-control phase of the program was determined through stability in study behavior as evidenced by parent-recorded data and the time constraints of the academic calendar. Parent-control was continued for from five to thirteen school days before self-control began.

Assessment covered a number of areas. Data recorded during baseline served as a reference for behavior change during intervention. Data recorded during the parent-managed program in Groups A and C were a reference for changes occurring when students assumed program management. Stability of two group members' behavior when a third began a new program phase was reference for assessing experimental effects in all four groups. Finally, academic performance based on report card grades compared the twelve experimental group students to the twenty three comparison group students.

Procedures

BASELINE DATA RECORDING Parents were taught to record data on their child's study behavior. During a home training session, worker and parents recorded data simultaneously. Comparing records determined parents' readiness to keep data independently. Parents' observations were conducted once every 30 minutes over the two and one half hour period they estimated their children would be studying. Duration and environmental setting of study behavior was kept on forms shown in Figure One.

Date 3/14 Time 7:15	Time 7:50	Time 8:10	Time 8:30	Time 9:10
Studying? YES ✓ NO ___	Studying? YES ✓ NO ___	Studying? YES ___ NO ✓	Studying? YES ___ NO ✓	Studying? YES ✓ NO ___
Place or Activity Study Area	Place or Activity Study Area	Place or Activity T.V.	Place or Activity Telephone	Place or Activity Study Area

FIGURE 1. Data Sample from Home Recording Checklist. The complete checklist included space for five days data, the date, and the students' names. Approximately every 30 minutes the parent observed the student. If the student was studying, YES was checked and the place in which the student was studying was noted. If the student was not studying, NO was checked and the activity in which the student was involved was noted.

In this example the student was studying during the first, second, and last observation periods. The place in which the studying occured was also noted. The third and fourth observations revealed that the student was not studying, but was watching T.V. and talking on the telephone.

INTERVENTION Because Goldiamond (1965) found using a specifically designated study area successful in increasing studying, a similar procedure was incorporated in this program. Siblings, television, records, and clutter were not allowed in the study area; the area was to be adequately lighted and have a chair and writing surface. Another component of the program was a home token economy system (Kazdin, 1977b). Even though students had the opportunity to choose their own reinforcers, the system was fundamentally the same for all students. The social worker used a reinforcer survey (Tharp & Wetzel, 1969) to devise individual reinforcer menus. A problem arose when some parents stated they expected children to do school work and did not understand why they should be paid. In these instances, the social worker explained that it would be nice if students worked for the sake of learning or because they were supposed to; but, the data showed they were not studying! Therefore, it was recommended the token economy system be tried for a short period to find if it could help the student begin working. Once the student began independent work, the token system would be systematically withdrawn. Since intermittent rewards maintain behavior change longer than do continuous rewards (Greenwood, Sloane, & Baskin, 1974; Kazdin & Polster, 1973; Skinner, 1953), gradually decreasing the frequency of planned reinforcement was an explicit program goal.

The kind and amount of scholastic performance necessary to obtain reinforcement was delineated in a point earning list. Typically, privileges of watching television, using the telephone, or playing with siblings or friends were contingent upon studying for a minimum amount of time. A process of negotiation involving parents, students, and the social worker was utilized for the assignment of point values to privileges and specific items on the reinforcement menu. The negotiation period emphasized academic behavior consisting of improving grades, maintaining good grades, and increasing study duration and frequency.

Attention to improving study skills was as much a part of the program as the token system. For use with all reading assignments, students were taught a modification of the SQ3R study program (Robinson, 1949). The program covers Survey, Question, Read, Write, and Review and consists of five steps: surveying the passages for headings and sub-headings; transforming headings into questions; reading the material; writing notes and answering questions devised in step two; and reviewing notes.

As with most teachers, those in the target school had heavy work loads; a minimum of extra effort connected with this program was thus requested of them. In addition to grading work students completed, the only additional task requested of teachers was to sign daily report card and assignment records, depicted in Figure Two. If a teacher did not assign homework, the student was to write "no homework" and the teacher signed the form in the same manner as when homework was

DAILY REPORT CARD AND ASSIGNMENT RECORD

Each day the student must fill in homework assignments in the appropriate squares. After the assignment has been recorded the student must have the teacher sign the assignment card to verify its correctness. If there is no homework assignment, that too should be certified. Teachers should record any grade achieved for the day, on tests, quizzes, and homework.

Date: 3/20/79 **Student's name:** TOM GILROY

	Teacher's Signature
Math — Assignment: WORKBOOK PAGES 23+24	J. Jenkins
Social Studies — Assignment: NO HOMEWORK	J. Bender
Science — Assignment: PART 2 OF NOTEBOOK	C. Mundy
English — Assignment: SPELLING LIST	M. Roger

Each subject row also has a Grades section with blank boxes:

Hmwk.	Test	Quiz	Papers

Any additional teacher comments are welcome.
Thank you for your help!

Tom is getting all his work in on time. He is doing much better.

FIGURE 2. Daily Report Card and Assignment Record. Students filled in homework assignments daily for each subject area.
Teachers verified assignments.

assigned. Students earned the same number of points for a signature for no homework as for the completion of homework assignments. This procedure was implemented to encourage completion of classroom assignments and appropriate use of class time allowed for homework completion. At home, assignment forms were used by students and parents to ensure that all homework had been completed. Whether or not the students had specific homework assigned, they were expected to spend a minimum amount of time studying before having access to privileges. Minimum amounts of time were negotiated during token economy system developments.

Finally, the social worker negotiated, witnessed, and specified responsibilities in a contract signed by parents and students (e.g., Figure Three.) All parties were given copies of the contract.

PARENT-CONTROL Intervention procedures were implemented within a parent-control structure by groups A and C. Parents recorded data on studying using time-sampled observations as during baseline. To gain access to privileges, receive material reinforcers, or progress to self-control, students had to demonstrate that they had completed assignments, had assignment forms signed by teachers, and showed all earned grades to parents.

SELF-CONTROL Groups B and D used intervention within a self-control structure. Monitoring and recording observational data were under student control, with parents making only periodic checks. Observational data recording by students was facilitated through the use of a wind-up timer: five times during a designated study period, students set the timer for ten to twenty minutes. When the timer sounded, it signaled the point at which students recorded whether or not they were studying. The timer also cued parents to check self-monitoring reliability. Frequency of parents' checks was determined by percentage of agreement between them and their children. If there was 100% agreement, parent checks decreased to four times the first week, three times the second, twice the third, and once weekly for the rest of the program.

The award and redemption of points were controlled by parents. Students initially showed their parents all completed work. As students evidenced change in study behavior, parental supervision was reduced. Nonetheless, all students were cautioned that if teachers or parents saw academic performance regressing, their parents would once again take control of the program. The importance of social reinforcers was explained to parents: they were told that if they verbally praised their children whenever they found them studying, they would increase the likelihood of future study behavior. The social worker then modeled how to give verbal praise. Many parents did not believe that praise or earning

FAMILY CONTRACT

We, the undersigned, understand procedures of the point and bonus program and will abide by them. HELEN LINOT agrees to earn at least 6 points for everyday privileges and as many bonus points possible for bonuses.

Parents of HELEN agree to present bonus awards when earned and limit everyday privileges when 6 points have not been earned.

Helen Linot
Student

L. Linot
Parent 1

Richard Polster
Witness

Tony Linot
Parent 2

Date 3/26/79

FIGURE 3. Family Contract. Sample contract each family signed to indicate their understanding and willingness to comply with the program.

points and good grades were important to their children. It appeared that parents had such poor histories of success in helping their children change study behavior that they had resigned themselves to continued failure. Indeed, one mother was quite surprised when her child decided not to accept the tape recorder earned through studying and improved grades. It was a learning experience for both parent and child when the student remarked, "I don't want the tape recorder; getting good grades is enough reward."

TERMINATION The program goal, students gaining independent study habits, was approached by the social worker systematically through decreasing frequency of contact with families. He did tell all families that he could be reached by telephone at any time if the need arose. Only two calls were received during the duration of the program—both placed by students who had recently begun their program—and concerned point exchange. One student wanted to know if he could watch television before he finished the required minimum amount of study time; the other wanted to borrow points for the studying he intended to do the next week. Because these requests breached contractual agreements, they were not granted.

Case Study

The progress of one student illustrates how one program was designed, implemented, and evaluated. Louis L. was a seventh grader clearly in need of immediate help. His academic profile showed an Iowa Test score of 4.8 (C+) and a grade-point average of 1.1 (D-). Louis had failing grades in mathematics and spelling and D grades in social studies, reading, composition, and science. In addition to Iowa scores indicating that he was capable of getting C grades, Louis's teachers said he could perform at a higher level. Teachers also reported that the student spent most class time socializing and that he rarely finished assignments in class or handed in homework.

Louis's mother warmly greeted the social worker at the first home visit. Ms. L said she was "happy to have help available and would try anything to help her son improve his grades." The worker showed her how to consistently record baseline data, and set a time for the next visit. When the worker returned he found Ms. L's data indicated that Louis devoted many hours to watching television. Informed of this, Louis agreed and said he did not really like all the shows he watched, but once he turned on the TV he watched all evening. And his school work suffered accordingly.

The social worker explained the home-study program to Louis and his mother. Louis liked the idea of being rewarded for completing his school work and improving his grades. Ms. L, on the other hand, was skeptical. She and her husband had previously offered to pay Louis if his report card grades improved; this tactic was not successful. The social worker explained that the consequences in that arrangement were too far removed from the everyday study behavior needed to improve grades. He convinced Ms. L. to start the program and then decide if participation was worthwhile. Louis's mother was happily surprised when her son actually followed the program and increased his studying. A fundamental contingency in Louis's program allowed him to only turn on television after completing homework. This daily contingency may have been a primary factor in his success.

Postintervention changes in Louis's study habits included: increased homework completion, increased reading for fun, increased work on mathematics and other extra projects, and decreased television watching during his free time. School behavior changes paralleled these positive results: Louis's teachers reported that although he was far from a scholar, he had decreased classroom socializing and was working more. Louis's grades also improved. For the first half of the school year his grade-point average was 1.1 (D-); in the second half his grade point average increased to 4.5 (C+). Louis was no longer an underachiever: the difference between Iowa Test Scores and grade point average was only 0.3. Louis expressed pleasure with improved grades and the portable radio his parents gave him as a result. His changed academic status also meant that he did not have to attend summer school—an obvious added pay-off.

Results

STUDY BEHAVIOR Given this perspective of one student's successful experience, results of the entire program describe the composite success of many students and families. Changes in study behavior for the four experimental groups are shown in Figure Four. During the parent-monitored phase, students in groups A and C increased studying to 51% of the times they were observed, a nineteen percentage point increase over baseline. All students except one maintained or increased studying when they changed from parent- to self-monitoring. Students in experimental groups B and D with no parent-monitoring increased studying to 92% during self-monitoring, a sixty-eight percentage point change over baseline.

Figure Five shows study-behavior change for two students who improved most and least. Gina, improving most, moved from 14% at baseline to 100% during self-monitored intervention. She had a corresponding grade point change of +1.84, representing a move from D+ to B-. Gary, showing least improvement, studied an average of 53% during baseline observation; in the parent-monitored phase, he increased to 65%. Self-monitoring, however, resulted in a decrease to 57%, corresponding with a -.06 change in grade point average. The difference between Gina's and Gary's performance may be attributed to the

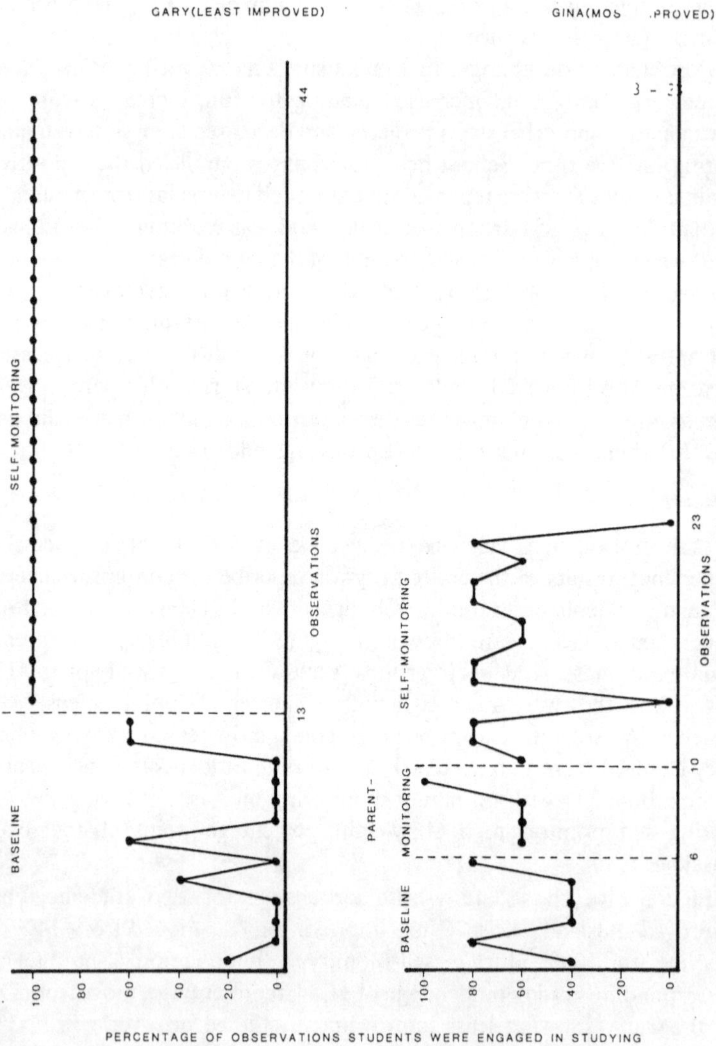

FIGURE 4. Observed studying for students improving most and least. Broken lines indicate termination of one phase and the beginning of the next.

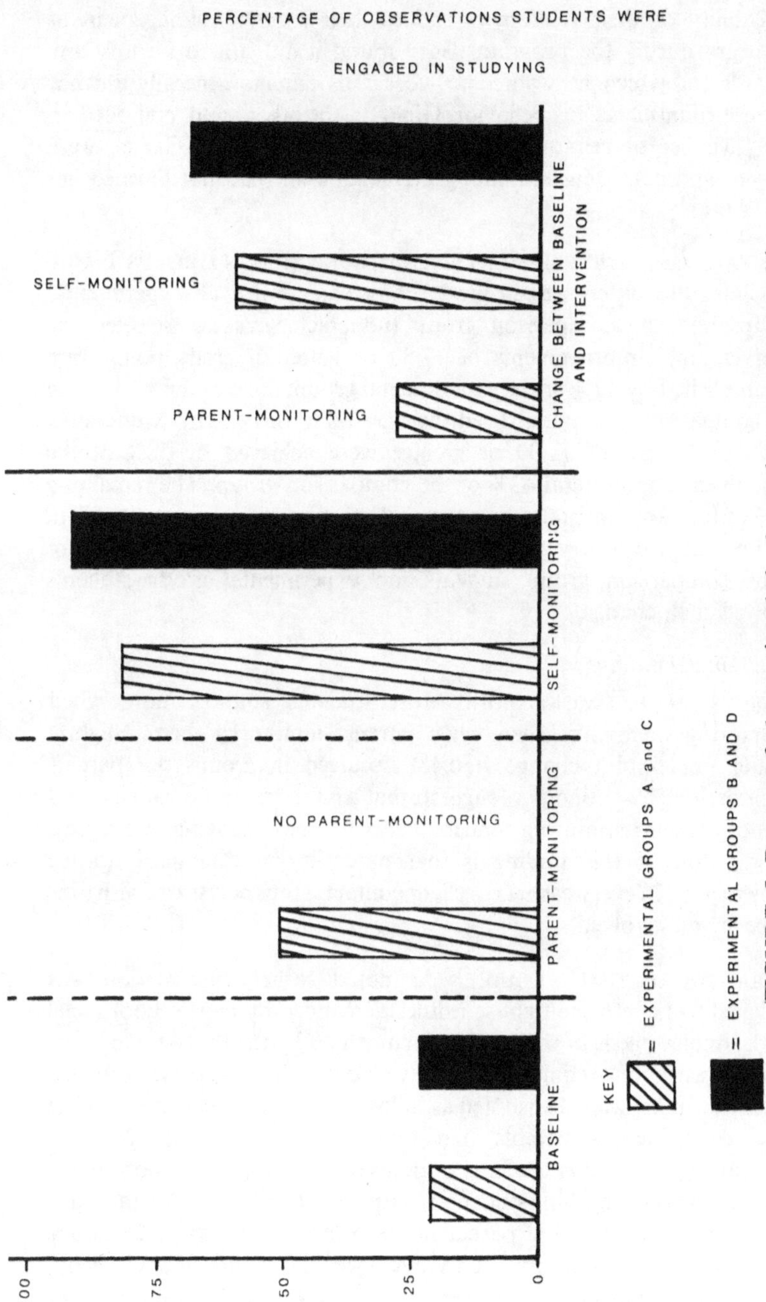

FIGURE 5. Percent of observational checks students were engaged in studying during baseline, parent-monitoring, and student-monitoring. Also shown are changes between baseline and intervention.

availability of their reinforcers and to their parents' management of privileges during the program. Gary found it difficult to identify any rewards for which he wanted to work. His parents generally did not attempt to influence his behavior. Gina, on the other hand, compiled an extensive list of reinforcers. Her parents, quite unlike Gary's, were diligent and consistent in limiting privileges if she had not finished her work.

COMPARISON OF EXPERIMENTAL AND COMPARISON GROUPS Figure Six illustrates differences in grade point changes for all experimental groups and the comparison group (underachievers not selected for intervention). Improvements of +2.50 or better in grade point were accomplished by 17% of the experimental group; none of the students in the comparison group improved their grades to this extent. Moderately positive changes of +1.00 or greater were achieved by 58% of the experimental group and 43% of the comparison group. The remaining 25% of the experimental group and 39% of the comparison group fell in the no-change category. Albeit negative grade-point changes occurred for some comparison group students, no experimental group students showed such change.

Additional Findings

SELF VS. PARENT-MONITORING Most students studied more when monitoring themselves than when parents monitored them. Slightly greater grade-point changes (+0.43) occurred in groups not parent-monitored. These findings suggest that the extra responsibility and freedom of self-monitoring contributed to increased studying. A practical ramification of this finding is that parent-monitoring need not be implemented in every case. Less client contact is thus necessary, with time saved by all involved.

SOCIAL WORK TIME REQUIRED As noted earlier, intervention was designed to fit into the tight schedules demanded by most school social work. Achievement of this goal is documented by the thirty-three hours of social work time required to serve twelve experimental subjects. Hours of client contact were distributed as follows: four hours teaching baseline data collection to parents, ten hours teaching parents program procedures, eight hours teaching students to take program responsibility, and eleven hours teaching students to implement programs. Average time spent with families using parent and self-monitoring was 3.25 hours; clients using self-monitoring only averaged 2.25 hours of social work contact. Thus, one hour per student was saved when only self-monitoring procedures were employed. Also worthy of consideration is additional time potentially saved: students working at their ability levels will likely demand less from teachers.

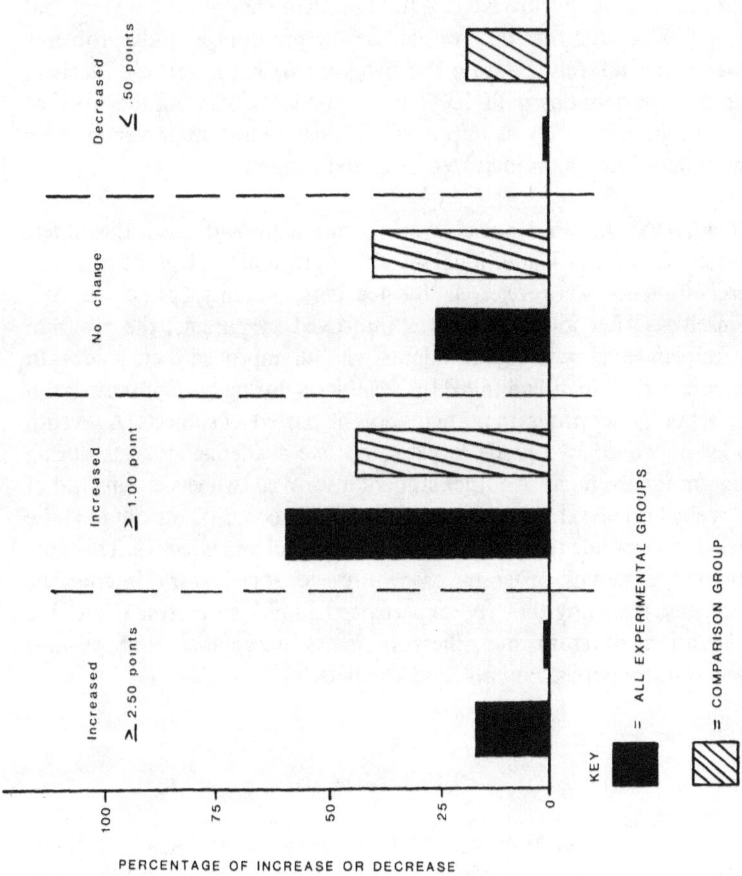

FIGURE 6. Grade point changes for experimental and comparison groups.

CONSUMER SATISFACTION Based on Reid and Epstein's (1977) client satisfaction survey, a post-intervention consumer satisfaction questionnaire was developed and distributed to teachers, parents, and students. Over 75% of the students and parents and half the teachers returned questionnaires. Of the students, 88% found the program helpful in motivating study behavior. The same number thought they studied more because of the program, rated the program as being of considerable benefit, and said they would use the procedure in the future if they experienced trouble with studying. Parents returning questionnaires also rated the program positively: 75% thought their child studied a great deal more; 100% stated that they would use the program if study problems arose in the future; 75% saw the program to be beneficial. Teachers shared these opinions with 100% of respondents, viewing the work of most program students as improved. Rating in-class attentiveness, 67% saw students' attention increased after the program.

REPLICATION Another social worker modified and used this intervention program with additional seventh, eight, and ninth grade students. Here, students were referred by teachers, parents, principals and themselves. After intervention was improved by parents, the program was implemented with eight students who all improved their grades. In one case, a freshman had failed three subjects during his first semester in high school; after program participation he passed all subjects. A seventh grader improved two grade levels in all five academic subjects during program involvement. Another student improved two levels—instead of the typical one level per year—on Iowa Test scores. These data led the worker to conclude that the program was helpful and effective. The same worker has taught program procedures to social work interns she supervises, reporting they too experienced similar successes. Use of the intervention program by others indicates acceptance and positive evaluation by pupils, parents, and teachers.

DISCUSSION

Successful program results appear to be in part due to mutually understanding relationships between social worker and school personnel. When first presented to the social service and administrative staff, the program was received enthusiastically. At a meeting with seventh and eighth grade teachers, however, some teachers responded negatively to the idea that students could change study habits. Thus, of six teachers with students in the project, three were fully cooperative, one generally cooperative, and two cooperative apparently because the principal supported the program. Not surprisingly, complaints about extra work were frequently expressed by these two teachers—even though the only additional effort was signing students' daily assignment forms.

Subsequent interactions suggested that changing the program would have made little difference in teacher attitude. When students demonstrated they could be trusted to do their assignments and no longer had to have teachers sign assignment forms, the same two teachers expressed concern that students were not asking them to sign forms. At this time the worker established himself as a listening post, no longer attempting to effect program changes because of teacher complaints. Ironically, these teachers were among those with the most positive over-program benefits.

Doubtless, establishing positive and cooperative relationships with teachers is essential to school-based intervention. School personnel should be viewed as program collaborators and consultants. By enlisting their advice, observations, insights, and opinions, we found teachers could become cooperative allies. Frequently overworked, highly pressured, and with limited time for contact with colleagues, teachers should be told their extra efforts are appreciated by the school principal as well as by the social worker.

Parent involvement, crucial to study-behavior intervention, can yield problems. Adolescents in particular often do not want parents monitoring their lives; thus, students must be consulted before parent participation is invited. After students consent, parents usually need to learn to attend to desired behavior. Modeling verbal praise, encouraging parent praise, and reinforcing their praise helps increasing parent use of social attention. In families with intact marriages, parents should also be encouraged to reinforce each other for praising their children.

A serendipitous program consequence was decreased negative parent/student interactions over academic performance. The program clearly specified the amount of study needed; program contingencies supported study behavior. As a result, parents rarely admonished their children for not studying. Rather, most postintervention parent interactions concerning school evidenced positive comments on improved study patterns.

Issues for Further Research

Since the only variable systematically evaluated was the necessity of parent-monitoring to precede self-monitoring, subsequent programs might test the potency of other intervention components. Not addresed here, for example, was homogeneity of the experimental group. Students were primarily from lower to upper middle economic strata, socially appropriate at home and school, and interested enough to agree to participate. It would be helpful to know if the program can be used in lower socioeconomic families where reinforcers for studying may be more difficult to obtain. It would also be useful to know if students with classroom behavior problems or those exhibiting initial reluctance to take part in the program could participate and benefit. Changes would likely have to be made to test the program with other populations to increase its generalizability.

Modifications might also be necessary to use the program effectively with younger children. Implementing the program with such students could have several advantages. Parents often have more control over fourth and fifth graders than they do over seventh and eight graders. Another advantage of working with young students would be helping them learn effective study habits as soon as they started receiving homework in school: students may not have to unlearn bad study habits or experience the beginning of a cycle of failure. A final issue for future research is maintenance of change. How long is the study program used after the social worker withdraws assistance? Equally important is how long improved grades are maintained after program participation has ended. Clearly, long-term follow-up is needed to address these and other relevant issues.

4

Social Competence in Adolescence

Lewayne D. Gilchrist

Recent research documents the relationship between social functioning and youths' long-term adjustment (Roff, Sell, & Golden, 1972; Van Hasselt, Hersen, Whitehill, & Bellack, 1979). A host of studies link poor social skills to specific problems frequently encountered in work with adolescents: delinquency (Freedman, Rosenthal, Donahoe, Schlundt, & McFall, 1978; Sarason & Ganzer, 1971), substance abuse (Newman, 1970; Roy & Schields, 1979; Smart, Gray, & Bennett, 1978), and sexual experimentation without contraception (Mindick, Oskamp, & Berger, 1978). In addition, social skill deficits play a part in the sometimes painful difficulties many teenagers face dealing with such normal tasks of adolescence as shifting relationships with parents and other adults, resisting peer pressure to engage in behavior that violates emerging personal values, developing satisfying opposite-sex relationships, and finding and keeping a job.

Although recent literature abounds with behavioral approaches to the improvement of social skills, surprisingly few studies focus specifically on teenagers. To explore issues and procedures helpful to clinicians designing and evaluating social skills training programs for adolescents, this discussion addresses defining social skills, applying social skills training to specific problems of adolescence, group and individual skills training formats, training techniques appropriate for adolescents, and guidelines for practitioners.

WHAT ARE SOCIAL SKILLS?

Social skills are difficult to define in concrete, useful terms. Few, if any, social actions are appropriate for all individuals in all circumstances. Opinions therefore, differ regarding the most useful way to conceptualize social skill, particularly for children and youth. Social actions judged "skillful" vary markedly with the nature of the situation, characteristics (e.g. age, sex, status) of the participants involved, and the prevailing social and cultural norms (Bellack, 1979; Eisler, Hersen, Miller, & Blanchard, 1975). It is, therefore, not surprising that as yet no commonly accepted definition of "social skill" exists.

One approach to a general description of social skill, offered by Marsha Linehan (personal communication), asserts that it is individuals' ability to obtain what they want in social situations without damaging their own integrity or the interpersonal relationship(s) involved. An expansion of Linehan's definition comes from Rinn and Markle (1979) who divide youths' social skills into four classifications: 1) self-expressive skills (expressing feelings and opinions, accepting compliments); 2) other-enhancing skills (agreeing with another's opinion, praising others); 3) assertive skills (making requests, disagreeing, refusing unreasonable requests); and 4) communication skills (conversing, interpersonal problem-solving, negotiation). These researchers define "social skill' as

> a repertoire of verbal and nonverbal behaviors by which children affect the responses of other individuals (e.g. peers, parents, siblings, and teachers) in the interpersonal context. This repertoire acts as a mechanism through which children influence their environment by obtaining, removing, or avoiding desirable and undesirable outcomes in the social sphere. Further, the extent to which they are successful in obtaining desirable outcomes and avoiding or escaping undesirables ones *without inflicting pain on others* is the extent to which they are considered "socially skilled," (Rinn & Markel, 1979, p. 108).

By broadening the scope of the interpersonal context beyond "peers, parents, siblings, and teachers" to include dating partners and adults in a variety of roles—employers, customers, law enforcement authorities, etc.—this definition remains applicable with adolescents.

Most social-skills training programs concentrate on improving verbal and nonverbal components of overt social behavior such as speech content, eye contact, voice volume, posture, gestures, and facial expression. A growing number of researchers, however, stress the importance of thoughts, perceptions, and other covert mental events that affect social performance (Mahoney 1974; Eisler, Frederiksen, & Peterson, 1978; Bellack, 1979). The work of Spivack, Platt, Shure, and their colleagues (Platt, Spivack, Altman, Altman, & Peizer, 1974; Spivack, Platt, & Shure, 1976) provides evidence that there are cognitions or mental steps in thinking about social encounters that correlate with children's successful resolution of interpersonal problems. They call these cognitions "means-end thinking," a construct similar to the model for adult problem-solving proposed by D'Zurilla and Goldfried (1971). They state that for a wide age-range of children,

> it is necessary to understand how well [a child] thinks about and works through the interpersonal situation. It is this process, manifest in a set of cognitive skills, that defines his social problem-solving capacity. It is the manner in which he proceeds that largely determines the quality of the outcome. It is *how* he thinks it through rather than what he might think at any given instant, that becomes the important issue in understanding the likelihood of long-range social success or failure (Spivack, Platt, & Shure 1976:4).

Meichenbaum and Goodman (1971) and Meichenbaum (1977) suggest that the ability to self-praise and to use covert verbalizations ("talking to one-self") as a means of organizing and regulating behavior are additional, important cognitive skills for youth.

Other researchers concur that social skill can be thought of, at least in part, as a system of covert or internal skills affecting self-control and problem-solving abilities across all social settings and circumstances. Other facets of this covert skills system include adolescents' knowledge of social norms, sensitivity to partners' responses, anxiety, information-processing capability, and ability to correctly label others' behavior and to accurately predict consequences of interpersonal actions (cf. Bellack, 1979; Mahoney, 1974; Schinke, Gilchrist, & Small, 1979). This cognitive conceptualization of social skill proves useful when dealing with the issue of posttraining generalization and maintenance of new behavior—a thorny problem for all behavioral training. The social realm is broad, constantly varying. Teaching flexible, generalizable strategies such as these appears to have greater long-term utility than rehearsing discrete acts. Increasingly, recommendations include wider use of cognitive and self-control procedures to enhance transfer of change to extratherapeutic settings (Conway & Bucher, 1976; Rosenthal & Bandura, 1978).

For the present purposes, social skills may be thought of as overt and covert learned behaviors that maximize chances for obtaining positive reinforcement from social interactions while minimizing cost to self and others. For the practitioner, however, decisions regarding the focus of training programs (i.e., what social skills to teach) can be difficult for several reasons. Very few studies have yet attempted systematic description of normal adolescent social behavior—Freedman, Rosenthal, Donahoe, Schlundt, & McFall (1978), Minkin, Braukmann, Minkin, Timbers, Timbers, Fixsen, Phillips, & Wolf (1976), and Cox,

Gunn, and Cox (1976) are rare exceptions—and a helpful, empirically valid, prescriptive literature does not exist. To select relevant, maximally beneficial social skills for training, program designers must rely on their own, perhaps only partial knowledge, of adolescent peer cultures, developmental norms, and societal expectations, in addition to understanding social learning theory and specific skill training techniques.

As with any behavioral program, assessment of adolescents' current level of social performance is crucial. Ineffective social functioning can be the result of several factors: lack of behavioral skill (i.e. simply not knowing what to do), inhibiting anxiety (i.e. knowing the proper response but being unable to perform it), or maladaptive cognitive processes (i.e. faulty evaluation of self- or others' competency). Obviously, training programs should be based on understanding which of these factors is most salient in the case at hand. Unfortunately, assessment technology has not kept pace with the development of social-skills theory, and practitioners should be aware of limitations in current assessment procedures.

Effective social interaction is highly situation specific, yet direct observation of adolescents' real social performance is often impossible. Role-play tests, therefore, are the standard method for assessing social skills. The fact, however, that teenagers perform effectively (or ineffectively) in role-played or contrived assessment situations is not a guarantee that they do so in the natural environment (cf. Bellack, 1979; Eisler, Hersen, Miller, & Blanchard, 1975; Trupin, Gilchrist, Maiuro, & Fay, 1979). Asking adolescents to describe and evaluate their own social performance also may not provide valid diagnostic information. Curran and his colleagues have consistently found lack of correspondence between self-report and other more objective ratings of social skill (Farrell, Mariotto, Conger, Curran, & Wallander, 1979; Curran, 1979). Further, assessment of anxiety and the more elusive cognitive components of social performance may be particularly difficult due to a current dearth of empirically validated instruments for this purpose.

One final issue further complicates a straightforward choice of target skills for adolescent social skills training programs. Many adolescents are referred for skills-training by others who have judged their behavior inadequate by adult standards, although referred adolescents themselves may perceive no need for training. In this case, practitioners' ethical responsibility dictates careful consideration of the value of proposed skills for the individual youth apart from their value to authorities or other referral sources.

In summary, far from denoting a common set of discrete behaviors, the term "social skill" can be viewed, in the words of one investigator, "as an organizing principal for relating a variety of superficially dissimilar behaviors under a single megaconstruct" (Curran, 1979: 55). This same investigator warns that "we must be constantly vigilant lest we begin to regard [social skill] as a static, invariant dispositional-trait-like unit" (Curran, 1979: 55). Even severely impaired adolescents can acquire new skills to enhance their all important encounters with others. Youths already skilled in one area of social behavior may need considerable help in another. Social skills training represents a flexible, efficient, and direct approach to helping young people with a variety of presenting problems. Future years should see increased attention to empirical validation and advancement of social skill training theory and methodology focused on adolescents, a population currently underrepresented in an otherwise burgeoning literature.

SOCIAL SKILLS TRAINING AND PROBLEMS OF ADOLESCENCE

Limits to the applicability of social skills training are hard to identify. Guerney notes that since skills training is based on an educational rather than a healing model, it is equally useful for problem prevention and problem remediation. With skills training, "The only essential difference between prevention and remediation...is not a difference either of kind or of process, but rather one of *timing*" (Guerney, 1977:4). This section gives a brief overview of the application of social skills training to specific problem areas germane to work with adolescents.

Health

Promoting health by preventing unhealthy behavior has received increasing attention in recent years. Many adolescents engage in risk taking and injurious behavior because of social pressure from peers (Gilchrist, Schinke, Blythe, & Renggli, in press; McAlister, Perry, & Maccoby, 1979). To combat social pressure, social-skills training teaches adolescents verbal and cognitive strategies for handling difficult interpersonal situations. According to McAlister "researchers have found that a person can be made resistant to social influence if she or he is forewarned of the expected arguments and taught to refute them in advance, a process often called psychological innoculation" (McAlister, 1979:203). Based on this "immunization" rationale, several prevention programs have yielded promising results for reducing incidence of smoking (Blythe, Gilchrist, Schinke, & Burt, 1979; Gilchrist, Schinke, & Blythe, 1979; McAlister, Perry, & Maccoby, 1979) and drug use (Cheek, Tomarchio, Standen, & Albahary, 1973; Shrader, 1979). Empirical work on reducing alcohol consumption and abuse remains to be done.

Social-skills training programs promoting health usually consist of three phases: provision of information about harmful effects of the target substance, or behavior, cognitive skills training to help youths apply the information to their own lives and to recognize instances of social pressure, and behavioral skills training including guided practice of specific strategies for countering such pressure ("I'd really be a chicken if I smoked that just to impress you"). This cognitive-behavioral social-skills training approach has potential for helping youths deal with many personal-choice behaviors harmful to health including consumption of junk food and physical risk-taking such as reckless driving and responding to "dares."

Sexuality

One of the most important events in adolescence is the development of sexual identity and sexual functioning. Uneven growth patterns, however, can equip adolescents for physical intimacy but leave them without interpersonal skills to achieve and regulate intimacy. One result is frustration and failure in dating relationships; another is unplanned, unprotected, and sometimes unwanted sexual intercourse.

Dating interactions are particularly important in adolescent socialization. Anxiety and lack of a variety of social skills, however, create discomfort for many youths (Martinson & Zerface, 1970). In one interesting program at Achievement Place (Maloney, Braukmann, Maloney, Braukmann, Ayala, Fixsen, Phillips, & Wolf, 1975), nondating boys were trained to adopt selected verbal and nonverbal social skills used by boys judged successful at dating. These were: facial orientation, head nods, attention feedback, information prompts, and other short verbal responses. Training also covered conversation-entering and conversation-maintenance strategies. Following training, youths' subsequent social interaction with girls increased markedly.

Lack of crucial interpersonal skills has been implicated in incidences of unwanted sexual intercourse and inconsistent or non-use of contraception. Cvetkovich and Grote (1976) found a significant number of youth having intercourse because it seemed expected of them or because they could not say no. Mindick, Oskamp, and Berger (1978) describe adolescent non-users of contraception as significantly more susceptible to social pressure than consistent users. Building on the work of these investigators, Schinke, Gilchrist, Blythe, and colleagues developed and empirically tested a social-skills training program for promoting responsible sexual behavior and preventing unwanted pregnancy (Schinke & Gilchrist, 1977; Schinke, Gilchrist, & Small, 1979; Blythe, Gilchrist, & Schinke, in press). This program provides information about human reproduction and birth control, problem-solving training to help adolescents make effective decisions, and communication skills training for transforming decisions into action. The latter training focuses on such situations as bringing up difficult topics (e.g. "I think we should talk about birth control"), making clear and consistent refusals of unwanted demands, and negotiating to enhance mutuality. Results from two field tests of this model are promising: the three part program has resulted in more favorable attitudes toward contraception and increased use of birth control. Further, adolescents uniformly express enthusiasm concerning the program's value.

Social skills training has also been used to help more seriously conflicted youth achieve stable sexual identities. Barlow (1979) reports success using training with a seventeen-year-old male client who applied for sex-change surgery. In social interactions, the client manifested many behavior patterns identified as female by others. After several months of role playing and videotaped feedback, he began to replace these patterns with more traditionally male gestures and reported feeling more at ease and no longer ridiculed for his feminine style. Follow-up six and a half years after training revealed the client achieving excellent grades in college, involved in a long-term relationship with a women he intended to marry, and, in his own words, "completely reoriented sexually."

Delinquency

In a series of sophisticated studies, Freedman, Rosenthal, Donahoe, Schlundt, & McFall (1978) validate the conceptualization of delinquent behavior as situation-specific social-behavioral skill deficits. In these studies, male adolescents labeled "good citizens" or "leaders" manifested significantly greater skill in handling criticism, resisting peer pressure, overcoming boredom, and resolving conflicts with parents and authorities than did male adolescents identified as delinquent. Though not yet well documented with female offenders, this skill-deficit conceptualization forms the basis for several well-known treatment programs. Foremost and largest is Achievement Place in Kansas. One of many skills training programs at Achievement Place prepares pre-delinquents for encounters with police. Operating on the findings of Piliavin and Briar (1964) and others that prejudicial handling of juvenile cases is affected to a large extent by police officers' discretion, and that officers' discretion in turn is strongly affected by youths' social behavior, Werner, Minkin, Minkin, Fixsen, Phillips, and Wolf (1975) devised and evaluated a program to teach youths how to communicate effectively in one highly specific social situation—being questioned by police. Training focused on looking toward the officer (facial orientation), polite references to the officer's authority ("Yes, officer," "I think so, sir"), and expressions of understanding and cooperation ("I'll answer your questions if I can," "I'll try to keep my record clean"). Police officers viewing videotapes of pre- and posttraining performance of trained and untrained youth rated the trained youths significantly *less* likely to cause suspicion, be labeled troublemakers, be stopped again by police, or be taken into custody.

Sarason and Ganzer (1973) successfully applied modeling and behavior rehearsal to teach delinquents social skills involved in applying for jobs, resisting temptations to engage in antisocial acts, and asking for assistance from teachers. Stumphauzer (1976) reports success in a similar program.

Jobs

The transition from child- to adulthood is usually accompanied by a need for economic self-sufficiency. Thus, many teenagers are faced with the task of finding and keeping a job. Social skills training has proven helpful for teaching adolescents how to secure employment. Most work to date has emphasized employment application and interviewing skills. Braukmann, Maloney, Fixsen, Phillips, and Wolf (1974) taught predelinquent boys to interact effectively with a job interviewer and the interviewer's secretary by training appropriate posture, eye contact, personal appearance, social behavior (i.e. social graces such as thanking the interviewer), and volunteering of information about qualifications and reasons for wanting the job. All boys improved on all skills even when training was delivered by inexperienced college undergraduates who had no preparation other than written instructions on how to use the program's training materials.

Barbee and Keil (1973; Keil and Barbee, 1973) similarly used a social-skills training approach to teach ethnic-minority adolescents to present themselves effectively to prospective employers. Walker (1969) reports success in using cognitive and behavioral skills training to enhance adolescents' job search skills and job performance. In one of the rare social skills programs focusing on young women, Schinke, Gilchrist, Smith, and Wong (1978) taught teenage mothers to fill out job applications neatly, concisely, and accurately and to present themselves effectively in videotaped job-interview simulations. Training emphasized presenting succinct, positive summaries of past employment, highlighting specific strengths of academic experiences, and answering questions clearly, concisely, and pleasantly. Posttraining samples of employment applications and videotaped interviews were rated by three personnel specialists from the community, all of whom had jobs that entailed making hiring recommendations at the un- or semi-skilled level. These specialists gave a recommend-for-hiring rating significantly more often to young women given social skills training than to young women who had spent comparable time in group discussions of job possibilities.

Parent conflict

A major developmental task of adolescence is achieving independence from the family (Conger, 1977). This disengagement of parent and child generates confrontations of varying intensity depending upon the family's conflict-resolution skills. Several social-skills training programs have taught adolescents and their families effective problem-solving, negotiation, and communication skills. Alexander and Parsons (1973) taught delinquent youths and their families to ask for clarifications of unclear statements, to brainstorm for several alternative solutions to a conflict, and to allow each family member equal time in conflict negotiations. Youths in trained families subsequently evidenced less recidivism than did comparable youths in families receiving other therapy approaches. Kifer, Lewis, Green, & Phillips (1974) have reported success with a similar program.

Robin (in press) presents a well constructed, highly detailed program for combining cognitive and behavioral social-skills training with families. His cognitive skills training follows a four step problem-solving model: families are taught how to define a problem, generate alternative solutions, select a solution, and plan its implementation. Behavioral skills training teaches family members to "express ideas and feelings assertively but unoffensively and receive ideas and feelings expressed by others attentively and accurately. Negative communication habits such as accusations, interruptions, lectures, put-downs, overgeneralizations, commands, sarcastic expressions, and inattentive postures are replaced with positive communication habits such as verification of meaning, passive listening, active listening, I-messages, appropriate eye contact, and appropriate nonverbal posture" (Robin, in press).

SKILLS-TRAINING FORMATS

Skills in training with groups

In 1968 Lazarus limned important qualities of behavioral therapy, pointing out that groups make efficient use of practitioners' time and effort, potentially lessen clients' feelings of isolation, and offer a desirably wide range of experiences and opinions from which to draw during training sessions. For these and other reasons, social skills training in groups offers a number of advantages to practitioners. Goldstein and Wolpe describe the value of the group for diagnostic purposes:

> The group setting offers an opportunity for a far more thorough behavioral analysis than does individual therapy. When dealing with the patient in an individual session, the therapist is able to observe his behavior in relation to only one person—the therapist—which gives little knowledge of the patient's possible responses to other people (1972:129).

Shrader clarifies the effectiveness of groups with adolescents in particular, noting the "availability of peer prompting and reinforcement...the opportunity to employ modeling and behavior rehearsal techniques to teach specific skills in settings similar to those the client will experience in real life; and the opportuity for the client to receive feedback on his performance from someone other than a therapist whose opinion may be discounted" (1979:165).

Three types of social skills training groups exist. The first can be described as a heterogeneous mixture of individuals with diverse social difficulties. Individual behavior programs are devised for each group member who works at his/her own rate of speed to master this private program. Generally long-term and relatively unstructured, these groups are usually part of more comprehensive residential treatment or outpatient programs for adolescents with serious interpersonal problems.

Sometimes naturally occurring but usually contrived, an ongoing task or activity requiring interaction may form the basis for group meetings—playing a game, completing an art or woodworking project, negotiating a purchase using communal funds, organizing and presenting skits or role plays, and dividing scarce resources fairly, are examples (cf. Rose, 1972). Group members interact, receiving instructions and feedback on their performance from group leaders. When resources permit, group meetings can be augmented with individual sessions to provide adolescents with additional training and feedback.

It is the process within these groups that determines the content of training; that is, skills are taught when need for them is demonstrated. Gittelman (1965) and Giebink, Stover, and Fahl (1968) are well constructed and evaluated examples of such groups with adolescents. Frankel and Glasser (1974), Rose (1972), and Flowers (1979) provide additional general insights into this interactive group approach. Since skills teaching occurs in the context of ongoing interaction similar to the natural environment, theory suggests relative ease in group members' transference of learning to extratherapy situations. As Giebink, Stover, and Fahl (1968) relate, however, such transfer often does not occur.

The second type of skills-training group is characterized by short-term, highly structured sessions, focused on a limited and specific problem area, and based on the assumption that all group members have the same needs. Group content is not individualized; rather, the same curriculum and preselected skills are presented to and practiced by all group members simultaneously. Representative situations for discussion and role play are presented by group leaders, not group members. Skills may then be practiced in terms of clearly hypothetical, perhaps initially amusing or exaggerated, encounters. This approach may be necessary to introduce skills to adolescents who would not participate otherwise. Requiring little self-disclosure and minimal self-risk from members can be an advantage when group makeup (adjudicated delinquents) or subject material (sexual encounters) make unlikely the establishment of open, protherapeutic communication among members within given time constraints. Though easier to organize and implement than more individualized programs, the highly structured nature of this approach presents several obvious drawbacks. Unless careful screening occurs, training content may not meet all, or even some, group members' needs and the hypothetical nature of training may interfere with learning and generalization.

The third and most efficient type of skills training group represents a combination of the two preceding types. Shrader's Project Entry Program for drug-abusing adolescents (Shrader, 1979) is an example. In the first half of the Project Entry Program (four sessions) leaders present predetermined communication and negotiation skills to the whole group; they then introduce homework—logs, diaries, special tests—to personalize these skills. In the last half of the program (four sessions), members present specific problems they are currently experiencing and the group role-plays possible solutions.

Typically delivered as an eight- to ten-session program, this groups training approach combines the individualization of the first group type with the focus of the second, highly structured type. It is probably most effective when adolescent members already possess adequate communication skills and can interact productively with each other with little specific preparation. If this is not the case, a longer program should be planned.

Skills training with individuals

Although groups are the preferred format, social skills training with individual adolescents is feasible and frequently done. Kaufmann and Wagner (1972), for example, took advantage of a residential treatment setting to implement a multicomponent program for helping a fourteen year old, Ed, control his temper. Therapists first taught Ed new adaptive verbal and nonverbal responses to replace maladaptive ones. The therapy staff then arranged carefully timed provocative situations or "barbs" to be directed toward Ed in different settings over the course of several weeks. When Ed responded to a barb appropriately, he was rewarded with praise and material reinforcement in the form of tokens. As the client's skill level increased, the barbs and reinforcements became increasingly intermittent. Follow-up six months after program termination revealed no further interpersonal problems due to loss of temper.

Skills training with individual adolescents can be used to prepare youth for future group training programs. Occasionally, because of excessive anxiety, habitual disruptiveness, distracting personal mannerisms or other reasons, an adolescent may be initially unable to participate in group training sessions. For example, thirteen year old Steve experienced numerous social problems due to extreme passivity in confrontations with peers. When placed in an assertiveness training group with five boys of his age, Steve continually disrupted the group with talk and stories so off-task as to seem bizarre. Further evaluation revealed him to be an alert, highly imaginative youth who, when something triggered his imagination, could not express his thoughts so others were able to see the relationship between what he was saying and the triggering event. In individual sessions, Steve was trained to discriminate appropriate from inappropriate times to express his ideas and, when he did express them, to preface his remarks with a reference to the speaker or event in the present to which he was responding. Using his new interpersonal skills, on readmittance to the assertiveness group Steve impressed his peers as amusing, even colorful, and was no longer considered odd or disruptive. He then began to work with the group on his original assertiveness problems.

SKILLS-TRAINING TECHNIQUES

Most of the techniques described in this section have been developed in clinical laboratories for social-skills training with adults. Potentially powerful, many are currently used with children and adolescents; nevertheless, more systematic investigation is needed to document their potency with younger populations.

Modeling

Referred to less formally as vicarious learning, the concept of modeling supplies the foundation for almost all skills training: trainees observe the actions of others and incorporate these observations into their own behavior. Rosenthal and Bandura (1978) provide a comprehensive review of the extensive literature on modeling. Of particular pertinence to practitioners are findings delineating characteristics of effective models. Investigators recommend using models who are close to the trainees in age, sex, and social characteristics but have slightly higher status—(e.g. twelfth grade males modeling for tenth grade males). In addition, results are better if models demonstrate copying rather than mastery behavior—that is, instead of presenting consistently flawless performances, the more effective models begin by showing a skill level no different than trainees' own, verbalizing fears and strategies for proceeding, and finally achieving acceptable performance.

Practitioners also might profitably consider use of media for modeling purposes. Empirical evidence confirms that youth can acquire social skills from symbolic (filmed or otherwise recorded) as well as live models (O'Connor, 1969; Keller & Carlson, 1974). When resources permit, construction of a film or videotape for repeated demonstration of target skills may prove efficient, especially for large scale use.

Behavior rehearsal, coaching, and feedback

Rehearsal or guided practice of target skills is undisputedly an effective social-skills training technique (cf. McFall & Lillesand, 1971; McFall & Marston, 1970) Such rehearsal is usually accomplished through role play. Trainers and group members offer instructions (coaching) before or during rehearsal situations and provide praise (positive reinforcement) and suggestions for improvement (feedback) following performance. A plethora of assertion and interpersonal skills-training texts offer detailed suggestions for implementing behavior rehearsal (cf. Strayhorn, 1977; Gambrill & Richey, 1976; Lange & Jakubowski, 1976). Because virtually all adolescents prefer action oriented to didactic or observational activities, behavior rehearsal will doubtless remain central to most adolescent social-skills training programs. Prior to initiating behavior rehearsal, practitioners may need to teach adolescents constructive ways to offer reinforcement and feedback. Left-handed compliments ("You don't look as dumb as you did last time") are not reinforcing, and negative feedback is more palatable if stated as a suggestion for future practice preceded and followed by several positive comments. An example is, "I liked the words you used when you introduced yourself and your eye contact was great. Next time try talking a little louder. Overall, though, you looked very confident."

Allowing trainees to observe their own performance on audio- or videotape can facilitate learning new skills, although with groups this technique may prove too cumbersome and time consuming. It is particularly valuable, however, when working with individuals. In an example from the author's practice, audiotaping helped an eleven-year-old client make more effective requests. Though possessing generally effective communication skills, the client, Jonathan, habitually employed a whining, begging tone in requests to parents and peers, a mannerism which alienated his father and resulted in teasing at school. During training sessions, examples of his "begging" were recorded along with the author's modeling of straightforward, assertive requests. Tapes were replayed until Jonathan could discriminate and describe distinguishing features of both kinds of requests. Skits requiring many requests were then devised and audiotaped, with Jonathan and the author jointly critiquing his performance. As his skill level increased, use of the tape recorder was gradually eliminated.

For a more comprehensive discussion of behavior rehearsal, coaching, and feedback, see Rose (1977).

Homework assignments

Assigning tasks for trainees to perform outside training sessions serves two important functions. First, these assignments provide more opportunity for skills practice than limited training sessions allow. Second, assignments serve as a bridge between the relative comfort of the training group and the more demanding natural environment. Practitioners should never assume that adolescents automatically apply newly acquired skills outside the training situation. A standard means for achieving this transfer of learning is written agreements or contracts for independent performance of target behavior—going for a job interview, asking for a date, or refusing an unreasonable request, for example. Contracts are drawn up and signed by both trainer and trainee. Specified are performance goals, time limits, rewards to be collected when assignments are completed, and mild negative consequences—in cases of noncompletion—short-term removal of privileges, or forfeiture of a small amount of money. Adolescents report results of this homework performance in subsequent training sessions.

Another technique for increasing completion of extrasession assignments is the buddy system. Each group member is paired with a "buddy," usually another group member, who coaches, monitors, and offers reinforcement for good performance outside the group (Fo & O'Donnell, 1974; Schinke & Rose, 1976). Resting on the well established dictum that peers exert considerable influence on adolescents' behavior, this technique is especially promising for work with adolescents.

Token and group contingency systems

Opinions are mixed regarding the worth of distributing small material reinforcers (tokens) contingent upon good performance in training sessions. Whether redeemable for backup reinforcers or not, tokens *do* represent unusually powerful tools for quickly shaping desirable behavior (Kazdin, 1977b; Rose, 1977). They can, nonetheless, interfere with learning by distracting trainees, who may "go through the motions" to obtain tokens with no lasting behavior change taking place. Weaning adolescents away from token reinforcement can also present problems. In the words of Frankel and Glasser:

> One of the challenges of working with a token economy is to help clients begin using normal social reinforcers instead of tokens to control their own behavior. A second important issue is to help clients structure their contingencies in such a way that the behaviors they are learning with tokens will generalize to situations in which no tokens are present (1974: 167).

In the author's experience, tokens have proven valuable for establishing protherapeutic norms in groups of involuntary, immature, or highly distractable adolescents. The length of the training program, however, invariably increases due to time spent switching away from tokens to other less artificial motivational aids.

Another technique useful with difficult groups is the group contingency system. "Stated simply, the group contingency means that no one in a group receives a reward until each member achieves certain individual goals" (Frankel & Glasser, 1974: 165). As with tokens, the power of this technique is offset by clear limitations. Group contingencies can fail because one or more group members, for lack of ability, resources, for ethical or other reasons, cannot perform the required behavior, because the contingency generates too much group pressure—so punishing for some adolescents that they drop out of the group—or because some members enjoy noncomplying and punishing the entire group (O'Leary & Drabman, 1971). Clearly, practitioners should exercise caution when considering group contingencies.

Problem-solving training

Platt Spivack, Altman, Altman, and Peizer (1974) demonstrated significant differences in problem-solving abilities of "normal" and socially "deviant" adolescents. Based on the work of these investigators and others, problem-solving training teaches adolescents a framework for analyzing and resolving interpersonal problems. Youths learn to gather information and separate fact from opinion to accurately define interpersonal problems. They also learn to generate as many socially acceptable solutions as possible, evaluate short- and long-term consequences of proposed solutions realistically, and construct feasible plans for implementing solutions selected as best.

Problem-solving training can be applied as needed to a broad range of adolescent social concerns or narrowly focused on one problem area—countering peer pressure to use drugs, for example. The technique promotes effective self-regulation by "helping the individual to discover and implement whatever adjustment strategies are effective in a given situation"(Mahoney & Arnkoff, 1978:709). The technique's flexibility can thus enhance independent functioning, generally—an important training goal. In addition to considerable work by Spivack, Platt, and Shure (1976), favorable improvement in youths' social functioning following problem-solving training is reported by Small and Schinke (1979), Kifer, Lewis, Green, and Phillips (1974), and Trupin, Gilchrist, Maiuro, and Fay (1979).

Additional self-control and cognitive techniques

Kanfer (1970) delineates a three-phase model of effective self-control. Youths must first pay careful attention to their own behavior (self-monitor), then compare monitored behavior to preestablished goals or the behavior of others (self-evaluate), and finally reward themselves if behavior matches or exceeds the chosen standards (self-reinforce). Though infrequently reported, all three self-control skills—self-monitoring, self-evaluation, and self-reinforcement—can be systematically taught in adolescent social-skill training programs. For example, a program teaching dating skills might require adolescents to self-monitor by listing on a card the number of verbal exchanges they initiate during the week with potential dating partners. In group sessions appropriate conversational gambits are modeled and practiced. Self-monitoring outside the group continues and youths are instructed to rate themselves on selected aspects of their performance—comfort, fluency, length of the exchange, etc. As trainees report their self-evaluations in subsequent group sessions, trainers liberally praise all conversation initiation efforts, positive performance qualities, and accurate evaluations. Trainees then rehearse delivering similar reinforcement to themselves by subvocalizing reinforcing statements or awarding themselves tokens. With highly motivated adolescents, a less structured approach teaching simply the general self-control paradigm may be adequate but evidence is lacking that youth will apply this paradigm without specific programming. Further guidelines for practitioners employing self-control techniques can be found in Mahoney and Thoresen (1974).

Learning to relax is another form of self-control. Since anxiety often inhibits social performance, relaxation training may assume an important role in social-skills training programs. Rose (1972) presents a detailed protocol for teaching relaxation to adolescents. Other less time-consuming relaxation procedures include deep-breathing exercises and concentrating on mental images of peaceful scenes—both usually paired with the covert statement "I am relaxed."

As Berlin (Chapter Eight), Meichenbaum (1977), and others relate, verbal messages that adolescents give themselves can strongly influence their social behavior. These messages, called self-statements, may be evaluative ("That was a dumb thing to do") or instructional ("Go ahead—nobody's watching"). With guided self-monitoring, adolescents can be helped to identify maladaptive self-statements; more facilitative, positive statements can be supplied and rehearsed as replacements—"I'm good at this," for example, or "Wait, stop and think this through."

Positive self-statement training can be combined with another, related cognitive technique, covert behavior rehearsal (McFall & Lillesand, 1971). This technique involves helping youths imagine exactly what they would do to perform some social act—applying for a job, lodging a complaint, asking for a date, for instance. Mentally, clients rehearse all steps necessary to accomplish their goal until anxiety diminishes and they feel comfortable enough to attempt actual performance (cf. Rose 1977). Cradock, Cotler, and Jason (1978) report good results using this technique to help high school freshmen overcome public speaking anxiety.

SUMMARY AND GUIDELINES FOR PRACTITIONERS

Social skills training represents an opportunity for adolescents to experiment with new behavior in an accepting and supportive environment, with the added oportunity for clear and consistent feedback from peers and appropriate models as to the effects of these behavioral trials. Though currently underresearched, social skills training appears to be a potentially valuable therapeutic modality for work with adolescents. A summary of important training issues and guidelines for practitioners follows.

Selecting target skills

Selection of social skills to be included in a training program should be based on carefully gathered knowledge of clients' current social functioning. For many practitioners, however, large caseloads preclude opportunities for detailed assessment. Nevertheless, practitioners should be aware that blindly selecting skills because they seem "logical" is disadvantageous. Personal bias may enter such selections—practitioners' private and perhaps idiosyncratic view of appropriate social behavior is thus thrust on adolescents without regard for their differing age and social milieu. Despite initial training successes, Cox, Gunn, and Cox recognized such bias in their own work:

> Our enthusiasm was somewhat dampened by the realization that our training failed to account for the developmental component which interacts with skill attainment. We became increasingly more concerned that we were trying to teach adult-level responses to children who had not attained the maturity to allow for maximum benefit from training. In addition, we realized that many of the social responses we were so rigorously teaching were not based on any empirical data based on popular, successful children (1976:2).

When adolescent clients belong to different racial or ethnic groups than the trainers, such biases in the selection of target skills may become destructive. To mitigate bias, as much as possible practitioners should rely on adolescent group members or adults with extensive exposure to given adolescent cultures to generate skills appropriate for training.

Whatever target skills are selected, practitioners must define verbal and nonverbal skill components as specifically as possible. Training programs should be built on these specific definitions. Programs based on loosely defined skills (e.g. "making effective refusals") will be less focused, less effective, and harder to evaluate than ones based on more detailed objectives, such as "increasing eye contact and adolescents' verbalization of 'No' and 'I,' decreasing use of smiles and distracting facial, arm, and leg gestures."

Establishing protherapeutic group norms

As with any therapeutic activity, practitioners cannot neglect process issues such as building rapport, promoting group cohesiveness and realistic expectations, and establishing productive norms. Practitioners should be aware that many adolescents are reluctant to self-disclose and find group training uncomfortable, at least initially. Time spent engaging in informal, get-acquainted "raps" may be crucial. Practitioners should also take care to structure learning tasks within the group so all members can succeed and avoid additional embarrassment. Before productive learning can occur, some adolescent groups may need instruction in giving feedback appropriately, avoiding scapegoating, and remaining on-task and attentive. Selective praise and attention can help shape desired conduct. Should stronger measures be required, fines can be imposed for negative or off-task behavior. Token or group contingency systems represent other means of control though practitioners should be familiar with earlier noted limitations of these techniques.

Occasionally, practitioners may encounter groups with strong preestablished norms reinforcing deviant behavior and punishing appropriate performance. Considerable time may be needed to prepare these groups for productive work. In addition to techniques already mentioned, practitioners can enlist aid from a person the group considers to have high status—an older adolescent, an athlete, a valued teacher, or a well-known personality from the community—to model and endorse productive group participation. This technique also increases enthusiasm and participation among adolescents who, though not disruptive or deviant, have low motivation.

Another potential problem in social skills training is boredom with repetitive practice. Adolescents may require numerous in-group practice sessions to attain competence; to hold interest, practitioners should creatively vary rehearsals so adolescents continually practice target skills but in constantly changing circumstances and with different partners.

Selective use of audio- and videotape is also helpful for maintaining interest.

Transferring skills to the natural environment

To simply provide training and then hope that adolescents will use their new social skills outside the training setting is unrealistic (cf. Stokes & Baer, 1977). As previously noted, homework assignments and behavioral contracts are useful tools for moving beyond training confines. Another technique involves training parents or other significant figures in the adolescent's environment to reinforce or continue teaching new skills once the group has terminated. Trupin, Gilchrist, Maiuro, and Fay (1979) and numerous others report increased maintenance and generalization of children's social skills following training both parents and adolescents. Practitioners can also promote generalization by emphasizing it directly during training. Allowing adolescents to log or brainstorm lists of situations where target skills might be used is one example. Systematic instructions to try skills outside of training coupled with liberal reinforcement of attempts to do so should be used in all social skills training programs and may by itself induce some generalization with mature, well-motivated groups.

Evaluating effectiveness

Clear demonstration of program effectiveness is not only reinforcing to client and practitioner, it may be required for program longevity. Although it is beyond the scope of this chapter to detail the array of assessment tools and research designs available to practitioners (see Campbell & Stanley, 1963; Jayaratne & Levy, 1979; Hersen & Barlow, 1976), such evaluation should be an important component of every social skills training program. Program planning should include assessment probes—for example, written quizzes, specially rated role plays, or field trips to try out new behavior in new settings. When possible, significant others in the adolescents' environment—parents, teachers, parole officers, peers, siblings, or dating partners—can report their perceptions of trainees' progress. Trainees can periodically rate themselves for anxiety level, negative self-statements, number of arguments, number of conversations initiated, and so on. Data thus compiled provide bases for making constructive changes in ongoing and future training sessions.

In conclusion, social skills training provides several advantages to practitioners. The rationale underlying the skills-training approach is clear and direct, facilitating support from community sources, legislators, administrators, parents, and youths themselves. Social skills training techniques are flexible and adaptable to widely varying populations, settings, and organizational requirements. Further, the skill-building approach permits the quantification and unambiguous evaluation that has become crucial in this age of accountability (Newman & Turem, 1974; Schinke, 1979 b). Worthy of future investigation are packaged media presentations and self-taught programmed materials especially for large scale use. Employment of paraprofessionals and particularly peers as group leaders also warrant practitioners' consideration. The future of social skills training with adolescents should see many exciting modifications and extensions of techniques outlined in this review.

5

Contracts in Foster Care

Theodore J. Stein
and
Eileen D. Gambrill

Most American children grow up in the care of their natural parents. But, a significant number—approximately 420,000—(National Association of Attorneys General, 1976) are raised in foster homes because their natural parents are unable or unwilling to care for them. Substitute care is meant to be short term (Child Welfare League of America 1975); it is expected that each child will be provided with a permanent home, by being reunited with biological parents, adoption, legal guardianship, or planned, long-term care. Sadly, many children "drift" in unplanned long-term care. Estimates of the percentage of children with no formal treatment plans run as high as 50-77% of all in foster care (Sherman, Nueman, & Shyne 1974). Contributing to the drift of children in placement is the fact that natural parents receive fewer services from child welfare workers than either the child or the foster parents (Mass & Engler, 1959; Jeter, 1963; Gruber, 1978; Stein, Gambrill, & Wiltse, in press).

Better procedures for ensuring continuity of care for children in foster placement are sorely needed. One vehicle for achieving such continuity is the written contract. Contracts can be made between parents and child welfare workers, between two or more clients, or between child welfare workers and other service providers. The unique contribution written contracts make is that they clarify the expectations of the parties involved concerning goals—such as restoration of a child to natural parents—and specify the objectives necessary for attainment of that goal. Further, contracts clarify responsibilities to all involved parties, identify consequences for progress toward objectives, and provide a time frame for pursuing goals. Finally, contracts provide a context for gathering assessment information and for arranging parent-child visits.

This chapter shows how some social workers have successfully wed various contracts to provide more responsible child welfare services.

The concept of a written contract will probably be new to most clients. For clients to participate in negotiating, signing, and following through with written agreements, time must be spent explaining the purpose of contracts, the procedure for developing them, and their advantages: they put in writing clients' goals for their child, they identify difficulties to be resolved, and they describe steps to be taken to resolve difficulties. Clients' and workers' respective goals are described, the time frame for reaching the goal is noted, and the consequences for compliance or noncompliance with the conditions are set forth.

Why should clients view contracts as advantageous? Since contract goals are selected by clients, the process of working together begins by recognizing their right to participate in decisions concerning future living arrangements of their child. After the tasks required to attain the clients' goal are identified, clients are in a more informed position to decide whether or not to participate. Contracts acknowledge clients as partners in the casework process and inform them about counselor assistance in reaching their goals. Because clients are given a copy of the contract, they have a ready reminder of all agreements.

Contracts may be written between counselors and clients or between two or more clients. In any case, purposes and basic components of written contracts are the same. Counselor-client contracts in foster care may identify a client's long range-goal, such as having a child returned. Contracts between clients may clarify arrangements such as the division of household responsibilities. Some contracts are simple and short term—a contract specifying conditions for a two-week trial visit, for example; others may be complex—describing steps involved in problem-solving. Some contracts may be written mainly to describe the conditions necessary for assessment. Contracts may also be used to coordinate multiple services provided to a client. The following sections discuss and give examples of these three variants of the written contract in social work intervention.

RESTORATION CONTRACTS

Restoration contracts, in which workers agree to provide direct services, are generally written in two parts. The first, illustrated in Figure One,

RESTORATION CONTRACT

This contract is between Joan Phillips*, a child welfare worker for Alameda County, and Alice Murray, mother of John Murray, presently a dependent child of the Alameda County Juvenile Court. In keeping with Ms. Murray's wish to have her child returned to her care, Ms. Phillips agrees to recommend restoration at the next court review hearing contingent upon compliance with conditions listed in this contract. Ms. Murray understands that failure to comply with intervention efforts will result in a report of such failure to the juvenile court and a recommendation that John not return home. Further, this court report will state Ms. Phillips' intention to pursue legal guardianship with Mr. and Ms. Kramor, John's foster parents.

1. Ms. Murray and her son John agree to visit according to the attached schedule with Ms. Murray providing transportation to and from the foster home.
(a) Ms. Murray agrees to allow Ms. Phillips to observe two visits with John each month. Observation will occur for approximately thirty minutes. Ms. Murray will be informed in advance of visits during which observation will occur. The goal of observation is to identify any difficulties existing in parent/child interaction that might threaten restoration. Should any difficulties be identified, Ms. Phillips will discuss these with Ms. Murray and help to develop an interventive program.
2. Ms. Murray is to obtain full or part-time employment by July 18, 1978 and to allow Ms. Phillips to verify employment; or
(a) if employment is not obtained by that date, Ms. Murray agrees to apply for an AFDC grant no later than July 21, 1978.
(b) if full-time employment is obtained, Ms. Murray agrees to make arrangements for John's formal supervision after school. Ms. Phillips will assist Ms. Murray in identifying appropriate alternatives to meet this requirement. This goal and steps to attain it will be described in detail when and if full-time employment is obtained.
3. Ms. Murray agrees to comply with the court directive for a psychiatric evaluation prior to John's return. Specifically, she will make a diagnostic appointment with a psychiatrist of her choice by July 7, 1978. The evaluation must be made available to Ms. Phillips at least 30 days prior to the next court review hearing.

This contract will be in effect for 90 days, from June 30, 1978 through September 28, 1978.

______________	______________
Alice Murray	Joan Phillips
Mother	Child Welfare Worker
Date____________	Date____________

* All names are fictitious.

FIGURE 1

helps identify problems that might hinder restoration. As parent/child visits increase in frequency and duration and occur in new environments, problems not present under previous conditions may emerge. Thus, contracts provide frameworks for establishing assessment conditions. The sample contract shows the assessment phase of a restoration agreement between the caseworker and the mother of a ten year old boy foster placement for the past five years. It was developed during the second meeting with the natural mother.

The first paragraph identifies the parties involved. The mother's goal for her son's future is stated and the gains and consequences are described. Three objectives were identified when the contract was drawn up. The first focused on establishing a visiting schedule, described the worker's intention to observe parent/child interaction during a portion of these visits, and gave the purpose of such observation. The worker's obligation to share assessment information with the parent is also noted. A visiting schedule describing frequency and duration of visits for the three-month contract period and identifying assessment visits, was amended to the contract, and copies of both the contract and the amendment were given to the parent. The amendment shown in Figure Two illustrates the level of specificity achieved within the contracting framework.

Objectives two and three illustrate additional areas that can be included in an initial agreement. The mother's interest in seeking employment is noted in objective two. Failure to obtain work could not be construed as a sufficient reason for keeping a child in care. Hence, a contingency was added so the mother could apply for AFDC if she was unable to find work. Item 2b illustrates a worker requirement. Given the child's age, the worker thought formal arrangements should be made for after school supervision if the mother located full-time employment. Since attaining full-time work was hypothetical at the time the contract was written, it was not necessary to specify how this goal should be accomplished. It was sufficient to state that steps to attain it should be implemented when and if the mother located full-time employment. The court required a psychiatric evaluation of the mother as a condition for restoration. The procedure followed to meet this condition is shown in objective three.

If problems are identified during assessment, changes necessary before restoration are written into later agreements. If the caseworker assumes responsibility for direct intervention, these objectives and detailed intervention plans are described, as are caseworker and client responsibilities in achieving goals. When collateral resources are responsible for problem-solving, these objectives serve to identify resources to be employed, the client's intention to cooperate with the program, and the client's agreement that necessary information can be

VISITING SCHEDULE AMENDMENT

Month One:

Weeks One and Two: July 1 - 14, 1978
Visits will occur on Saturday afternoons between the hours of 2:00 and 4:00 p.m. There are no restrictions placed on where visits are to occur. Joan Phillips will observe during one of these visits according to conditions described in Goal 1.

Weeks Three and Four: July 15 - 31, 1978
Visits will occur on Saturdays for the entire afternoon. Ms. Murray will pick up John at 12:00 noon and return him at 5:00 p.m.

Month Two:

Weeks One and Two: August 1 - 14, 1978
Visits will occur on Saturdays for the entire day. Ms. Murray will pick up John at 9:00 a.m., and return him to the foster home at 5:00 p.m.

Weeks Three and Four: August 15 - 31, 1978
Visits will occur on both Saturday and Sunday for the entire day. On each of these days, Ms. Murray will pick up John at 9:00 a.m. and return him to the foster home at 5:00 p.m.

Month Three:

Weeks One and Two: September 1 - 13, 1978
Visits will occur for the entire weekend. Ms. Murray will pick up John at 9:00 a.m. on Saturday, and return him to the foster home at 5:00 p.m. on Sunday.

Weeks Three and Four: September 14 - 28, 1978
Visits will occur for four consecutive days. Ms. Murray will pick up John at 9:00 a.m. on Thursday, and return him to the foster home at 5:00 p.m. on Sunday.

If visits are maintained according to schedule, and any identified problems are resolved, Ms. Phillips will request an *ex-parte* order from the juvenile court, permitting John to remain in Ms. Murray's home on a continuous basis beginning with the last four-day visit of Week 4, Month 3.

FIGURE 2

obtained from the appropriate resource—in this case, a psychiatrist of Ms. Murray's choice.

When problems are identified, contracts are not rewritten, an attachment to the original agreement is written. Such an attachment is illustrated in Figure Three. This case involved a mother whose daughter had been in continuous foster placement for six years. Both mother and daughter wished to be reunited. During assessment, difficulty in discussing personal problems and in arriving at mutually acceptable conclusions was noted as a primary difficulty. Therefore, the need for a negotiation training program was written into the contract, and the actual program described in the contract as shown.

DECISION-MAKING CONTRACTS

Clients are sometimes unsure about plans for their children's future living arrangements. Decision-making contracts can facilitate the process of selecting options at the earliest possible time in a child's placement career. Such contracts contain all the basic components of contracts previously described, including arrangements for parent/child visiting. In addition, they identify possible alternatives for the youngster; give option consequences for natural parents, foster parents, and the child; and state procedures for worker/client discussions of alternatives.

The decision-making contract illustrated in Figure Four shows the goal of deciding between restoration or adoption. Adoption was listed as an option because, next to restoration, adoption is most likely to result in continuity of care for the child. Since the child had been in placement less than one year, moving her to a pre-adoptive home was viewed as reasonable if the foster parents were not interested in pursuing adoption. The adoption unit supervisor was confident that an appropriate home could be located. In addition, since child abuse had been alleged in the initial petition, there were grounds upon which to base a termination action if the mother refused to voluntarily relinquish the child.

When a child has been in one foster home for a long period of time, alternatives to restoration are determined in part by foster parents. In descending order, adoption, legal guardianship, and long-term care are the alternatives most likely to result in providing continuity in care. Each option should be discussed with biological parents, foster parents, and the child.

Regularly scheduled parent/child visits are considered essential for providing clients with the information necessary to reach an informed decision. Since parental indecisiveness might result from difficulties during parent/child visits, it is the worker's responsibility to help parents make visits positive experiences. The contract notes that discussions of alternatives for the child's future will not be held until the second month.

PLAN FOR GOAL 2: NEGOTIATION TRAINING

The objective of this program is to help Ms. Stevens* and her daughter Linda learn new ways of discussing issues in which there are differences of opinion, so that such differences can be resolved in a manner satisfactory to both persons. To accomplish this objective, Mr. Andrews, caseworker, agrees to meet with Ms. Stevens and Linda each Thursday afternoon between 3:00 and 4:30 p.m. Meetings will focus on helping Ms. Stevens and Linda state issues of concern so both parties understand the issues. Thus, Ms. Stevens and Linda will learn how to "pinpoint" behavior causing distress. Pinpointing involves describing behavior so two observers could agree that the behavior was occurring. In addition, Mr. Andrews will teach Ms. Stevens and Linda how to "paraphrase" what the other has said. Paraphrasing involves having the listener repeat, in her words, what she has heard the speaker say. The speaker responds by indicating agreement or disagreement with what has been said. Mr. Andrews will also assist Ms. Stevens and Linda to learn how to "trade" to resolve differences of opinion. Trading involves identifying what each party is willing to give or contribute to problem resolution.

Ms. Stevens and Linda agree to:

(1) Be present at their home during these scheduled meetings.
(2) To practice the tasks learned in negotiation sessions on a schedule established by Mr. Andrews in a designated room in the mother's home and at no other time and in no other place.
(3) In any practice area in which there is disagreement or difficulty, both parties agree to write down their view of the difficulty. This is to include identification of the stage of negotiation training (being specific, paraphrasing, or trading) that is problematic. Within the identified area of difficulty, each party should write down who was speaking, what was said, and her perception of the difficulty and how it could have been resolved.
(4) Mr. Andrews agrees to go over any issues that are listed and to assist Ms. Stevens and Linda in resolving these.

* All names are fictitious.

FIGURE 3

FIGURE 4

DECISION-MAKING CONTRACT

The object of this contract is to reach a decision regarding future living arrangements of Anna Motlow*, daughter of Evelyn Motlow, presently a dependent of the Alameda County Juvenile Court. Two placement alternatives have been discussed: Anna may be restored to the home of her mother, or adoption may be pursued.

To facilitate decision-making, the following will occur: For the first month of this contract there will be regularly scheduled visits between Ms. Motlow and Anna, with caseworker observation of parent-child visits to take place during each visit. Beginning with the second month, Ms. Collins, caseworker, and Ms. Motlow will discuss placement alternatives. Discussions will take place once weekly, for approximately one hour. Visiting between mother and daughter will continue during this time on a schedule established at the end of the first month. Placement alternatives and implications are listed below.

RESTORATION: The result of this outcome would be that Anna is permanently restored to her mother's care. For this to occur, any problems identified during assessment have to be resolved. Ms. Collins will develop and implement a plan to assist in problem resolution. Should this outcome be selected, another contract with the objective of restoration will be written. This contract will identify any conditions that have to be met prior to restoration, such as a schedule of accelerated visits with continued caseworker observation. If difficulties are identified during these visits, Ms. Collins will develop and implement a plan to resolve them. This contract would include Ms. Collins' agreement to recommend restoration of Anna to her mother.

Ms. Collins agrees to discuss feelings and/or concerns of Ms. Motlow in any area related to this outcome. Discussion will occur during the scheduled meetings noted at the end of paragraph two.

ADOPTION: Should adoption occur, Anna would become the legal child of her new parents. All legal rights and responsibilities currently existing between Ms. Motlow and Anna would be transferred to the new parents. The legal relationship between Ms. Motlow and Anna would be terminated.

Should Ms. Motlow select this outcome, it is expected that she will sign papers voluntarily relinquishing Anna for adoption. The Department of Social Services will assume responsibility for placing Anna. If Ms. Motlow decides on this option, the legal implications of the decision will be put in writing.

Should Ms. Motlow fail to reach a decision by the end of the contract period, it is the intention of Ms. Collins to take action to legally terminate parental rights.
This contract is in effect for a period of 90 days, beginning October 12, 1978 and ending on January 10, 1979.

Signed:

____

Evelyn Motlow

____

Anna Motlow

____

Lisa Collins

____

Date

* All names are fictitious.

This provides time to devote full attention to the parent/child relationship. Outcomes for parent and child are stated in the first sentence of each alternative listed in the contract.

There are at least two advantages to listing each alternative and its consequences: first, parents are given information for reaching an informed decision. Second, a non-threatening atmosphere for discussing sensitive issues such as adoption is created because parents expect the topic to be raised. Discussion of adoption often puts parents at ease, possibly giving them permission to select this outcome. If restoration is chosen, a new contract is negotiated.

Service Coordination Contracts

When collateral resources are involved in foster care cases, methods must be arranged to coordinate service delivery. The respective tasks of each party should be clearly described. Without a coordination method, duplication of services may occur or conflicting advise may be given. Failing to prepare and exchange information required for court reports is another potential difficulty.

Contracts may be employed to coordinate service delivery among multiple resources. Figure Figure represents a contract illustrating task divisions among three resources: a public health nurse, a psychiatrist, and a caseworker. The contract's objective is stated in the first paragraph, and all three parties tasks are described subsequently.

CONTRACT FOR COORDINATION OF SERVICES

This contract is entered into among Sylvia Allen* child welfare worker for Alameda County; Elaine Rose, psychiatrist in private practice; and Ann Newton, public health nurse, Alameda County Public Health Department. Each of these parties is a service provider in the case of Mary Lee Altman, infant daughter of Sheryl Altman. The objective of this contract is to establish a framework for coordinating service delivery. Goals to be attained by each party and the means for attaining them are identified below. A procedure for exchanging information is described and time limits for goal attainment are noted.

1. Ms. Newton, Public Health Nurse: Ms. Newton agrees to assess the natural mother's knowledge and skills in selected areas related to infant care. Areas of concern are the client's knowledge of proper nutrition for an infant, her skill in menu planning, in bathing,

diapering and dressing an infant. In addition, she agrees to assess the mother's ability to discriminate between physical conditions requiring medical attention and those that the mother is able to remedy herself (e.g. diaper rash). If deficits are identified in any of these areas, Ms. Newton agrees to develop and implement a plan to teach new skills or increase present skills to a level deemed acceptable for the infant's safety.

2. Dr. Rose, Psychiatrist: Dr. Rose agrees to conduct a psychiatric evaluation with Ms. Altman. The objective of this evaluation is to address the question of whether Ms. Altman is able to resume full-time care of her infant daughter.
3. Ms. Allen, Child Welfare Worker: Ms. Allen will be responsible for assessment of parent/child interaction in all areas she deems appropriate that are not covered by Ms. Newton or Dr. Rose. Ms. Allen agrees to gather, summarize and report to the court all information supplied by Ms. Newton and Dr. Rose. If problems arise in terms of achieving objectives, Ms. Allen agrees to call and chair any necessary meetings to resolve them. Ms. Allen will telephone Ms. Newton and Dr. Rose once each week during the contract period to monitor compliance with the conditions set forth in this document.

While it is recognized that work with the natural mother may extend beyond the assigned tasks, all parties agree: (1) not to extend their work into any area specifically assigned to one of the other parties; and (2) to give priority to fulfilling those objectives for which they were brought into this case. If problems arise that hinder goal attainment, Ms. Newton and Dr. Rose agree to attend any meetings scheduled by Ms. Allen. Further, Ms. Newton and Dr. Rose agree to submit final reports to Ms. Allen by August 16, 1978. This contract is in effect for a period of 60 days.

Signed: ______________________________

Sylvia Allen, M.S.W., Child Welfare Worker Date

____

Ann Newton, R.N., Public Health Nurse Date

____

Elaine Rose, M.D., Psychiatrist Date

* All names are fictitious.

FIGURE 5

Important elements of service coordination contracts include agreements that each party will restrict its activities to the tasks described in the contract; that they will give priority to meeting these obligations; that any barriers they encounter interfering with fulfilling responsibilities will be reported to the caseworker; that they will attend meetings to develop ways to remove barriers; and that they will submit reports to the worker at specified times.

AMENDING CONTRACTS

One purpose of a contract is to arrange for collection of assessment information, for example through observing parent/child interactions. If problem areas are identified, additional goals must be specified. This process is described in writing in the contract. When additional objectives are added, contracts must be amended.

Changes occurring in a specified objective may also require contract amendment. For example, a client who has stated an objective of gaining employment prior to having a child restored, may instead decide to apply for an AFDC grant. The worker must then determine if this is acceptable. Time limits may be reduced if observation indicates that parent/child interaction is satisfactory and visiting can be increased more rapidly than originally planned. On the other hand, time limits may be extended. A parent may complete four of five contract objectives and request an extension for completion of the last. The addition or changes of objectives might require an increase in original time limits. In these authors' work, clients have been offered second and third opportunities to fulfill contract objectives before workers take action on noncompliance consequences. When this occurs, an amendment is attached to the original contract, stating why time deadlines are being extended.

If amendments are made it is not necessary to rewrite the entire contract. A footnote can be added to the original contract stating which of the objectives has been changed and describing changes. The footnote is initialed by all concerned parties, and some notation, such as an asterisk, used to indicate which of the original objectives is being amended. For example, when parent/child visits have to be cancelled, the time period for fulfilling the contract can be extended and an amendment and additional visiting schedule prepared. Figure Six illustrates one footnote procedure. The new visiting schedule would be similar to the schedule shown in Figure Two. An asterisk would be placed beside the objective related to visiting as well as beside the final sentence in the original contract in which time limits are specified.

Perhaps the most difficult task in forming effective contracts for workers and for clients in writing specific objectives. Educational experiences within social work tend to encourage the use of global, vague goals, whereas exactly what will be different when an objective has been met should be described, so that two or more people will agree when the objective has been attained. To test the clarity of an objective, colleagues can be asked to describe what they would expect to see when the objective has been met. With clear objectives their descriptions will match expectations for change.

ILLUSTRATION OF FOOTNOTE
FOR CONTRACT AMENDMENT

*The visiting schedule is amended and the period of the contract extended to include two additional visiting periods. This is necessary since, due to illness of the children, two of the previously scheduled visits had to be cancelled. All of the conditions for observation and assessment as noted in the initial contract will pertain during these two added visits. This contract is extended until March 14, 1978.
Initialed by:

____ (father) ____ (social worker: Alameda County)
____ (child welfare worker: Alameda County)
____________________ date

FIGURE 6

MAKING CONTRACTS

Often, workers encounter impediments to making contracts with clients and other professionals. Some major impediments are identifying objectives, specifying treatment plans, time investment, and organizational resistance.

Identifying Objectives

Social workers often try to write specific objectives before they have gathered necessary information. For example, if a client reports that her daughter is "destructive," information is needed regarding the behavioral referents of this label before describing what the daughter will do if she is not destructive. The same label may mean different things to different individuals. Clients may be unable to describe the behaviors that led to labeling a child destructive, or to clearly identify the situations in which the behavior is displayed. In such cases, the contract objective should be to observe the youngster in situations thought to evoke destructive behavior. In this way, specific behaviors and contexts in which they occur can be determined. This information should enable identification of specific objectives.

Difficulties may arise when the impetus for writing an objective is a "sense" that something is amiss. In working clients, subjective hypotheses are invariably formed; these should serve as cues to gather additional assessment information. If assessment does not provide data supporting such hypotheses, specific objectives cannot be written. Differences in values between worker and client may be the source of such hypotheses, so it is important. Keep in mind that one should focus on difficulties that, if left unresolved, might result in a child being returned to foster care.

Learning to write specific objectives requires practice. The task seems deceptively simple at first. It is also important to learn to discriminate between inference and description. Inferences are abstractions from observed events. It is also important to distinguish clearly between objectives and the means of pursuing them (see for example, Mager 1975). One error workers often make in trying to specify clear objectives is to confuse objectives with intervention methods. Only after objectives are identified can informed choices of intervention be made. Initial objectives should be scanned to ferret out vague aims, to identify entries that mix objectives and method, and to decide whether each entry is relevant.

Specifying Treatment Plans

Plans that clearly describe how objectives are attained comprise an important part of contracts and contract attachments. An essential ingredient for documenting services offered is a clear description of exactly what was done, including a log of counselor-client contacts, objectives pursued during each contact, what actually occurred during the contact in terms of procedures employed, and the outcome. The failure to document step-by-step progress toward meeting objectives and services offered makes decision-making difficult.

Time Investment

Some workers express concern that writing contracts and attachments for each case is a formidable, time-consuming task, which is certainly true to the extent that learning any new approach requires time, but these costs decrease as experience increases, and there are many ways of saving time, such as standardized contract forms like the one presented in Figure One. The opening paragraph, with the exception of the last sentence, is standard for all cases with a goal of restoration. Likewise, a visiting schedule with the condition that observation will occur during some portion of each visit is contained in all such contracts. Other objectives may vary case by case, but forms containing common information may generally be prepared in advance. Space can be left to note objectives that cannot be standardized.

As workers become adept at using them, contracts save time. Attached to court reports they save time in describing case plans. Changes in treatment plans resulting from additional information do not necessitate rewriting contracts, as written amendments may be attached to the original contract. It is not necessary to specify the steps for attaining all goals in the initial contract. Some goals become relevant only if others are attained. For example, location of suitable housing will only be necessary if identified difficulties between parent and child are reduced; if such programs are not successful, the child will not be restored, precluding the necessity for a new living arrangement.

Organizational Resistance

As written agreements between child welfare workers and clients are novel to most juvenile court judges and referees, we strongly recommend that time be devoted to their education through meetings that explain the purpose of such documents and present written examples to allay initial resistance. In our experience, once judges understand contract use, they support the method. Clarity of the contracts' descriptive writing can be a major factor in their acceptability. Judges appreciate descriptive rather than inferential or professional terminology, and once accustomed to contracts, they become agreeable to modifying court reporting formats, even to the extent of accepting contracts in lieu of the lengthy narratives previously used.

An additional area of concern regarding courts is the contracts' legality. To the best of our knowledge, the legality of client/counselor contracts has never been tested. Concern over legal questions is best addressed by attending to the wording of contracts. For example, we cannot guarantee clients that the court will restore a child even if recommended by the worker. For that reason, when restoration is the goal, the contract states that this "would be recommended to the court"; clients are told that such recommendations may not be followed. It warrants mention that we have not encountered a single instance of judges going against the worker's recommendations when contracts were used. If use of the term "contract" causes problems in court, "agreement" can be substituted. As in all social work practice, workers should not promise anything they cannot deliver, and workers should not establish conditions for restoration judges will not honor. For example, failure to obtain employment is not a sufficient reason to maintain a child in placement. When such an objective is identified, it should include a viable alternative.

DISCUSSION

Time pressures are great in making permanent plans for children in care. Abundant data show that the length of time a child has been in care has value for predicting the likelihood of differential outcomes, be they restoration, adoption, guardianship or long-term care (Maas 1969; Fanshell 1971; Stein, Gambrill, & Wiltse, in press). Therefore, treatment plans should be developed and put in writing at the time evidence indicates placement will occur. This action involves collaboration between intake or protective service workers and workers carrying the case once a child is placed. Frequently, when staff operate in isolation from each other, the length of time a child remains in care is prolonged. Workers providing services after placement may disagree with or may not understand plans made by intake or protective service workers. Valuable time may be lost reassessing the family situation.

Early collaboration and contract formation has a further advantage. Workers have the opportunity to observe family interaction while the family unit is intact, an optimal situation for gathering accurate assessment data. Following placement, assessment frequently occurs under contrived conditions—for example, during brief visits and in environments other than those to which the child will return. Early contracted collaboration also has advantages to parents. They will not be subject to multiple periods of assessment and differences in workers' opinions as to what must occur prior to restoration. When workers operate independently, each may suggest different courses of action for child restoration. Forming contracts at the point of intake and using guidelines previously presented facilitates early planning and increases the likelihood of permanent plans.

Multiple resources will always be involved in planning, delivering, and evaluating child welfare services. Social workers must increase the range of available services and suggest deficits in community resources (Jenkins & Sauber, 1966; Shyne, 1969). Moreover, purchase-of-service agreements with community agencies is growing, and is reinforced by current Title XX provisions (Miller, 1978). The case-manager role further accords child welfare workers primary responsibility for marshalling community services rather than offering such services themselves (Public Services Administration, 1973). These trends in the field point to even greater burdens being carried by social work contracts. We hope the variants of contracts described in this chapter as used in foster care services help guide others in such future work. Weighing the strengths of contracts against impediments to using them betokens many more applications of the procedure throughout child welfare and allied social work practice.

6

Crisis Intervention with Youths

Edmund T. Dimock

INTRODUCTION

For many teenagers in our society, adolescense is a time of stress and alienation from the family. The sexual revolution, the drug culture, and conflicts with the "establishment" create problems for youth and parents. Most adolescents experience only minor problems; however, a few young people respond by engaging in criminal activities, developing emotional problems, or using drugs. Society responds quickly to such behavior through the courts or other criminal and social sanctioning bodies.

What about adolescents who respond by running away from home, not obeying parents, being truant from school, or violating curfew? Termed "status offenders" because the illegality of their behavior results from their nonadult status—or "predelinquent" because of the law-breaking connotations of delinquency—these youths are not included in conventional criminal-justice, mental-health, or social-service systems.

This chapter describes Youth Crisis Services, a program designed to specifically serve the status offender. Youth Crisis Services was launched as a joint venture between the Children's Home Society of California and mental health and probation departments in four northern California counties.

BACKGROUND

Status offenders in California are the legal responsibility of local probation departments. But, probation officers attempting to work with status offenders encounter impediments, largely due to limited community resources for adolescents and their parents. Youth Crisis Services attempted to help such families by diverting status offenders from the juvenile justice system into a voluntary community-based program.

Many referrals to Youth Crisis Services are adolescents who have run away from home. Even though angry and upset, most youths will return and stay home if the immediate crisis is addressed, if parents are willing to negotiate with their children;, and if outside intervention is available to assist the family. Many adolescents referred for services, however, do not return home. Some angrily refuse to meet with their parents. Others cool off and can eventually be reunited with their families. A more serious problem occurs when parents do not want children home until they "learn their lesson and can obey the rules." Such parents, viewing their children's behavior as willful, believe that successful parenting is the result of punishment and adherence to strict rules. These disagreements, more serious than those involving transient crises, generally take longer to resolve. When brief separation between adolescent and family is indicated, short-term intervention within a coeducational, community-based group home appears a viable resource.

Five hundred youths have been referred to Youth Crisis Services in over a three year period. Average age at time of referral for these youths was about fifteen years old; 48% of these referred were male. Family structure patterns showed 45% of the adolescents lived in single-parent families, 20% had a stepparent residing in the home, and the rest were living with relatives, foster parents, or in some other substitute-care arrangement. Most referred youths have experienced school problems. Referral sources assessed over two-thirds of the teenagers as potential school drop outs. Almost all youths have reported school as a major source of conflict for them and their parents.

DESCRIPTION OF THE PROGRAM

Because of its rural setting, Youth Crisis Services first encounters clients when problems are severe. Rarely do parents request services in the early stages of their child's behavior problems. Prevailing norms of keeping family difficulties from outside scrutiny and mistrust of the public welfare system likely influence decisions to not voluntarily seek professional help. Instead, adolescents come to the attention of our program after they have violated rules set down by the law or school. Most run-away and acting-out youths are referred from the juvenile court, and three counties involved with the program first refer clients at the time they are placed in substitute-care group homes.

In spite of such long delays in learning of family distress, every attempt is made to address and resolve crises so youths stay with or quickly return to their homes.

Youths unwilling or unable to return home are kept in the group home, which provides temporary housing and represents an important alternative. Adolescents are often so angry and confused they cannot tolerate the emotional closeness of a family setting. Especially for these clients, group homes are a neutral environment, providing distance between parents and the adolescent, thereby decreasing the need for the youth to run away and interrupting the pathological family network, while offering an opportunity for an emotional breather for the adolescent and family along with a structure that allows positive change (cf. Dimock, 1977). As with home-based services, the goal at the group home is to reintegrate youths into the family.

GROUP HOME INTERVENTION

Tangible Rewards

Tangible rewards are based on principles of operant conditioning in which: "Certain behaviors are...dependent upon the *consequences* of those behaviors to the actors. Some consequences will result in an increase or repetition of the behavior; some will not. The future rate, or frequency, or form of that behavior will be governed by the consequences attached to the behavior" (Schwartz and Goldiamond 1975:13). Behavior immediately and tangibly rewarded will likely happen again in the future.

In Youth Crisis Services' group homes, token systems are tools for helping adolescents become responsible. Residents receive points, later exchanged for tokens, for performing tasks according to standards jointly determined by staff and residents. Tasks, ranging from practical chores such as sweeping the front walk to social skills like calling home when late, are listed with point values on individual weekly point charts. Each task is defined in explicit terms on the bulletin board. Many chores are described in procedural steps, with standards and completion times given. Following are steps for stove cleaning:

Time: 30 minutes

Needed: Ammonia, water, sponge, and scraping pad

1. Lift all burners and take out pan underneath. Remove foil and discard.

2. Place burner pans in sink with ½ cup ammonia and water to soak.
3. Use sponge dipped in sink water to wipe entire top of stove.
4. Scrub burner pans with scraping pad until no trace of grease or stain remains.
5. Dry burner pans and line with new foil.
6. Replace pans under burner, replace burner.

Residents not participating in the system neither lose nor gain points, but are unable to purchase privileges. Residents may choose to do dishes and earn points, or choose not to do dishes and forego some privileges: the responsibility is solely with them. Points are tallied at a daily "chip time," the total being paid to residents in poker chips. Each resident has a unique color chip to prevent trades or bullying. Chips are used to purchase privileges such as television, snacks, telephone calls, or time away from the home. Privilege lists change with time and follow resident needs and interests.

Contracts

Contracting is an effective process for defining behavioral objectives and determining how they are to be achieved. Schwartz and Goldiamond suggest that the contract is not to be viewed in stilted legalistic terms, but as a *process* (1975: 94). The importance our society gives to the written written word lends strength to behavioral contracts.

Contracts are part of most interventions in Youth Crisis Services group homes. Used for resolving problems created by group living, all group home contracts embody four fundamentals: the activity that needs to be done, who will do the activity, how it will be done, and what will occur after the activity is completed. Contracts are written in simple language so they are understood by all participants. To encourage success, contracts emphasize positives. Contracts containing similar elements are critical to family intervention and are therefore detailed in that section.

FAMILY INTERVENTION

Working with families having an adolescent in crisis demands immediate intervention. Early assistance to parents and youths thus deals with the problems that precipitated the referral. Such crisis-oriented social work will usually reduce family tension to a point where youths will remain or return home. Moreover, early success is likely to increase family motivation for further change. Initial intervention, halting additional problems, may do little to repair long-standing patterns of family intervention. Workers must help family members identify behavior leading to the present difficulty. Because these may be unknown to youths and parents it is frequently necessary to structure the problem identification process. One way is to have each family member list likes and dislikes about their home life. Another is to ask individuals to write down what happens at home to make them angry or unhappy. When there is question or disagreement over the frequency of problem behavior, workers ask family members to keep track of how often and when the behavior occurs. The resulting baselines provide information for developing subsequent intervention strategies. It is also important to note responses following problem situations since behavior consequences influence future occurrences of behavior.

After the problem behavior is identified, Youth Crisis Services workers aid families in developing objectives. The question becomes: "How much change is enough?" Desired change is always negotiated by family members, with workers mediating. Objectives are qualified and stated in behavioral terms. To illustrate: "Jimmy must be in the house by 9 p.m. on nights before school." Non-specific generalities—"Be in the house on time"—are inadequate and stimulate misunderstandings.

Problems identified and objectives developed, workers next help families find acceptable, effective, and often unique intervention strategies: what works with one family may not work with the next. Families need to understand that there is no cure-all. Achieving desired change may require several strategies implemented over time. Thus, families are told that intervention plans need to be flexible for renegotiation.

Tangible Rewards

Like those applied in group homes, simple token or point systems can be useful in family settings. Arguments over chores and non-completion of homework are two situations appropriate for the structure provided by tangible points. Many successful systems use only check marks on a calendar to signify task completion. Tallied weekly, total marks determine the amount of a youth's allowance. Our experience is that families easily learn tangible reward systems, but discontinue them after leaving the program. Perchance use of home tangible reward systems is strengthened by the monitoring performed by workers. Whatever the reason, families infrequently continue these systems after termination with Youth Crisis Services.

Contracting

Unlike tangible reward systems, contracts maintain their viability after families leave Youth Crisis Services. Clarifying specific concerns and expectations, contracts are useful for reducing family conflict. Blame and scapegoating are diminished by contracting because each party is able to benefit. Parents view the process as helpful for gaining control over the situation; adolescent involvement with contracting reduces powerlessness felt toward the adult world.

Family contracts are especially useful where problems derive from parental difficulties in setting limits for adolescents, and can help modify parent's behavior as well as that of the adolescent. Likewise, contracts are indicated for families unable to give clear messages to one another because the communication process has broken down. It is important for the workers to involve all family members in the contracting process, leading to mutual "ownership" of problems, and thereby increasing the likelihood of the contract's success as a family product. Workers accordingly should function as objective consultants and ensure that contract terms address family problems and lay out reasonable consequences.

TWO FAMILIES

Case histories of two families illustrate the Youth Crisis Services approach to helping parents and adolescents in crisis.

Lori B.

After a fight with her stepfather, thirteen-year-old Lori ran away to her paternal grandparents' home. Lori refused to return home and was placed in a foster receiving home. The local probation department then referred the B. family to Youth Crisis Services.

Lori lived with her mother, stepfather, and Lori's four siblings on a small ranch. Problems with Lori started shortly after Mr. and Mrs. B's marriage four years ago. Mrs. B. believed Lori's poor behavior at home was an attempt to break up the marriage. Lori also started exhibiting regressive behavior, temper tantrums and inappropriate removing of clothing.

Lori, with her mother's permission, was voluntarily placed in a Youth Crisis Services group home; the same day, a very angry Lori met with her mother. She told Mrs. B. that she did not want to return home because of the continued fighting among family members. It was agreed that Lori would temporarily remain in the group home. During this initial meeting, the worker assisted in identifying problems of fighting at home, Lori's anger at Mrs. B., her inappropriate removing of clothing, and her refusal to return home.

Lori returned home the next day and immediately left for church camp. Unfortunately, Lori was injured at camp five days later and sent home. She remained at home less than one day and ran to her grandparents because of the "fighting." Lori and her mother agreed that she should return to the group home.

The group home's token system was modified to include "appropriately dressed outside of the bedroom" as an expected behavior for Lori. Staff supplemented points with verbal praise and suggestions to Lori about what to wear. This approach proved effective for helping Lori with this problem. In fact, the token system seemed to provide Lori with a structure missing at home. After seeing positive change in Lori's behavior, Mrs. B. developed interest in the group home's token system and appeared interested in using a similar system with Lori at home.

Lori's planned return home was preceded by a meeting to assist Mrs. B. and Lori develop a tangible reward system. Not as inclusive as the group home's token system, the home system dealt primarily with attention-getting behavior, chores, appropriate dress, and arriving home on time. Points earned granted Lori daily time to ride her horse and were exchanged weekly for an allowance. Unsure of the system's effectiveness with her other children, Mrs. B. agreed to use it only with Lori.

The home token system was expanded two weeks later to provide additional opportunities for Lori to demonstrate responsibility. Additional expectations were incorporated into the system rather than Mrs. B. having to constantly "remind" Lori. Weekly contact continued with Mrs. B. for one month to encourage the system's continued use.

Lori was still on the token system two months after termination, apparently giving Mrs. B. a means of setting limits for Lori, while reducing the incidence and intensity of arguements between them. Possibly, much of Lori's resentment towards Mr. B. resulted from his attempts to provide direction and control. The token system allowed Mr. B. and Lori to relate to each other in a different manner, and Lori's relationship with her stepfather improved when she returned home. Four-year follow-up data support these positive changes for Lori, Mrs. B. and Mr. B.

George L.

Thirteen year old George L. was referred to Youth Crisis Services for school attendance problems and serious behavioral problems at home. The attendance issue was partially resolved by helping George transfer to another school whose resources met his educational needs. George and his mother, however, resisted discussion about family difficulties and refused further service.

George seemed a rather lonely boy with few friends. His brothers had recently entered military service; shortly afterwards, he lost his beloved grandfather. His mother expected him to be content to stay at home, enjoying solitary activities during the day while she worked.

Two months after the initial contact, Mrs. L. requested additional services from Youth Crisis Services. A problem had developed after the school year that Mrs. L. could not resolve. George was never home during the day, and Mrs. L. was afraid he was getting into trouble. Mrs. L. showed no concern for George's need of peer relationships. George felt he was meeting his mother's demands by leaving notes for her, indicating his destination and time of return. Mrs. L., on the other hand, felt little control over George's activities as he did not seek prior permission.

The social worker met with Mrs. L. and George. It was obvious that both felt a loss of control over the situation. The worker suggested contracting to the family since expectations and limits were key issues. George and his mother were initially anxious, questioning a contract's utility. Their anxiety was reduced with the worker's exploration of the behavior each member wanted from the other and explanation of how contracting would increase the probability of that behavior occurring.

Mrs. L. said that it was her responsibility as a mother to know where George was during the day and what he was doing. Both George and Mrs. L. indicated that George had wanted a dog for the past six months but Mrs. L. had refused to purchase one as she did not feel George had "earned it." With this information, the worker, Mrs. L. and George prepared a written contract as illustrated below.

Effective Date: From June 30—July 4th

EXPECTATIONS: Mrs. L. will telephone George each day between 10:30—12:00. George will be home at that time and will have made his plans for the day so he can tell his mother where he will be, a telephone number where he can be reached, and when he will be home—no later than 9:00 p.m.

CONSEQUENCES: Mrs. L. will buy George a puppy after the above expectations have been met for 10 days. If he is not at home to receive his mother's call, the next day George will not be able to go out. On a day that he is restricted to the house, mother will telephone to ensure George is at home.

After two weeks, Mrs. L. reported that the contract was "working beautifully." She knew where George was, and she and he were now going to pet stores and deciding on what kind of puppy to buy. A positive attitude toward this and similar contracts has continued for three months following the initial contract. The contract procedure has been monitored by the worker. Mrs. L., since she spends less time fighting with George, finds him more enjoyable to be around and spends more time with him. George is responding to his mother's improved predictability. It appears that the contract has had the effect of improving the interpersonal relationships between Mrs. L. and her son.

PROGRAM IMPACT

Youth Crisis Services was designed to fill a service gap and saw little need for program evaluation. No procedures were systematically developed to assess service delivery or overall objectives. A major constraint to any subsequent evaluation has been the difficulty of coming up with measures for determining program success while involved in day-to-day service delivery.

Despite these limitations an attempt was made to assess consumer satisfaction—an important measure of program responsiveness. Social work staff sent questionnaires asking clients of their subjective satisfaction with Youth Crisis Services to over 100 adolescents and their parents served by the program during a one-year period. Disappointing returns showed only 37% of their parents and 18% of the adolescents responding. A scale of one (complete satisfaction)— to seven, was used to record responses. The question "Did you get cooperation and assistance from Youth Crisis Services staff?" received a mean rating from parents of 1.5 (standard deviation (*SD*) of 1.12). "Did the program do an effective job of helping your family?" received a mean rating from parents of 2.28 (*SD* = 1.8). "Did the program help you get along better with parents?" was given a mean rating of 2.53 by adolescents (*SD* = 1.68). In response to "Did the program help you get along better with teachers?" young people gave a mean response of 3.8 (*SD* = 2.3). Finally, "If you now use the procedure you learned in the program (contracting, tokens) with other people, are you happy with how these procedures work?" got a mean rating of 2.5 (*SD* = 1.7) from all parents and youths. A number of factors contributed to the consumer satisfaction measure not being used again. A major reason was the low number of responses. Many nonresponders could have been families most dissatisfied with Youth Crisis Services. A few staff were opposed to the consumer satisfaction questionnaire. Some were wary of biases affecting completion and return of questionnaires. Some Youth Crisis Services workers failed to see how results from the questionnaires could increase the effectiveness of the program. Questionnaires provided no method for determining why respondents were satisfied or not satisfied.

BENEFITS AND CONCLUSIONS

Probation departments in counties served by Youth Crisis Services have been extremely supportive. During the first eighteen months of operation, probation officers discussed the program with other agencies and at a regional probation association meeting. These efforts resulted in five other counties expressing interest in a Youth Crisis Services program. Subsequently, two counties contracted with Children's Home Society and a third county sought out another agency to provide a similar program. Two counties continue their interest and are seeking funding.

Youth Crisis Services programs have also grown by incorporating additional target populations. In one county, the probation department requested that Youth Crisis Services be expanded to include delinquent adolescents in juvenile detention. In another county, the local community mental health program transferred its children and adolescent clinic to Youth Crisis Services. Representatives from Youth Crisis Services now participate in planning efforts to improve community services for adolescents. Staff members serve on community boards, representing services to adolescents and speaking up for their unique needs. When California decriminalized status offenders, representatives from Youth Crisis Services were sought out for their expertise to serve on planning bodies concerned with developing alternatives to secure detention for the status offender.

The community makes the final determination of whether or not a program like Youth Crisis Services will be funded from year to year. Programs that violate community expectations or fail to respond to community concerns will not be financially supported. Programs striving to provide service harmonious with the community milieu stand a better chance of being funded in the future. The six year tenure of Youth Crisis Services attests to the community's willingness to support services to adolescents within such a framework.

7

Treatment of Child Abuse

Robert F. Schilling, II

INTRODUCTION

Child abuse, a long-standing problem, claims increasing public and professional attention. Noted in the social work literature by Carstens in 1921, this problem recently came to national awareness, largely through efforts by healthcare workers, as the "battered child syndrome" (Kempe, Silverman, Steele, Dregmuller, & Silver, 1962). Subsequent years have seen a proliferation of child abuse reports, but how extensive is this phenomenon? Likely only a small percentage of the total abuse is reported, albeit many abuse complaints are not substantiated (Nagi, 1975). State reporting bureaus, receiving an estimated 167,500 reports of child abuse annually (Nagi, 1975), may miss far more cases than they find: recent research by Gelles (1978) suggests nearly two million children may be abuse victims each year. Much of the published literature deals with ameliorating child abuse; however, little is written on systematic child abuse intervention. Moreover, the extant literature offers few guidelines for obtaining relevant and objective data for critical decision-making. This chapter examines child abuse from a social learning perspective and outlines an intervention model based on behavioral methods and systematic collection of data.

SETTING

The methods of intervention described in this chapter result from five years' direct experience with abusive and dysfunctional families, gained at Children's Home Society of Washington, a private welfare agency with residential, foster care, and counseling services in eight locations throughout the state of Washington. Working in a branch office with a catchment area of 100,000 people, the author's caseload consisted mostly of white, lower-middle-class families referred by Childrens' Protective Services. In Washington, Childrens' Protective Services is administrated by the State Department of Social and Health Services. Although CPS workers do provide counseling in some instances, their primary mandate is investigation of complaints about maltreatment of children. Moreover, CPS workers acknowledge their investigative role often precludes the possibility of establishing a helping relationship with abusing parents. Thus, CPS refers families to community agencies such as Childrens' Home Society.

Contrasted to the overall analytical framework of Childrens' Home Society, this branch office operated in a less traditional manner. Such an approach, along with the office staff's collective value opposing any single solution to human problems, allowed the author the freedom to use a range of intervention methods. Although behavioral practitioners were only beginning to turn their attention to child abuse (Tracy & Clark, 1974) the author's behavioral training influenced this approach even with the first abusing families referred to the agency. Gradually a behavioral model of service delivery evolved. Before discussing the model, it is useful to briefly review suggested causes of child abuse and the contributions of other behavioral practitioners in the child abuse field.

CHILD ABUSE CAUSALITY: IMPLICATIONS FOR INTERVENTION

An extensive, often conflicting body of literature attempts to define the etiology of child abuse. Most studies are either anecdotal (see for example Steele & Pollock, 1974)—using only subjective measures of classification—or descriptive—using characteristics applying to non-abusing parents also (Jayaratne, 1977). A pervasive theme throughout the literature explains child abuse as a function of parental psychopathology, though Gelles (1973) argues convincingly against the inconsistency and narrowness of these theories. Several researchers have suggested that abused children are more likley to have physical handicaps, cognitive deficits or unusual personality characteristics (Friedrich & Boriskin, 1976, Roberts, 1979). Although the literature often suggests child abuse is broadly distributed throughout society, Pelton (1978) successfully attacks this previously held belief. Since lower socioeconomic groups are over-represented in most incidence studies, sociological and cultural deviance theories receive some support (Garbarino and Crouter, 1978). This issue will likely be a subject of continuing debate, but it seems likely that cultural and socioeconomic factors may prove important causal influences in child abuse. Other investigators, to be discussed later, advocate a social learning model of child abuse causality. Finally, other minor themes include life change (Conger, Burgess, & Barrett, 1979) family stress (Elmer, 1979) and social isolation (Wayne, 1979).

Although articles ascribing psychological factors to child abuse causality are usually anecdotal or descriptive (Steele & Pollock, 1974) standardized instruments have also been used to determine behavioral and personality characteristics of abusing parents (Paulson, Afifi, Thomason, & Chaleff, 1974). Doubtless these efforts are of some heuristic value, and may yield important predictive data, but they provide limited information regarding intervention. A more useful departure from standardized testing was undertaken by Burgess and Conger (1977). Employing a family interaction code similar to that developed by Patterson, Ray, Shaw, and Cobb (1969) and subsequently used in a vareity of settings (Schinke & Wong, 1977a), the investigators observed abusing and non-abusing families. Abusing families were found to be less skilled in physical contact and more apt to be verbally negative and coercive than controls. Although these are initial findings based on a small sample, Burgess and Conger's approach may have immediate implications for intervention.

The difficulty of determining child abuse causality is succinctly stated by Bybee: "At this time there is not a single, empirically validated, causal model for abuse and neglect. Each of several models account for some violence toward some youth some of the time. The results from many studies of different theoretical orientations can be viewed as evidence that there is a complex and interdependent network of factors affecting (that is, increasing the probability of) violence toward youth within the family system" (Bybee, 1979: 166). Given that child abuse has only recently been subjected to scientific scrutiny, advocating any one cause or solution seems unwise. A more reasonable course is continued exploration in the areas of causation, prevention, and early intervention.

Empirical investigations have now begun to test if existing hypotheses of child abuse are supported by research findings. As Jayaratne observes, "the literature suggests that parental inadequacy and misinformation are major contributing factors to child abuse. Where the studies in the literature fail is in the examination and delineation of different parenting styles between abusing and nonabusing family systems" (1977:8). Despite continuing speculation about predispositional determinants of child abuse, it seems prudent to assume abusing parents and their child victims are not constitutionally different from the general population. Intervention models based on behavioral methods are entirely consistent with this assumption. What behavioral approaches are found in the child abuse literature?

BEHAVIORAL INTERVENTION

Behavioral strategies as diverse as stress innoculation, assertiveness training and social-skills training (Resick and Sweet, 1979) have been suggested, but only a few investigators have actually attempted techniques beyond the operant procedures common to parent training programs. Sanford and Tustin (1973) employed respondent conditioning in modifying an abusing father's aggressive response to his daughter's loud noise. In treating an abusing mother, Polakow and Peabody (1975) used group sessions to develop social and interpersonal skills, emphasizing assertive behaviors. Cognitive restructuring of irrational childrearing beliefs was used by Reavley and Gilbert (1976) with a mother afraid of harming her child. One program combines all these strategies along with parent training techniques (Kinney, 1978).

Most case studies and program descriptions using behavioral methods (see for example Mastria, Mastria, & Harkins, 1979; Tracy & Clark, 1974; or Jensen, 1976) employ various parent training procedures to alter parent-child interaction. As Shorkey (1979) notes: "...assessment and treatment focus on the identifiable and observable behavior of parents in their current interactions with their children." Relying on quantitative assessment, behavioral practitioners formulate individual goals with abusing families. Intervention techniques include behavioral rehearsal, modeling, prompting, social reinforcement, extinction, discrimination training and shaping.

In an unpublished report, Reid and Taplin (1978) suggest that parental inconsistency and high rates of aversive behavior are key elements leading to abuse. They found more mothers and children, but not fathers, exhibiting aversive patters—nagging, negative physical contacts—in abusive than in non-abusive families. Having established that certain aversive behaviors are causally linked to abuse, and having demonstrated that these behaviors occur more frequently with abusive families, Reid and Taplin argue persuasively that decreasing aversive behavior lessens the probability of recurring abuse. Training families in pinpointing, recording, negotiating and providing consequences (Patterson, Reid, Jones, & Conger, 1975), the authors found aversive behavior decreases significantly for mother and children. Although these results remain tentative due to methodological limitations, Reid and Taplin's efforts are perhaps unique in clearly specifying salient outcome measures. Moreover, their work is well grounded in theory and reflects their empirical approach to intervention.

Having briefly reviewed the behavioral literature dealing with child abuse, what elements common to all of these approaches are noteworthy? Behavioral methods offer several advantages for social workers dealing with child abuse: 1) emphasis on observable events and behavior; 2) effectiveness in facilitating rapid change—necessary for abused children to remain at home; 3) emphasis on the recording of observable data, to enhance professional decision making; 4) the fostering of social program accountability. Perhaps more than any other child welfare specialization, children's protective service workers emphasize observable behavior change. Thus, children's protective workers and behavioral practitioners share a common perspective in delivering services to abusing families. The following section describes a behavioral model useful to children's protective workers and other child abuse practitioners.

A Behavioral Model Of Child Abuse Intervention

INITIAL INTERVIEW Considerable efforts have been devoted to establishing the science of social work interviewing and fundamental counseling techniques (Kadushin, 1972; Linehan, 1977). Detailed review of these efforts is beyond the scope of the present chapter; but several points warrant reiteration. Briefly explaining the agency is always useful, since clients often do not clearly understand its function. Clarifying the purpose of the interview helps dispel misconceptions. For example, clients may believe they are going to be "tested" or otherwise evaluated for mental competency or adequacy as parents. Social workers should not assume that referral sources given clients accurate or complete understandings of the purpose of referral. Brief exchange concerning mutual expectations is especially important when parents are angry, confused, threatened or reluctant to accept social work services.

Having clarified the purpose of the interview, workers should discuss allegations of abuse. At this time, parents and children can express their views on allegedly abusive incidents. Workers may then observe initial indicators of whether or not the family is abusive and if family members are willing to accept the child abuse as a problem. Careful note-taking provides a basis for documenting this initial posture. Should the family not return, these notes may serve as the only record of the family's unwillingness to participate in assessment and intervention.

Families will frequently admit a child was spanked too hard, explaining circumstances were beyond their control. For example, one mother stated: "Sure, I left a bruise mark on my son's face, but that was only because he moved his head." This opportunity allows workers to learn conditions leading to the incident. Whether or not the abuse is recurring, situations promoting abuse are likely to have occurred many times. In this instance, the mother responded: "I do lose my patience with that kid, but you wouldn't believe the number of times I told him to stay out of my things! The minute I get on the phone, he runs right to my desk." Clients are then encouraged to expand on the other stressful situations. Whenever possible, workers express understanding for the difficulties of being a parent, but do not condone abusive behavior. Emphasis is on the client's expressed thoughts and feelings; requisite skills are empathizing, listening, and paraphrasing (Danish and Hauer, 1973; Ivey and Authier, 1978).

Shortly after the midpoint of the interview, usually lasting about ninety minutes, the worker begins to negotiate a written contract (Seabury, 1976). Certain contractual elements such as length of treatment, are often pre-determined by the referral source and will be non-negotiable. These elements should be included in the contract along with negotiable particulars. The contractual process begins with a brief review of what has transpired during the course of the interview. The signing of written agreements, marking the end of the initial contracting process, often coincides with the termination of the first interview.

Case Example: In the following example, the worker is nearing the end of the initial interview with the Miller family. Parents are in their mid-thirties; children are aged eight, ten, and thirteen.

> Worker: We only have a few minutes left, and before we discuss the contract I mentioned earlier, I thought I would go over the major points discussed tonight. You were referred here by Mr. Johnson of the Children's Protective Service, who alleges that David has been spanked to the point of bruising on at least two occasions. You differed with this, saying the bruises occured only once, and emphasized that you were not in the habit of beating your children. Both Mr. and Ms. Miller and David agreed that the situation leading to the spanking, namely arguing between Mr. Miller and David, occurs many times each day. Everyone agreed that this was a serious family problem, and was one of the reasons why you thought your family life was unhappy. We also talked about other problems such as David's table manners, and Mr. Miller's lack of responsibility with children.
>
> As I recall, everyone agreed that decreasing the amount of quarreling between David and Mr. Miller would be a desirable goal. I suggest we work on this area and perhaps one or two other areas during our six meetings in the next month. As you know, this is the number of sessions required by the Children's Protective Service. I also think it will be an adequate period of time to see if your family can change some of the problems we discussed. While I'm talking, I'm writing down the points to be included in the contract: 1) the number of sessions to be held during the next four weeks; 2) arrangements for altering our scheduled appointment time; 3) fees; 4) assignments, which are

> mutually agreed upon by family members and me; 5) an understanding of the private and privileged aspects of our meetings, including my responsibility to provide Children's Protective Service or the court with an evaluation of the progress made by your family during our meetings; 6) rules for discussion during our sessions; 7) follow-up arrangements after we stop meeting.
>
> Let's go over the contract together in detail, and please understand that we can change this to suit your needs. Do speak up if you don't understand any items or don't agree with any terms.

At this point, some family members are usually receptive to the contractual process; others seem hesitant. Workers should explore the reasons behind silence; reticence may be an indicator of future non-participation in the intervention. After they have signed the contract, family members each keep a copy.

As in most behavioral intervention, contracts in child abuse counseling represent a building block for later work. Contracts reduce misunderstandings between clients and workers, and notify the family that their performance is being monitored. Thus, contracts identify explicit consequences for non-performance. Contracts also document family cooperation and progress (see Gambrill, Chapter 5). The Miller family interview demonstrates how an initial intake session leads to a contract. In short, a helping relationship, founded on basic social work skills, must be established before subsequent intervention can proceeed (Kadushin, 1972; Rogers, 1961; Truax & Mitchell, 1971).

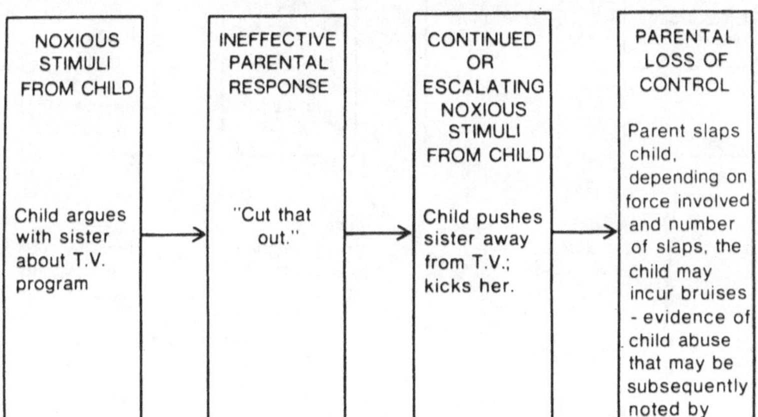

FIGURE 1

BEHAVIOR CHANGE Although a small number of abusing parents may purposefully injure their children, most experts agree child abuse typically invovles a loss of control in a given situation. For instance, social workers providing child abuse services frequently hear such statements as "I just couldn't take his screaming any longer" or "I was so angry I couldn't think." If abuse is an unplanned, unthinking loss of control in a stressful situation, teaching self-control should lessen the probability of recurring abuse. Loss of control—operationally defined as responding to noxious events with physical punishment inflicted without forethought—involves a chain of events: 1) noxious stimulus from child; 2) ineffectual parental response; 3) continued or escalating noxious stimuli from child; 4) parental anger or loss of control, all schematically depicted in Figure One.

The paradigm becomes infinitely more complex as other variables are considered. For example, if the day at school was particularly trying, the child may whine sooner or louder than usual. The child will likely be less inclined to respond to the parent's initial rebuke. Moreover, the child's whining will be tolerated less if the parent is in the midst of a marital argument (see Figure Two). Of the many possible variables contributing to loss of control, some are likely to occur with greater intensity or frequency. Workers must discover as many of these influencing variables as possible.

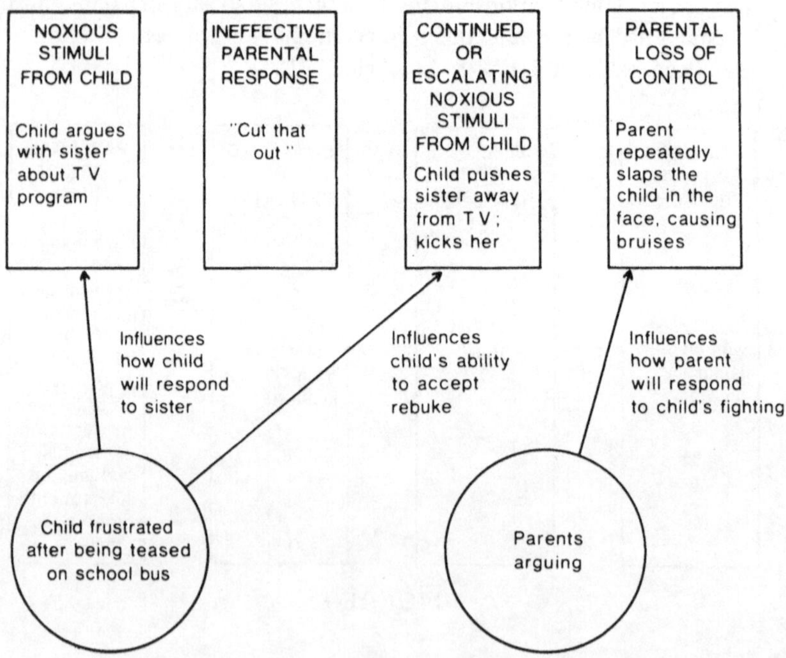

FIGURE 2

CASE EXAMPLE This process of discovery begins during the first interview and continues through a series of increasingly refined behavioral assignments. Returning to the Millers, we learned that dinner was a tension-laden activity, with verbal disagreements, threats, and name-calling frequently leading to physical punishment. Forming a tentative impression of mealtime events, the worker suggested that family members provide additional data based on the next few days: Parents and daughter Susan agreed to write a brief paragraph each night concerning mealtime events. At the second counseling session, the worker and the family began to specify individual elements of what at first appeared to be a continuous family argument.

By the end of this session, family and worker realized that mealtime arguments typically began with a discussion of David's table manners or his habitual teasing of sister. In addition, both Mr. and Mrs. Miller learned about their own feelings just prior to the meal, describing themselves as "uptight," "on edge," or "waiting for something to happen." Mr. Miller admitted he had little tolerance for David's poor table manners and acknowledged increasing frustration over frequent bickering between David and his sister.

On the worker's recommendation, David and Mr. Miller agreed not to eat together until they could arrive at a mutual understanding of dinner table decorum. They ate alone or with the family on alternating nights. Although it did not attack any of the basic problems within the family, such a move avoided verbal abuse and possible physical abuse during a time of known stress. Learning to avoid predictably volatile situations—as with the Millers—families begin identifying other situations leading to abusive consequences. All members are responsible for learning family social cues; but abusing parents, above all, must recognize cues affecting them. Thus, David and Mr. Miller learned to recognize potentially explosive circumstances and then followed the "eating-separately" regimen. When Mrs. Miller reports David again teasing his sister and whining about mother's refusal to give him a snack before dinner, Mr. Miller anticipates that these elements may produce a volatile situation; accordingly, he may choose to work on the car rather than watch television in competition with the children's bickering.

Learning to recognize available cues and using obviating strategies—initial steps in a larger scheme of behavior change—is important for several reasons. Unless abusive behavior is eliminated immediately, children cannot remain with parents. Identifying antecedent conditions also enables parents to begin lasting, more complex behavior change. Further, eliminating or decreasing abusive behavior is in itself desirable.

Gaining an understanding of the Millers at mealtime, the the worker suggested another behavioral assignment. Mother and the oldest daughter, Susan, seen as neutral figures in this instance, were instructed to unobtrusively count the times David used his napkin, talked with food in his mouth, and said "please." The worker called the family several times during the week, ensuring that Mrs. Miller and Susan understood the assignment and were collecting data. The following session, Mrs. Miller and Susan reported data showing David's table manners improving markedly David proudly announced he had discovered mother and sister watching his manners; monitoring alone was enough of an incentive for him to change his habits (see Figure Three). Nonetheless, the worker assigned another week of dinner-time monitoring to see if David could maintain newly acquired table manners.

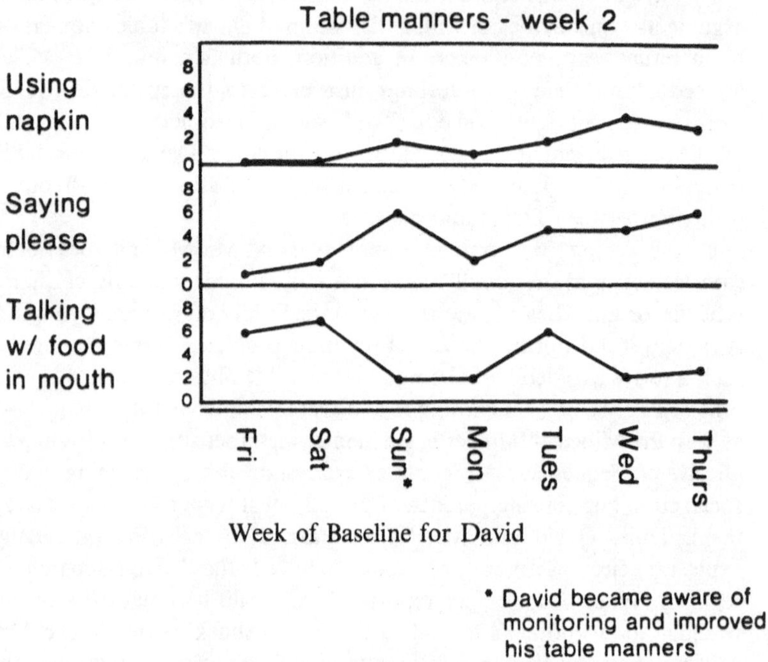

FIGURE 3

Having achieved some immediate success with David, the worker engaged Mr. Miller in a behavior-change project. Mr. Miller admitted frequent arguments with Susan concerning bedtime, agreeing that his requests were at best tactless. The worker suggested that father and daughter independently record the bedtime scenario in journal format for one week. Refusing to keep a journal, Mr. Miller agreed to tell his wife what to write. During a later session, discussion of the two journals revealed that Mr. Miller was unaware of his gruffness; Susan learned she habitually ignored her father until he raised his voice. Both agreed the issue was not the bedtime hour, but the way the matter was resolved. The worker facilitated a discussion of ways of avoiding the problem at bedtime routine. Acceptable ways of announcing bedtime were discussed, with these elements included in a father/daughter contract. This contract proved a successful way of handling another family conflict.

None of these interventions dealt directly with the maladaptive relationshiop between David and Mr. Miller. Each behavior change project, however, increased the possibility of successful intervention involving both family members. David demonstrated he could make positive changes, and his father was able to acknowledge them. Mr. Miller became aware of how insensitive he could be to his daughter's needs; this discovery may have increased his awareness of David's feelings. Observing Mr. Miller's capacity for change with Susan, the worker learned what methods might likely be effective in later intervention. Certainly, Mr. Miller held strong beliefs about child rearing; but he could change his behavior, especially if Mrs. Miller offered tactful reminders. It was also clear that Mr. Miller disliked complex monitoring schemes, preferring to let others record events.

During the fourth session, the worker suggested that David and Mr. Miller again eat together with the family. Mr. Miller practiced asking David firmly but politely not to talk with food in his mouth. Although he still found it difficult to praise his son for expected behavior, he promised to offer at least one compliment during each evening meal. Mrs. Miller and Susan consented to monitor Mr. Miller's mealtime remarks—both critical and positive—and David's manners (see Figure Four).

After reviewing the individual progress made by David and his father, the worker focused on another family problem, feeding the dog. "David, as I recall you and your dad often got into an argument when the dog wasn't fed by a certain time. Sometimes you would get a hard spanking. Do you and your dad agree that was often how things happen?" The worker allowed father and son to tell their respective interpretations of how the dog got fed in the past. He then reviewed data collected on this chore during the past week. "Let's see, it says here the dog was fed by Mom or Dad after you went to bed every night except two." David admitted he had forgotten on five nights, despite reminders from mother. Mr. Miller expressed a feeling of vindication, having previously agreed not to nag about the daily chore for the entire week. He agreed with the worker that in the past physical punishment had been ineffective in getting David to feed the dog on his own. Discussing several non-physical strategies for dealing with the problem, the worker suggested no TV or outside play after supper until the dog was fed and that David have a

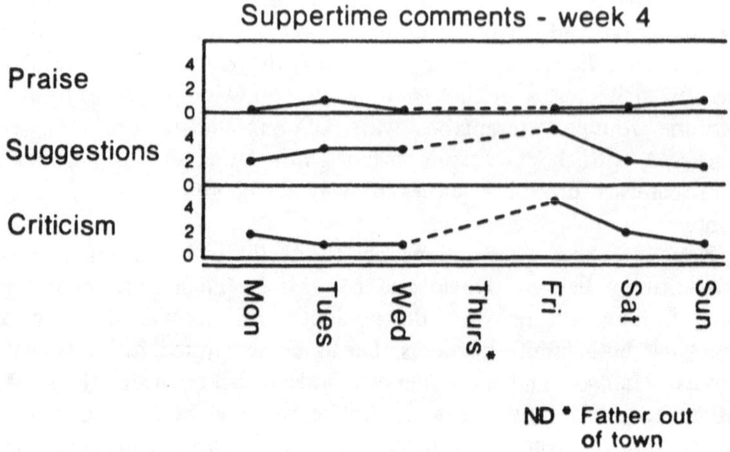

FIGURE 4

chance to gain something as an added incentive. After more discussion, all agreed David could earn a later bedtime for feeding the dog on three successive evenings. Both parents agreed not to nag or complain about having to feed the dog if David failed in his duty.

The worker began the next session by reviewing data collected on dog feeding over the previous week. "Hey David, you fed the dog five out of seven nights. That's a big improvement!" Mr. Miller added that David had earned one late bedtime and just missed earning another. Both parents said they had become aware of how often they thought of nagging David about feeding the dog. Mr. Miller had praised his son for doing his chore on two evenings, but said it seemed insincere to use praise except for a task done especially well. Acknowledging the parents' complaint that the dog food was spilled on several evenings, the worker noted this area as one requiring improvement. He suggested, however, that present expectations not be raised for another week.

In the next few weeks the Miller family and the worker negotiated a new contract of six more sessions over three months. Although the family successfully completed several more behavior change projects, progress did not continue in an uninterrupted pattern. Warnings about expectations of uninterrupted progress notwithstanding, the parents were most distressed following an unsuccessful week when everything seemed to go wrong. The worker emphasized such setbacks were only temporary obstacles, not causes for despair. If a child tires of a given program, it may be because intervention, once novel, is no longer exciting. Parents must remain open to changing contingencies if they no longer achieve desired results. The worker counseled the Millers to use their newly acquired observational skills to analyze their own behavior before discarding previously used contingencies. Moreover, the best of programs may temporarily collapse when the family responds to disruptive events such as an injury, loss of income, or friction with relatives. The family was advised to resist former maladaptive behavior patterns by recalling significant progress they had made.

In the weeks remaining in the contract period the worker encouraged the Millers to design and implement their own behavioral interventions. He praised their efforts, reinforcing attempts to again manage their family. During the final session the worker read his letter to the children's protective agency; the parents were obviously pleased and offered no criticism. The worker re-stated his belief in their ability to maintain possitive relationships, but added that he would be available if future help were needed.

Several further points, not covered in the previous case example, warrant mention. Throughout the intervention, particularly during the initial phase, social workers must be readily accessible. Telephone contact must be provided clients in crisis or needing reassurance. Moreover, working toward non-abusive relationships among family members requires a pragmatic rather than moral approach. Mr. Miller was typical of abusive parents frequently controlling children through aversive means (Tracy & Clark, 1974). Many abusing parents agree that physical punishment has not been effective in making children behave in a desired manner. Lacking viable alternative discipline methods however, parents are not often eager to give up physical punishment (Davoren, 1975; Bordin-Sandler, 1976). Thus, non-physical alternatives must be presented as practically useful, without moralistic overtones (Bordin-Sandler, 1976).

The Miller case presents a relatively uncomplicated course of intervention. With other families intervention is not so smooth; the data not as compelling; the decisions not so straightforward (Nagi, 1977). Families sometimes make immediate progress, then reach a plateau. In other instances families only partially engage in the helping process, missing appointments or failing to complete assignments. How and when do workers decide that families have little chance of making necessary changes? At what point does the agency cease contact? Such questions demand rational decisions based on clinical data.

Data-Based Intervention

Data collection is an integral part of behavioral intervention. Beginning at intake, the worker gathers data on observable events or on evidence of previous events (Linehan, 1977; Mastria, Mastria, & Harkins, 1979).

Subjective elements included in assessment are so labeled. Workers ask behaviorally specific questions of interested parties—physicians and the referral sources—separating subjective from objective information. Data-based recording methods are also used in client interviews; whether clients were late, where family members sat, which members participated, all are relevant for planning. Careful attention is given to the parents' explanations of alleged abuse, which are recorded immediately after the interview. Thorough assessment includes history of early childhood development to identify possible deficiencies in development and to assess parental understanding of normal development. Children are viewed carefully for abrasions or bruises during close contact before and after the interview, ideally by another staff member in a play environment. Since examining areas under clothing can be frightening to children and offensive to parents, closer examinations are best left to hospital or children's protective personnel not working with the family on a regular basis. Less certain but more easily observed indicators of continuing abuse are children's responses: abused children may move their heads or bodies quickly when an abusing parent moves close to them. In families where children are too afraid or too young to speak out during the interview, such non-verbal signs provide important clues.

After intake and initial assessment, social workers continue to gather quantifiable and observable data from other sources. Children's Protective Services, physicians, and other referral agencies provide adjunctive information. Teachers are in good positions to observe children's progress and signs of continuing abuse. Other agency personnel—including clerical staff—observing the family can provide additional information about family interaction. Again, workers stress observable data without excluding subjective sources.

Data provided by clients during assessment and intervention are important indicators of progress. Expected to record family behavior patterns, clients agree to supply information by signing behavioral assignments. When failing to record events families are not complying with intervention. Certainly a point for discussion, such failure is evidence of lack of client progress. But completed assignments, including recorded data, demonstrate commitment to change even when intervention is not successful. Interestingly, few clients fabricate or distort the recording of behavioral assignments. Families not completing assignments usually cancel appointments or offer excuses. One speculation is that faking data requires as much effort as recording actual events.

Behavioral Recording Aids: Case Record Accountability

Behavioral practitioners in social work and other disciplines have an enviable record in the area of data-based recording: the literature has many charts, graphs, and logs suited to many applications. Such aids are especially germane to direct practice involving child abuse since the severity of the problem and implicit legal ramifications require scrupulous accountability.

For example the Problem Oriented Recording System (PORS) effectively sorts objective and subjective elements in referral reports and interviews (Weed, 1971). Although complete discussion is beyond the present chapter's scope, PORS should be given serious consideration as part of a behavioral recording system. Some agencies use a dual system, combining elements of data-based recording with a problem oriented format (Raveneberg, 1978; Wood, Callahan, Alevizos, and Teigen, 1977). Precise data-based recording is not entirely compatible with problem oriented records. As Franks and Wilson (1976: p. 286) note: "The level of precision achieved in describing problem behaviors in PORS does not approach that of the carefully conducted behavioral analysis." PORS is nevertheless far superior to conventional narrative recording.

One mechanical aid found valuable is the self-carbon memo. Using this, workers can write contracts or behavioral assignments during the interview. Parents, children, and worker sign the document, each keep a copy. This method obviates needless record keeping and serves to record the intervention contract and behavioral assignments. The worker's copy becomes the focal point of the family session; it serves as a reference when clients call seeking assurance or further clarification of agreed upon tasks.

Commerical behavior-recording aids are available (Cautela, 1977; Stuart & Stuart, 1975) but workers may prefer to design their own devices. A variety of universal forms may prove invaluable as applications of such instruments are virtually unlimited. Ideally, a photocopy machine should be readily available, as families often prefer to keep completed data sheets after discussing them with the worker. Whether original or photocopied, data sheets augment other case record material such as PORS recording, contracts, assessment inventories, psychological tests, physician reports and previous social histories.

Legal and procedural issues are becoming increasingly important in child abuse. Reviewing the changing status of parental rights, Derdeyn (1977) states that both federal and state statutes give parents an implicit right to service. In proceedings to terminate parental rights, courts are requiring child welfare agencies to show proof of efforts to rehabilitate families. Thus, agencies must prove parents guilty of certain acts against their children, and demonstrate their efforts to work with the family. Behavioral practitioners rapidly accumulate data points on which to base decisions, reports, recommendations, and court testimony. These data strengthen the worker's case, whether for deprivation hearings or for letters recommending action by children's protective services.

Data-based recording facilitates decision-making and leads to action should children need to be removed from their homes. At Children's Home Society, data-based recording has also helped formerly abusive parents regain legal custody of children. For example, a children's protective worker once opposed returning legal custody of a child even though the child had been returned home several months previously. Discussion with the children's protective worker revealed that this judgment was based more on subjective beliefs about the child's mother than on demonstrable facts. After receiving a report containing subjective clinical impressions and a list of successfully completed behavioral assignments, the caseworker quickly returned legal custody to the family. An additional benefit of this outcome was to strengthen the worker's relationship with the family.

No area within the profession requires accurate record keeping more than the sensitive and often volatile area involving cases of child abuse. Client access to records, combined with growing concern over malpractice suits, underscores the necessity of documenting agency efforts and client progress in child abuse cases (Green & Cox, 1978).

Cautionary Note on Using Behavioral Methods With Abusive Families

Any treatment modality contains features inappropriate for certain clients—behavioral methods are no exception. Consider the time out procedure that involves removing children from present surroundings and placing them in a non-stimulating environment, usually for about five minutes. Although time out is an extremely effective alternative to more aversive punishment and has few known side effects, the procedure does not enhance the possibility of learning new competing behaviors (Plummer, Baer, & LeBlanc, 1977). Further, an easily applied method of temporarily removing a noxious stimulus, time out is subject to over use. Parents routinely using aversive methods of control may readily employ—and overuse—time out. For example, one father demonstrated his mastery of the technique during the interview. He was swift, matter-of-fact, and otherwise appropriate in using time out, but his child was guilty of only giggling. Obviously, continued use of time out with such behavior will have adverse effects.

Another example of misunderstanding behavioral methods is that of the abusing parent who gave glowing approval to Patterson's *Living With Children* (1976). "That book proves what I've been saying all along: children are like animals—when they do what you want, you're nice to them; when they mess you up you ignore them. Take my daughter, now when she's good I let her sit on my lap, but when she disobeys I won't talk to her for a couple of days. Pretty soon she gets the idea." This parent asserted that behavior modification was "dog training" and supported such beliefs about child rearing. Clearly, this parent misinterpreted social learning theory; in fact, he further justified harmful child rearing beliefs by incorrectly translating behavioral techniques.

A parent disinclined to give up physical punishment may fault any alternative intervention suggested. An added liability with behavioral methods is necessary data collection, which may in turn help parents prove the inadequacy of non-physical alternatives. The author recalls a mother who dutifully collected data during the intervention phase of a behavior-change project. Intervention was a miserable failure, and the mother triumphantly exclaimed that the data proved spanking was the only way to rear children. Perhaps intervention was ill conceived; perhaps the mother sabotaged the plan. In any case, the mother refuted alternate non-physical methods of discipline.

Behavioral methods are powerful tools. As these case vignettes illustrate, these tools must be applied with understanding of family circumstances and childrens' developmental needs. The ethics of teaching behavioral techniques with clients who may misuse them is an area to be explored. Until more is known about the consequences of work with abusive families, social workers must proceed with caution. Nevertheless, behavioral methods offer the most efficacious means of evaluating intended or unintended results.

Evaluating Child Abuse Intervention

Children's Home Society records show behavioral intervention effective in ameliorating child abuse. Although some abusive families could not be engaged or did not show significant change, they represented only twenty-eight percent of families served during the four years for which Children's Home Society has outcome data. Intervention was most effective in helping parents recognize potentially dangerous situations and learn to avoid them. Rarely did families again resort to abusive punishment; many gave up corporal punishment altogether.

Although these results are encouraging, the absence of control groups precludes unrestrained endorsement of behavioral methods described here (see Gorsuch, Chapter 17). Individually tailored outcome measures used in this clinical setting were designed to judge single case interventions, rather than program effectiveness. Kazdin (1978b) states, "The ultimate test of generality of findings among subjects or any other condition is replication." Although the behavioral interventions were administered to many successive families, the kind of service varied to the extent that specifying an intervention strategy common to all cases becomes impossible.

Finally, as with most programs (Zukerman, Ambuel, & Bandman, 1972) the present model suffers from a lack of follow-up data. Agency responsibility ended when the final progress reports on the abusing family was sent to Children's Protective Services. Thus, behavioral methods described here appear effective in modifying abuse, but long term effectiveness remains unknown.

CONSUMER SATISFACTION In child abuse intervention there are several distinct groups of consumers: parents, children, children's protection agencies, and in some instances, the courts. Parents, typically resisting counseling, are at first skeptical about being helped. Once social workers demonstrated they were not concerned with establishing guilt, parents frequently expressed willingness to engage in counseling. The tasks of agency staff were easier most likely because they did not initially investigate abuse allegations. Like Davoren and her colleagues they "were...in...the fortunate position of being rescuers, at least during early contacts with out-patients. We could side with them against the world and understand them rather than be part of that misunderstanding world" (Davoren, 1974:144). Many parents said they were relieved to find social workers acting as advocates after painful experiences with investigating authorities.

Although agency staff did not initially investigate alleged abuse, they were bound to report evidence of continued abuse. Staff were open with clients about roles as informants and helping agents. This honesty appears both ethical and effective in alleviating client mistrust of the practitioner. Case records indicate most families came to perceive workers as advocates. By worker reports, however, fully one fourth of abusive parents continued to mistrust and resent them as authorities or intruders. Anecdotes from case records suggest failure to deal with client mistrust risks irreparable damage to the helping relationship. As Truax and Mitchell (1971) state, effective clinicians must demonstrate non-possessive warmth, including trust. The critical element of trust, often compromised when workers take on conflicting roles of helper and informant, merits further research.

How did children view the helping process? Some were relieved to be "rescued" by the social worker; older children especially used the protection of the family interview to voice feelings about mistreatment. In counseling sessions, for example, one boy sat so the worker was between him and his stepfather. Some children said they resented counseling; others conveyed dislike by conveniently disappearing when parents were about to leave for a scheduled interview. Thus, based on limited anecdotal evidence, children's perceptions of intervention are largely unknown.

Children's protective workers have expressed satisfaction with the service provided by Children's Home Society, however, since referral alternatives are few, lack of criticism does not necessarily indicate complete satisfaction with child abuse intervention. Involvement with the courts has been limited; for that reason it is difficult to determine how satisfied attorneys and judges have been with the intervention. Assumptions that behavioral methodology increases the likelihood of a just court decision remain untested.

Client satisfaction, receiving increased attention in all areas of social work, is particularly crucial in child abuse intervention. If abusive families are disaffected by their experiences with social workers, they will probably not turn to human service professionals if future difficulties arise. Unfortunately, consumer satisfaction data is limited to anecdotal reports, case records, and returning clients. Systematic assessment of consumer satisfaction would be a logical addition to this practice model.

Barriers to Instituting Behavioral Methods in Child Abuse Intervention

The child welfare system appears neither more nor less eager to embrace social learning theory than are other social work systems. Professionals associated with Children's Home Society made few objections to using behavioral methods with abusive families. Possibly, such families are less desirable than are more motivated clients who presumably better use insight therapies. More important is the fact that child abuse is usually manifested in discrete, observable behaviors that must be curtailed rapidly. Behavioral specificity has always been a part of child abuse intervention. Behavioral methods have thus been more readily accepted by child protective workers. Discussing social learning rather than behavior modification may not have changed many opinions about behavioral methods; but such discussion enabled staff to overcome initial mistrust often encountered by behavioral practitioners (Reppucci & Saunders, 1974). Nevertheless, child welfare's strong analytical traditional is a potential obstacle to instituting behavioral methods.

The child protection bureaucracy's lack of aggressiveness in pursuing legal sanctions is another area undermining behavioral methods in child abuse intervention. Workers at Children's Home Society observed that protective service caseworkers would swiftly remove abused children if significant evidence of maltreatment existed. Too often, the shock effect of this move was the only corrective measure. The child was then returned to the family with the understanding that counseling would continue. After the family failed to follow through with a mandated course of action caseworkers frequently refused to turn to the courts because the case "was not strong enough." Evidence of casework progress was rarely used by those deciding to take further legal action. Behavioral workers will be less inclined to record intervention efforts if such documentation is ignored by child protection authorities.

Lack of judicial follow-through is not unique to child abuse cases. Most workers are aware that the courts are overburdened. Equally clear to families, however, was that child protection authorities did not carry through on contingencies to take further action. Although Children's Home Society workers emphasized the importance of consequences, this emphasis was negated by the state's inability to exercise them. To a large extent, this situation is an unavoidable byproduct of a legal system stressing parental rights—sometimes at the expense of children's welfare (Goldstein, Freud, & Solnit, 1973; Fay, 1975).

Guidelines for Practice

The model described evolved from earlier experiences with non-abusing dysfunctional families. Recognizing that abuse may often be a response to the same faulty interactions experienced by many troubled families, the author found a basic behavioral approach effective with abusing parents. After four years, no compelling evidence indicates abusive families require an entirely different intervention mode. Experience with abusing families. however, suggests guidelines for successful intervention.

To avoid misunderstandings about the intervention process, all participants in the child abuse model are informed about what is to follow. Children's protective agency workers must know that criteria for "success" do not include acceptance of abuse allegations. Families should know what is involved in a counseling model based on learning rather than intrapsychic factors. They are told that they are to try new behavior patterns, and that they are to observe and record family behaviors. Parents learn that periodic progress reports are provided the children's protective agency; they are aware that they can read these reports. Common sense and empirical research support the efficacy of clients understanding the intervention process in advance (Heitler, 1975).

Communication and cooperation between intervention workers and children's protective workers is always desirable (Nagi, 1977). For example, the worker providing intervention counseling must clearly understand the nature of the alleged abuse, the concerns shared with the family, and the family's initial response. If this information is not conveyed accurately, the ongoing worker may unknowingly cause the family to feel anger, betrayal, or confusion. Similarly, faulty communication later on in the intervention may result in the two workers aiming for different objectives, again unfairly compromising the family. Finally, neither worker should be surprised by the other's response upon termination, albeit there may not be agreement about the final conditions surrounding this phase of service delivery.

Workers involved in child abuse intervention must recognize that child protection often involves two adversaries: child protection authorities and abusing parents. Other participants in this system, lawyers and agency workers, are also engaged in a struggle to decide issues affecting clients. Behind substantiated allegations of abuse looms the threat of legal sanctions such as removal of the child, permanent or temporary loss of custody, or criminal proceedings. When workers understand the legal system they can influence that system: they need to be informed and active participants in the child protection legal bureaucracy. By alerting all involved in the intervention procedures—sending copies of behavioral contracts to defense attorneys, children's protective workers and prosecutors, for example—social workers become expert at documenting attempts to engage the client and improve family relationships. But, they should not lose sign of the fact that legal sanctions usually remain unexercised threats.

NEEDED RESEARCH

At least two areas of child abuse demand further research. The first is defining and explaining child abuse and its causes (Giovannoni & Becerra, 1979). Albeit social workers are not currently able to accurately describe factors causally associated with child abuse (Jayaratne, 1977; Welner, Welner & Robbins, 1977), a few promising instruments are being tested. Schneider, Hoffmeister, and Helfer (1976) have suggested that their recently developed instrument, the Michigan Screening Profile of Parenting (MSPP), might be used to detect potentially abusive parents. The MSPP consists of fifty statements with Lickert scale responses ranging from strongly agree to disagree: e.g. "At least one of my children reminds me of someone I don't like." The MSPP is a significant attempt to correlate previous experiences with current parent-child interactions. Emphasizing the developmental nature of their work, the investigators proscribe the use of the MSPP as a clinical predictor; however, they encourage other professionals to inquire about using the MSPP in other settings.

A formidable effort has been undertaken by Disbrow, Doerr, and Caulfield (1977) who developed a battery of tests to identify potentially abusing parents. Using systematic interviews, questionnaires, videotaped observations, and physiological measurements, the investigators originally collected data on hundreds of variables. By discarding many unclear variables, and by employing factor and discriminant analyses, these variables were reduced to seventeen indicators. Correlating these indicators with measures of abuse, the researchers correctly identified eighty-four percent of previously neglecting or abusing parents. Like Helfer and his colleagues, Disbrow, Doerr, and Caulfield are now in the validation phase of their research. Although they request others not to use their measures without permission, Disbrow and her colleagues suggest that parts of their battery might be administered during the early postpartum period, and that other scales be used as the child develops.

Previously mentioned investigation by Burgess and Conger (1977) has important implications for establishing behavioral predictors of child abuse. Findings indicate abusing families tend not to interact on a physical level—information that may be useful for persons making judgements about probable abuse.

Conger, Burgess, and Barrett (1979) measured recent life changes and perceptions of physical and emotional well-being. Initial findings based on a small sample indicate abusing parents may experience more life change and less physical and emotional well-being. Paulson, Schwemer, Afifi, and Bendel (1977) found three of twenty-three scales on the Parent Attitude Research Instrument were statistically significant. Further analysis using multivariate tests demonstrated that the screening instrument correctly classified abusing mothers and controls only sixty-five percent of the time. The authors caution against simplistic acceptance of "significant" results often reported for individual test variables, when in fact the overall significance level for all tests may be quite different. This is of no small importance, given the many researchers attempting to identify correlates of child abuse.

Far from being able to describe salient factors associated with child abuse, social workers are farther still from measuring intervention outcome. A survey of some 103 variables measured on hundreds of instruments found only a few measures acceptable for use in summative evaluation of demonstration projects (Seaberg, Gillespie, Long, & Conte, 1975). Although a lack of outcome criteria is not unique to child abuse intervention, the consequences of relying on ineffective programs are potentially much greater in this area of social work practice. Consider, for example, the ill-defined criteria for even the most basic decisions in child protection (Nagi, 1977). Under what circumstances are children removed from their homes? When are they subsequently returned home? When has a family successfully completed their counseling contract? When is a limited risk of reinjury outweighed by other constraints such as backlog of other cases? Recent discussion (personal communication) with child protective supervisors and workers revealed these and other related issues are decided more by intuition than by any systematically collected data. Clearly, in child abuse intervention much remains to be done in the areas of research, program evaluation, and data based practice.

Empirically based approaches to child abuse intervention must be accompanied by contributions to the child protection literature. Practitioners able to generate research and theory about child abuse can no longer leave this responsibility to academicians. As Cain and Klerman (1979:23) note, social workers "...should view the development of meaningful theories from systematic observations and the basing of practice and programs on sophisticated research and theory as part of their obligation to clients." Efforts to develop valid instruments, sound theories, and effective practice should continue. I hope practicing social workers vigorously involve themselves in this quest.

SUMMARY

Public and professional interest in child abuse has resulted in a number of causal theories and interventions. Behavioral approaches are employed primarily because they emphasize observable behavior change—the salient objective of any child abuse intervention. Data-based practice, closely tied to behavioral methods, facilitates decision-making and ensures that abusing families clearly perceive the changes expected of them. Equally important, data-based practice helps workers be more accountable to supervisors, collateral agencies, and the courts. A generic behavioral model appeared effective in one agency. Nevertheless, lack of group control or follow-up made positive claims tentative.

A number of examples and techniques are discussed in this chapter. Still, these are offered as only one set of useful strategies aimed at remedying child abuse. The particular behavioral methods described here are secondary to the issues of empiricism and accountability, crucial in the protection of children. Social workers who structure their practice with these integrally linked goals in mind will provide quality service to both parents and children.

II

Behavioral Methods With Adults

BEHAVIORAL METHODS WITH ADULTS

Certainly, all behavioral procedures noted in the foregoing section are applicable to social work with adults. Tangible and social reinforcement, observable outcome goals, and contingency contracts are germane for any client group and presenting problem. Nonetheless, the attributes and struggles of adulthood demand special consideration. Their developed cognitive ability lets adults assume major responsibility for their own treatment. Likewise, this ability limits intervention. Adults can easily not comply with the behavioral regimen, elect to drop out of treatment, or intentionally or inadvertently undercut efforts intended for their own betterment. Adults significantly influence their personal environments and so can uniquely tailor intervention. Just as readily, however, they can perpetuate and maintain damaging patterns and lifestyles. An asset in all behavioral work with adults is that their years give them skills to cope with surviving childhood handicaps or maladjustments, howsoever these may unduly restrict them. Regardless of intellectual and physical wherewithal, adults shoulder the burden for their economic security.

The six chapters comprising this section take up such issues in the orchestration of behavioral social work for adults. The sophisticated potential and the accompanying problems of thought processes in adulthood are highlighted in the treatment of excessive self-criticism. Cognitions and behavior are associated with assertiveness and with heterosexual functioning. Adult problems that surround substance addiction raise the challenge of social work with clients who derive powerful rewards from bad habits. Habilitation with mentally handicapped persons exhibits the economic payoffs of behavioral training for those excluded from competitive employment. Redressing the inequities that fall to older persons in institutional care manifests how social workers can improve the lot of a growing, disenfranchised minority.

Across these clients and troubles are commonalities that gird behavioral social work with adults. For example, each chapter emphasizes rehearsal of new behavior. Sharon Berlin uses rehearsal to help woman learn to be less self-deprecatory. In small groups, clients imagine problem situations and come up with statements to combat negative thoughts. After voicing self-statements, clients silently think to themselves of new adaptive response. Women in Cheryl Richey's assertiveness groups gain desired skills through rehearsal while other clients act as coaches and antagonists. Wayne Duehn and Nazneen Mayadas preface rehearsal sessions by showing women and men ways to relieve sexual dysfunctioning by talking to themselves, visualizing sexual activities, saying positive thoughts aloud or in whispers, and covertly rehearsing self-statements.

Betty Blythe pits rehearsal against ingrained cigarette smoking. She further relates the technique to social work intervention responsive to alcohol abuse and to overeating. Developmentally disabled clients prospered when Rick Grinnell and Alice Lieberman facilitated their rehearsal of nonverbal and verbal behavior. Later, clients are able to employ these responses during interactions with job interviewers. Ray Berger outlines a stepwise approach to give nursing home residents greater control of a regimented environment. Admirable in Berger's program is the preassessment of clients' social competence. Together these six chapters portray a remarkable concinnity of social-learning methods. The authors and their data paint an exciting future for behavioral social work with adults.

8

Women and Self-Criticism

Sharon B. Berlin

Self-criticism is the process of negatively evaluating ones' attributes, motives, and actions. Psychological constructs of self-criticism and low self-esteem refer to similar phenomena: self-criticism is a discrete act of negative self-evaluation; low self-esteem describes a global, pervasive sense of worthlessness. Habitually evaluating self-performance as inadequate and negatively appraising personal and physical characteristics lowers overall self-opinion, ultimately resulting in low self-esteem. Determining whether chronic self-criticism leads to low self-esteem, or whether the pervasive sense of worthlessness is impetus for self-criticism is academic; of more clinical relevance is recognizing that these phenomena occur concomitantly, each influencing the other.

Depression refers to episodic low-mood experiences, a syndrome or cluster of symptoms, or to a disease entity with specificable cause, course of illness, prognosis, and treatment (Becker, 1977; Weissman & Paykel, 1974; Mendels, 1970). Depression as low-mood or more serious affective disorder involving several symptoms may be implicated in the self-criticism, low self-esteem cycle. Certainly, people can talk or think themselves into gloomy low moods or into states of anxious arousal (Beck, 1976). Negative self-attribution also appeares to be a major component—if not a precipitating condition—of the depression syndrome (Beck, 1974; Lewinsohn, 1975; Seligman, 1975). Transiently common to most people and sometimes helpful, self-criticism warrants clinical attention when it usurps the ability to feel adequate, experience pleasure, and take corrective action.

Self-criticism is particularly prevalent among women. Data from state and county mental hospitals, community mental health centers, and needs assessment surveys show rates of treated and untreated depression disproportionately higher among women than men across all age groups (Goldman & Ravid, in press). Epidemiological studies from the United States, England, and Scandinavia show more women than men reporting symptoms related to depression. Estimates are that twenty to thirty percent of all females experience moderately severe depression episodes at some point in adulthood (Goldman & Ravid, in press).

Explanations offered to account for sex differences in rates of depression include hormonal imbalance, genetic predisposition, women's greater readiness to acknowledge subjective distress, and the powerlessness of traditional female roles (Klerman & Weissman, in press; Spitzform, 1978). Assimilation of social attitudes has also been widely implicated: compared to men, women learn to expect less success, express less confidence in their abilities, and take more personal responsibility for frustration and failure (Maccoby & Jacklin, 1974; Bogo, Winget, & Gleser, 1970; Jacklin & Mischel, 1973). Although knowledge of the etiology remains tentative, most agree that the causes of depression are complex and hetereogenous (Akiskal & McKinney, 1973; Becker, 1977).

Because depression is a serious and growing mental health problem, the last decade has witnessed increased efforts to develop appropriate intervention strategies. In addition to pharmacological approaches (Bielski & Friedel, 1976), relatively new psychological strategies based primarily on behavioral and cognitive-behavioral conceptualizations show promise in remediating depression symptoms (Fuchs & Rehm 1977; Rush, Beck, Kovacs, & Hollon, 1977; Shaw, 1977). Little attention, however, has been given to developing and empirically testing intervention methods for related and equally insidious problems of chronic self-criticism.

Describing one approach to this problem, the present chapter outlines the development and evaluation of a cognitive-behavioral intervention package for women who self-criticize excessively. Intervention focused on helping female clients learn to be more aware of self-criticism, to evaluate its validity, to modify inappropriate self-criticism, and to achieve individual performance goals. Behavioral techniques allow clients to modify unrealistic performance standards, inaccurate interpretations of events, and selective attention to negative outcomes. Also included in this chapter is a discussion of the theoretical and empirical literature forming intervention rationale, a description of study process and findings, and implications for practice.

Supporting Literature

Intervention was based on a cognitive-behavioral perspective, viewing emotional experiences and overt action shaped by personal and environmental events. Contrasted with traditional learning-theory precepts that behavior is controlled solely by environmental consequences, cognitive-behavioral theorists suggest environmental occurrences are simply information sources, differentially attended to, interpreted, evaluated, retained in memory, and used to guide behavior. Environmental events are mediated by cognitive processes (Bandura, 1977a; Mahoney, 1974; Meichenbaum, 1977). Because such processes are learned, they are modifiable through behavioral procedures of modeling, rehearsal, reinforcement, and environmental practice (Goldfried & Davison, 1976; Kazdin, 1974a, 1974b).

Conceptualizing human functioning in terms of cognitive processes has stimulated the development of many new intervention strategies. Data supporting cognitive-behavioral theory has been primarily derived from clinical and analogue trials. Albert Ellis (1962), among the first to devise clinical procedures to modify cognitions, focused on "irrational ideas." Ellis's emphasis on the irrationality of subjective distress and unconditional self-acceptance has been faulted by some (Bandura, Adams, & Beyer, 1977; Mahoney, 1974) and outcome studies of his Rational Emotive Therapy (RET) have produced unclear results (Mahoney, 1977). Nonetheless, many RET components have been profitably incorporated into more recent and effective approaches (e.g., Beck, 1976; Meichenbaum, 1977).

Contributing substantially to cognitive-behavioral intervention procedures, Meichenbaum (1977) has trained clients to "talk to themselves" in a self-guiding fashion. Meichenbaum's self-instructional approach is based largely on research (Klein, 1963; Mischel, 1975; Patterson & Mischel, 1976) investigating children's self-verbalization as facilitating task mastery. Reasoning that overt and covert self-speech helps people learn new tasks and cope with difficult problems, Meichenbaum's clinical paradigm includes three steps: 1) problems are defined to make them amenable to intervention and to increase client sense of control and expectations for positive results; 2) clients observe their own maladaptive thoughts and behaviors to increase occurrence sensitivity; 3) new awareness of self-criticism becomes the cue for incompatible thoughts and adaptive behavior.

Concerned with anxiety reduction, research by Goldfried and associates (Kanter & Goldfried, 1976, Goldfried, Linehan, & Smith, 1976) has yielded support for cognitive-behavioral intervention. Goldfried explains anxiety as a function of thoughts and self-appraisals made prior to and during anxiety eliciting situations. Evidence shows beliefs about negative behavioral consequences—especially others' negative reactions—correlate highly with social anxiety (Goldfried & Sobocinski, 1975). Rational restructuring interferes with such maladaptive beliefs by: 1) presenting the rationale that feelings are affected by how people appraise situations and by their coping abilities; 2) assessing client assumptions and self-statements about anxiety arousing situations; 3) analyzing self-statements to decide if they are realistic projections of probably outcome; 4) teaching clients to modify irrational statements using anxiety reactions as cues for the more accurate assessment of situations and coping skills; and 5) helping clients practice this sequence through imaginal rehearsal.

This intervention paradigm has been found effective in reducing interpersonal anxiety (Kanter & Goldfried, 1976) and test anxiety (Goldfried, Linehan, & Smith, 1976). Also applying the model to assertiveness training, Goldfried (1976) suggested unassertive behavior is often maintained by concern with reactions of others, rather than by skill deficits. Supporting this analysis, Schwartz and Gottman (1974) showed cognitive restructuring superior to behavioral rehearsal in increasing assertiveness. Similarly, Glass and his associates report rational self-statements effective in improving heterosexual interactions among college students (Glass, Gottman, & Shmurak, 1976).

The efficacy of cognitive-behavioral techniques has also been established in the treatment of depression. Rush, Beck, Kovacs, and Hollon (1977) report that clinically depressed clients receiving cognitive-behavioral intervention showed greater improvement than did clients receiving tricyclic pharmacotherapy. Based on Beck's concept of depression as resulting from negative cognitions (1974), intervention consisted of teaching clients to recognize connections among cognition, affect, and behavior; monitor negative thoughts; examine evidence for and against distorted cognitions; and substitute reality-based interpretations for distorted negative cognitions. Since most previous comparative studies found pharmacotherapy more effective in reducing depression symptoms (e.g. Covi, Lipman, Derogatis, Smith, & Pattison, 1974; Friedman, 1975; Klerman, DiMascio, Weissman, Prusoff, & Paykel, 1974), the Rush, Beck, Kovacs, and Hollon (1977) effort represents a landmark study.

Comparing Beck's cognitive approach to behavioral skills training, nondirective counseling, and no intervention for reducing depression symptoms among college students, Shaw (1977) reported cognitive therapy superior to all other conditions. Differences between the cognitive and behavioral training dissipated, however, at the time of a one-month follow-up. When Taylor and Marshall (1977) compared cognitive therapy, behavioral skills training, a combination of both, and no intervention with depressed college students, results indicated cognitive and behavioral training equally effective, with combined intervention most effective. Finally, Fuchs and Rehm (1977) used cognitive-behavioral procedures to decrease depression among moderately depressed women.

In summary, theoretical and research literature leads us to three conclusions:

1. Cognitive information appraisal influences behavior.
2. Self-critical behavior results from information deficiencies and distortions.
3. Cognitive and behavior change occurs by manipulating information sources and by modifying information appraisal.

Drawing on these conclusions, intervention for the current study was designed to change women clients' negative self-attribution by altering unrealistic expectations, reducing distorted appraisals, and facilitating successful performances. Resulting clinical strategies were to increase client awareness of self-criticism, evaluate self-criticism validity, substitute incompatible self-statements for self-criticism, and instigate performance changes in the natural environment.

METHOD

Setting and Clients

The study was carried out at a private, nonprofit social work agency; the clients, fifty adult women responding to written advertisements. Women making telephone inquiries were given additional information and ruled out in screening if they were younger than twenty, involved in another form of therapy, taking psychotropic medication, or indicated that self-criticism was not a major psychological or life problem. Such applicants were then offered information about more appropriate resources. Of seventy-nine women involved in pre-intervention assessment, fifty-four agreed to participate in the project; fifty-two completed intervention; fifty completed the entire study. Table One presents descriptive information on the final sample of fifty women.

Procedure

Intervention took place in groups of eight to ten, meeting weekly for six sessions, led by female co-leader teams—three graduate social workers and one M.A. psychologist—all with previous experience in individual and group counseling. To ensure consistent intervention, leaders received eight hours pretraining and were provided with detailed procedural manuals.

Table 1

Client Characteristics (N=50)

Mean Years of Age	34.8	**Marital Status**	
Race		Never Married	15
White	49	Married	25
Non-White	1	Divorce/Separated	9
Mean Years of Education	15.6	Widowed	1
Occupation		**Level of Depression†**	
Student	12	Major	4
Homemaker	6	Minor	17
Professional/Academic	9	Minor with Anxiety	27
Clerical	10	None	2
Business/Accounting	7		
Unemployed	1		
Other	5		

† According to Research Diagnostic Criteria for Affective Disorders (Spitzer & Endicott 1975).

Research Design

The intervention's impact was evaluated through a pretest-posttest control group design. Screening and assessment procedures completed, clients were matched on pretest responses and randomly assigned to one of three experimental conditions: cognitive-behavioral, attention-placebo, or wait-list. The attention-placebo condition controlled for expectation effects, the contact with group leaders and members, and self-monitoring; the waiting-list condition isolated effects of life events, experience of volunteering for a research project, and screening and assessment procedures. At pretest, posttest, and 6-week follow-up, clients participated in assessment of self-criticism, depression, self-esteem, and anxiety. After follow-up assessment, wait-list clients received intervention. Also debriefed at this time, attention-placebo condition clients were given opportunity to participate in cognitive-behavioral training.

Cognitive-behavioral training

These groups encompassed training components of underlying rationale and problem conceptualization, increased awareness of negative personal attributions, evaluation of self-criticism, substitution of incompatible covert statements, and overt performance. Each of these are next described.

Self-Monitoring Checklist

NAME__________________

DATE __________________

	A.M.		P.M.										
	10	11	12	1	2	3	4	5	6	7	8	9	10
1. Overeating	☐	☐	☐	☐	☐	☐	☐	☐	☐	☐	☐	☐	☐
2. Physical Appearance	☐	☐	☐	☐	☐	☐	☐	☐	☐	☐	☐	☐	☐
3. Negative Comparisons	☐	☐	☐	☐	☐	☐	☐	☐	☐	☐	☐	☐	☐
4. Undisciplined / Disorganized	☐	☐	☐	☐	☐	☐	☐	☐	☐	☐	☐	☐	☐
5. Lazy / Nonproductive	☐	☐	☐	☐	☐	☐	☐	☐	☐	☐	☐	☐	☐
6. Immature / Infantile	☐	☐	☐	☐	☐	☐	☐	☐	☐	☐	☐	☐	☐
7. Unintelligent	☐	☐	☐	☐	☐	☐	☐	☐	☐	☐	☐	☐	☐
8. Indecisive	☐	☐	☐	☐	☐	☐	☐	☐	☐	☐	☐	☐	☐
9. Unassertive	☐	☐	☐	☐	☐	☐	☐	☐	☐	☐	☐	☐	☐
10. Too Aggressive	☐	☐	☐	☐	☐	☐	☐	☐	☐	☐	☐	☐	☐
11. Irresponsible	☐	☐	☐	☐	☐	☐	☐	☐	☐	☐	☐	☐	☐
12. Selfish	☐	☐	☐	☐	☐	☐	☐	☐	☐	☐	☐	☐	☐
13. Jealous	☐	☐	☐	☐	☐	☐	☐	☐	☐	☐	☐	☐	☐
14. Incompetent	☐	☐	☐	☐	☐	☐	☐	☐	☐	☐	☐	☐	☐
15. Other (Specify on back)	☐	☐	☐	☐	☐	☐	☐	☐	☐	☐	☐	☐	☐

Directions: Each hour from ten a.m. to ten p.m. reflect back on the previous hour to determine if you have self-criticized. If you have, make a mark in the box corresponding to the appropriate reason for criticizing and time. A recurring criticism constitutes only one criticism even though it may last the entire hour. If the criticism overlaps into the next hour, count it twice; once, for example, in the ten o'clock space and once in the eleven o'clock space. You may criticize yourself for several different reasons during a given hour. In this case, make several marks corresponding to reasons within one hour. You may take up to three days a week off. Try to be as accurate as you can.

FIGURE 1

Group leaders first explained that self-criticism is understandable and controllable. They noted that self-criticism stems from discrepancies between personal standards and behavior, that chronic self-criticizers usually have high, perfectionistic expectations, that they tend to make inaccurate interpretations about self-performance, and that although sometimes deserved, self-criticism can become a generalized, automatic response influencing feelings of anxiety, depression, or lethargy. Clients were cautioned not to criticize, deny, nor immediately "talk themselves out of" unpleasant feelings since emotions can be legitimate sources of information, useful in planning responses. Such possible benefits of self-criticism as sympathy and avoidance of external criticism may perpetuate a deleterious cycle. Throughout this explanation, group leaders elicited client responses and personal examples. Finally, the purpose and sequence of each intervention component was outlined.

To increase clients' awareness of the occurrence and nature of negative self-attributions, group members were directed to record self-critical thoughts or overt statements using the self-monitoring checklist reproduced in Figure One. At the end of every hour from 10:00 am - 10:00 pm, clients were to recall at hourly intervals whether they had been self-critical. They were then to mark boxes corresponding to their reasons for being self-critical.

The training to rationally evaluate self-criticism helped women determine if their criticisms resulted from inadequate performance or from high standards. For rational evaluation, groups were divided in half and met separately. Women summarized criticisms of the previous week, articulated personal expectations, and determined whether to adjust standards or behavior. Assisted by leader questions and promptings, a woman might be asked: "What do you think is a good way to handle this situation?" "Given, the circumstances, given who you are, what is the best you can do?" "What keeps you from doing your best?" As each woman analyzed negative self-evaluations, group members offered assistance and support by asking for clarification, giving feedback, and sharing similar dilemmas and possible solutions.

Following rational evaluation, clients modified self-critical statements. If poorly performed behavior needed changing, criticism was replaced with appropriate self-instruction. If criticism resulted from unrealistic expectations, standards were revised. Learning this procedure was assisted by viewing videotaped models, participating in covert and overt reheasal, and engaging in monitoring of modified self-statements. Videotaped modeling showed women models in brief scenes criticizing themselves, reconsidering the criticism, and speaking more realistically and constructively. Covert and overt rehearsal included relaxation, imagining self-criticism situations and substitution sequences, and sharing imaginal experiences. After inducing relaxation (Jacobson, 1974;

Modified Self-Statements

NAME: ______________________ DATE: ______________________

TIME	SITUATION	CRITICISM	INTENSITY	STANDARD	MODIFIED SELF-STATEMENT

EXPLANATION: 1. Every hour on the hour from 10 a.m. to 10 p.m. reflect back on the previous hour to determine if you have self-criticized during that time. 2. If you have, briefly note the CRITICISM, the SITUATION in which it occurred, whether the criticism was the result of an unrealistic STANDARD or a problem BEHAVIOR (mark "S" or "B"), and the INTENSITY of the criticism—how you felt as a result. Rate the intensity on a scale of 0=neutral feelings to 10=extremely distressed. 3. You may take up to three days off per week. 4. If you *cannot* fill out all the columns every hour, at least note the criticism and intensity of feeling. Then go back later and fill out the other columns.

FIGURE 2

1978), leaders asked members to imagine situations in which they commonly self-criticized, to become aware of self-critical thoughts, evaluate criticisms, and replace them with more constructive evaluation or instruction. Following imaginal rehearsal, members recounted experiences to the group. Modified self-statement monitoring, recorded hourly on prepared forms (Figure Two), involved noting self-criticisms and situations in which they occurred, the intensity of criticism, whether criticism represented undesirable standards or behavior, and more reasonable self-statements replacing criticism.

Performance assignments were instituted to improve behavior when self-criticism was appropriate and required specification of one to three problem areas. Using forms to rate their problems shown in Figure Three, clients listed problems, necessary action, and constructive self-instruction to replace criticism. Women also completed measurement portions of the form with estimates of problems severity and importance. Problem severity was rated on a scale of 1—100; problem importance was given a percentage weight. A total score was calculated by summing products of severity and importance ratings for each problem and then dividing by the number of problems. In group, members reported on task achievement, consulted with leaders and other group members about strategies to overcome obstacles, and revised tasks, self-instructions, and the problem list.

Attention-placebo training

Intended to be credible while avoiding the specific cognitive-behavioral techniques under examination, the attention-placebo groups incorporated modified versions of previously described intervention rationale and criticism self-monitoring. Not included were components of self-criticism evaluation, substitutions of incompatible self-statements, and performance assignments. Additional components in the attention-placebo condition were various self-monitoring formats, graphing of self-criticism frequency, and group discussion.

During the first and last weeks of intervention the same self-monitoring checklist used in cognitive-behavioral groups was employed. To determine applicability of other self-monitoring formats, attention-placebo group members also used less structured forms, golf stroke wrist counters, and daily journals. Each self-monitoring format was rated by group members on a scale of one to ten for its usefulness, feasibility, and accuracy. After monitoring, attention-placebo-condition clients plotted daily numbers of self-criticisms on frequency graphs. Graphs were displayed via overhead projectors as women reviewed weekly self-criticism activity. Group leaders focused self-criticism review by asking about trends in occurrence, nature and significance of criticism, and increases in self-awareness. Providing a context for self-criticism review, leaders introduced weekly discussion topics including origins of self-expectations, vulnerability to criticisms from others, self-criticism of physical appearance, and comparisons of the self to others. Discussion covered personal dilemmas, resulting self-criticism problems, and offers of advice, encouragement and support. Leaders clarified problem dimensions, intentionally not suggesting ways to modify self-criticism.

Individual Problem Rating†

Name ______ Date ______

Problem List	Self-Instructions	Seriousness (0 ___ 100) (not very) (serious serious)	Importance (Portion of 100%)
1. ______			
Current target ______			
2. ______			
Current target ______			
3. ______			
Current target ______			
4. ______			
Current target ______			

†Adapted from Seaberg and Gillespie (1977)

FIGURE 3

Wait List

Clients on the waiting list participated in pretest, posttest, and follow-up assessment only. They received cognitive-behavioral training after follow-up assignments.

Assessment Measures

SELF-CRITICISM ANALOGUE TEST. Women were individually audiotaped at pretest, posttest, and six-week follow-up while describing recreational activities, work and work habits, family relationships, social life, and abilities and talents. Using ten-second intervals, two raters scored tapes for positive and negative self-references, other statements, or silences. Interrater agreement ranged from 67—100% with an 85% mean; intrarater agreement ranged from 90—97% with a 93% mean.

BECK DEPRESSION INVENTORY (BDI) A twenty-one-item, self-report measure, the BDI reflects perceptions of cognitive, affective, somatic, and motoric manifestations of depresion (Beck, 1967). Total scores range from 0—63, with higher scores indicating greater severity of depression.

SELF-OPINION RATING SCALE (SORS) Used as an index of self-esteem, the SORS was constructed by combining feaures of two simliar measures reported by Sherwood (1962), Robinson and Shaver (1973); and Jacobs, Berschied, and Walster (1971). Clients rated themselves on twenty-four descriptive traits using a seven-point scale. Scores ranged from twenty-four (extremely positive self-opinion) to 168 (extremely negative self-opinion).

FEAR OF NEGATIVE EVALUATION (FNE) Developed by Watson and Friend (1969), this thirty-item true/false scale was used because pilot work showed self-critical women highly sensitive to the possibility of negative evaluation from others.

SELF-CRITICISM FREQUENCY As part of the intervention, monitoring self-criticisms was undertaken by clients in cognitive-behavioral and attention-placebo treatments. Because of evidence on self-observational unreliability (cf. Lipinski & Nelson, 1974; Kazdin 1974c), attempts were made to enhance monitoring accuracy by using a more structured, brief reporting format during weeks one and six when scores were used for measurement. For all self-monitoring, clients had the option of taking up to three days off each week and were encouraged not to self-monitor on days they might be distracted.

EXPECTATION OF IMPROVEMENT Quantifying perceptions of intervention credibility, this scale was completed by cognitive-behavioral and attention-placebo groups during first sessions before and after leaders explained intervention. Using a seven-point scale, women rated expectations that self-criticism problems would improve.

ESTIMATE OF OUTCOME Cognitive-behavioral and attention-placebo clients used a variant of the outcome scale developed by Carr and Whittenbaugh (1965) to rate their improvement, remaining distress, and control over thoughts and feelings at the final session. The adaptation of their scale is depicted in Figure Four.

Estimate of Outcome†

On the following questions, think about your self condition *now* as compared with before your group experience.
Thank you very much for your cooperation.

1. In your opinion, what has been the outcome of group counseling so far? Check the alternative that best describes your situation.

________	significantly improved	________	slightly worse
________	moderately improved	________	moderately worse
________	slightly improved	________	significantly worse
________	no change		

2. Do you feel more or less distressed (anxious, depressed) than before?

________	much more	________	slightly less
________	more	________	less
________	slightly more	________	much less
________	no change		

3. Are you more or less able to control thoughts and feelings than before?

________	much more	________	slightly less
________	more	________	less
________	slightly more	________	much less
________	no change		

†Adopted from Carr and Whittenbaugh (1965)

FIGURE 4

RESULTS

The major hypothesis of the study that clients given cognitive-behavioral training would show more pre- to posttraining improvement on measures of depression, evaluation-anxiety, self-esteem, and self-criticism than would clients given attention-placebo training or those on the wait list. Relative differences were evaluated by determining which groups improved and by comparing changes to determine if one group improved more than others. Results are summarized according to each outcome variable.

Depression

Statistical and visual analyses, portrayed in Figure Five, indicate cognitive-behavioral and attention-placebos condition clients improved their Beck Depression Inventory scores. Differences among the three conditions was slight and non-significant at posttest. By the six week follow-up, differences between cognitive-behavioral and wait-list conditions appeared. There were no differences between the cognitive-behavioral and attention-placebo conditions.

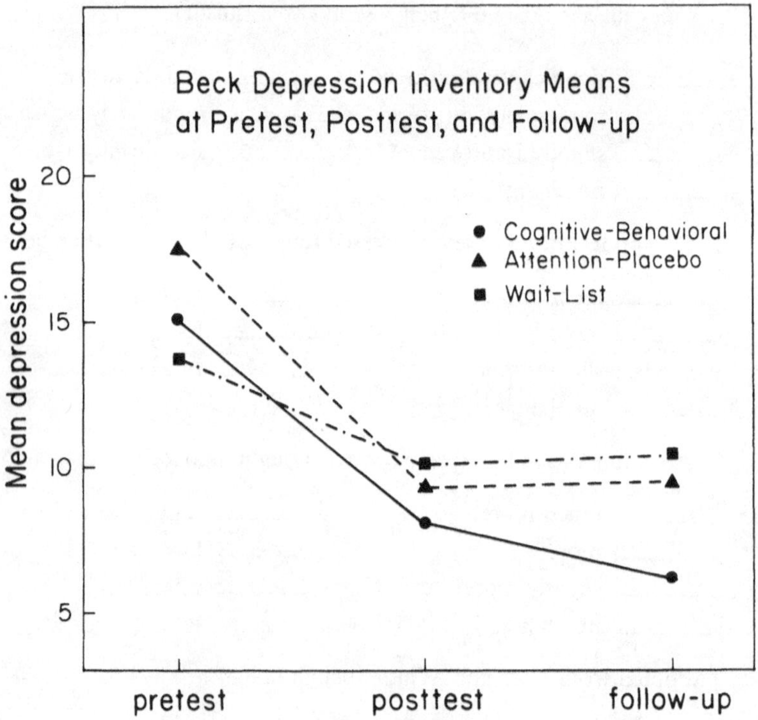

FIGURE 5

Evaluation Anxiety

As illustrated in Figure Six, there were decreases in evaluation anxiety—measured by the Fear of Negative Evaluation Scale—for cognitive-behavioral and attention-placebo clients at posttest. Although reduction in anxiety was less for wait-list clients, differences were found between pre- and posttest clients. Cognitive-behavioral and attention-placebo clients improved more than did wait-list clients at posttest: cognitive-behavioral clients showed more improvement than did wait-list clients at follow-up. There were no differences between cognitive-behavioral and attention-placebo clients at final assessment.

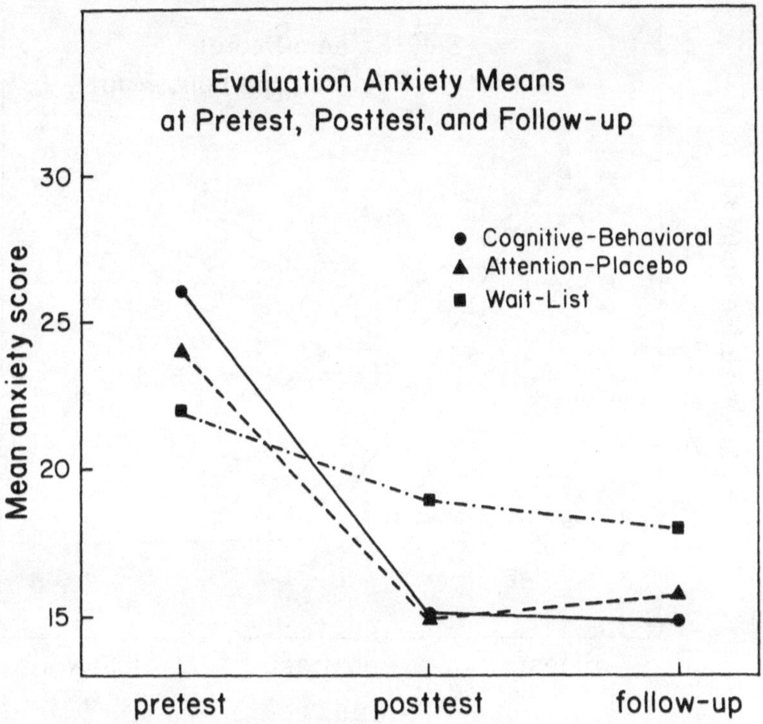

FIGURE 6

Self-Esteem

Cognitive-behavioral intervention had a positive effect on self-esteem as measured by the Self-opinion Rating Scale and shown in Figure Seven. Clients in this condition reported more sensitive self-opinions at posttest and at follow-up than at pretest. As predicted, improvement was greater than that achieved by wait-list clients. Although attention-placebo intervention affected less improvement, self-opinion scores from pre- to posttest also differed compared to wait-list clients, with attention-placebo clients showing greater, albeit nonsignificant, improvement. Differences between cognitive-behavioral and attention-placebo clients were not significant at posttest or follow-up.

Self-criticism

Results from Self-criticism Analogue Tests are graphed in Figure Eight and indicate that cognitive-behavioral and attention-placebo intervention helped reduce negative self-references. Neither intervention was superior to the other nor to the wait-list condition on this variable.

Regarding daily self-criticisms, analysis of pre- to posttest changes

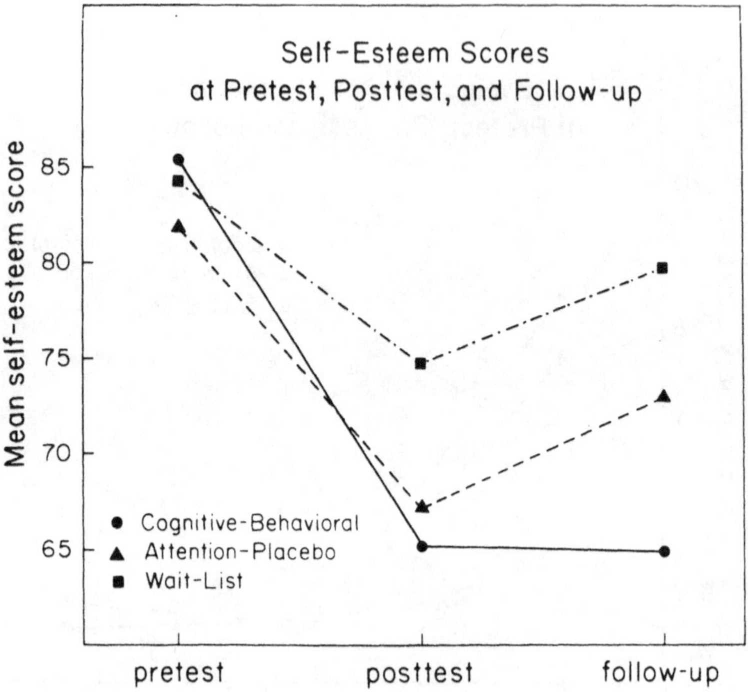

FIGURE 7

from weeks one to six were done between cognitive-behavioral and attention-placebo conditions. These data revealed clients in the former condition reduced self-critical statements more than did those in the latter condition. Comparisons across time are shown in Figure Nine.

In summary, data suggest that cognitive-behavioral intervention helped clients reduce self-criticism. As indicated by several measures (Beck Depression Inventory, Fear of Negative Evaluation, Self-opinion Rating Scale, Self-criticism Analogue Test—categories of work, recreation and social life), cognitive-behavioral intervention was more effective than no intervention. Fewer measures (Self-opinion Rating Scale, daily self-criticism average) showed cognitive-behavioral intervention more effective than attention-placebo groups.

Additional results on just clients in the two training conditions give further credence to the relevance and value of intervention.

Individual Problem Rating

As previously noted, cognitive-behavioral-condition clients specified behavior they wanted to change and rated problems according to severity and importance. These written problems were kept on the forms shown in

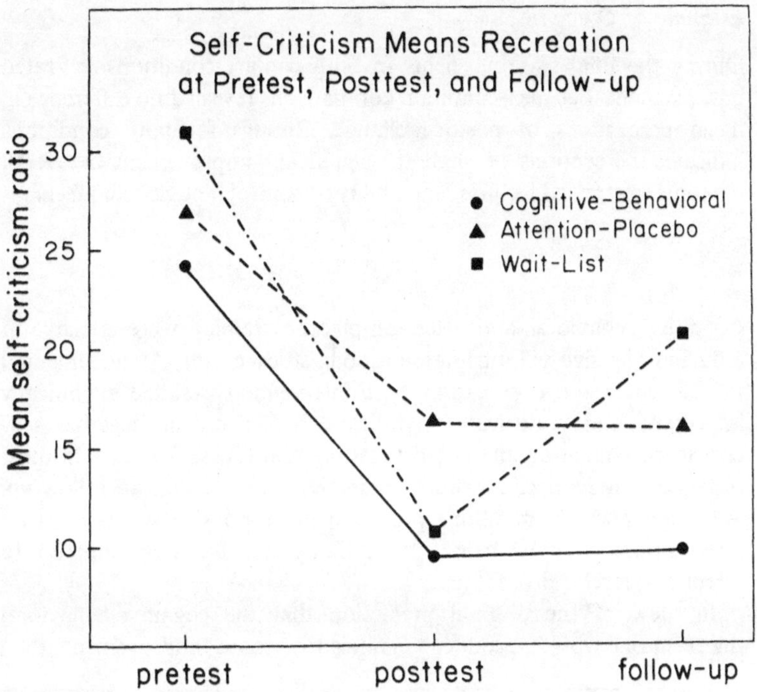

FIGURE 8

Figure Three. Analyzing data on these forms indicated reduction in problems clients reported from weeks three to six.

Self-Observation Evaluation

Clients in attention-placebo groups evaluated self-monitoring procedures by rating relative feasibility, utility, and accuracy, and of the six procedures employed, found wrist-counters the most feasible, useful, and accurate. The every-hour version of the open form was seen as least feasible; the time-sample version was least useful and accurate.

Expectations for Improvement

At the beginning of the first intervention session, women in cognitive-behavioral and attention-placebo conditions rated expectations for becoming less self-critical. Comparison of expectation scores between the two conditions indicated no differences. To check whether clients found the rationales for the two interventions equally credible, at the end of the first session participants again rated improvement expectation; mean ratings were comparable.

Estimate of Outcome

During the final session, clients in both contact conditions self-rated improvement. Between-condition comparisons revealed no difference in mean perceptions of positive change. Ratings for both conditions indicated perceptions of slight to significant improvement in overall outcome, distressed feelings, and ability to control thoughts and feelings.

DISCUSSION

Cognitive-behavioral and attention-placebo training were effective in reducing negative self-attribution among study clients. As documented by self-report and observation, both interventions resulted in clinically important and statistically significant reductions in negative self-criticisms, evaluation anxiety, depression, and low self-esteem. In most instances, these declines were maintained or greater at follow-up. Although both interventions produced more positive effects than no intervention, cognitive-behavioral training was generally superior to attention-placebo procedures.

In view of the original prediction that the cognitive-behavioral intervention would produce significantly more improvement than

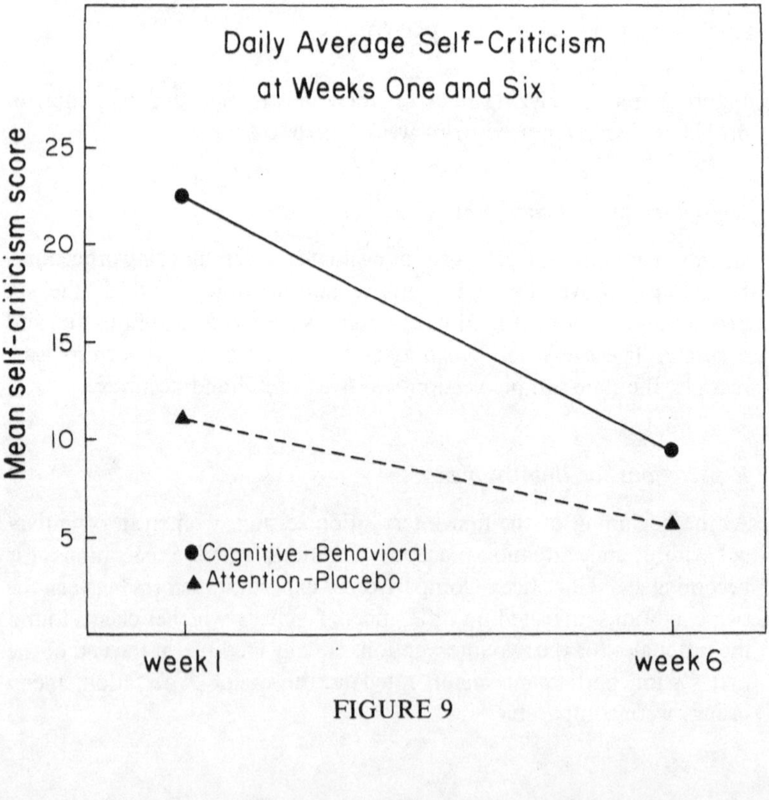

FIGURE 9

attention-placebo intervention or no intervention on all dependent measures, several questions can be raised: Why wasn't cognitive-behavioral intervention more effective? Why was the attention-placebo intervention as effective as it was? Why did the wait-list group improve at all? For practitioners considering using cognitive-behavioral techniques, related questions are: Do the added benefits of the cognitive-behavioral intervention justify the increased cost in time and materials? How can intervention be enhanced? Who benefits most?

Cognitive-Behavioral Intervention

Regarding cognitive-behavior training, perhaps too many techniques and procedures were introduced. Indeed, group leaders reported feeling rushed during sessions and exhausted after teaching many different techniques during most sessions. The many topics to be covered at each session also made it difficult to thoroughly discuss some issues raised by group members. In attention-placebo groups, it was possible to be more flexible in responding to individual situations and to encourage greater participation. Such flexibility may have influenced positive change for attention-placebo group members.

Because self-criticism was the original presenting problem for all clients, that self-reported criticism was reduced more in cognitive-behavioral than in attention-placebo groups is meaningful. Results showing self-critical statements of cognitive-behavioral clients during the first week fifty percent higher than those of attention-placebo clients suggests excessive self-criticizers may have been over-represented in the cognitive-behavioral group.

Attention-Placebo Intervention

Specific to attention-placebo training, one explanation for changes shown by these clients is that they implemented the active ingredients of the cognitive-behavioral intervention package: noting self-criticisms, evaluating these statements, and replacing them with more constructive messages. A group of attention-placebo clients responding to a debriefing questionnaire rated self-monitoring as the most useful intervention. Clients also reported that awareness of what they said to themselves helped them view many statements as unreasonably harsh or not useful, leading to subsequent modification of such statements.

Wait-List Condition

Factors possibly influencing change in the wait-list clients were effects of volunteering, assessment, and ongoing life events. Within-condition improvement on a few variables showed positive trends. Changes may reflect daily life experiences or experimental demand. Further, processes of initial screening and assessment may have influenced client scores. Many women regarded screening interviews as an opportunity to talk in detail about very personal issues. Although interviews were to be structured and brief, on some occasions client needs took precedence over interview objectives. Expectations that help was forthcoming for wait-list clients may have been powerful and positive motivators (cf. Rotter, 1978; Mahoney 1977b; D'Zurilla & Goldfried, 1971).

Modifications of Cognitive Behavioral Intervention

Based on this experience, clinical applications of the cognitive-behavioral intervention package might profit from several modifications. The number of sessions might be increased from six to eight so each meeting would cover fewer techniques at a slower pace. Six weekly and two final bi-weekly sessions might be optimal. One leader can readily manage a group of five or six; otherwise the group should be expanded to at least eight members and employ a second leader, so that the group may be divided when procedures require individual attention.

Problem-conceptualization and intervention rationale should be carefully explained, incorporating client reason for self-criticism. The task is to translate or reframe explanations for self criticism-into terms facilitating remedies. Making the rationale clear and plausible does not imply over-simplication: clients struggling with life-long problems do not like being told, "Really the solution is very simple."

Self monitoring may be resisted. Assignments should be simplified and clients given clear understanding of purposes. Especially important is explaining how increased awareness of criticisms is of benefit. During the present project, clients were offered monetary incentives (a one dollar refund for each week of "good" self-monitoring) and allowed to take off up to three days each week from self-monitoring. Clients in the attention-placebo groups clearly endorsed the most simple self-monitoring methods—wrist counters and checklists. This suggests a revision of the open forms used in cognitive-behavioral intervention. Although the open form was constructed so self criticism recording would serve as cues, it may not be essential to write out future self statement modifications. An alternative would be to continue using a simplified form with a column added to check whether or not criticism was modified. Also important is instructing clients to give themselves encouraging feedback each hour: another column might permit recording these positive messages.

Videotaped models may not be essential. Of greater importance is client understanding of what is meant by modifying self-criticism. Therefore, leaders must provide a variety of examples, modifying their own lapses into self-criticism and those of clients. Examples should not be too easy; they should include wavering, revising, and struggling in the think-out-loud process of criticizing, evaluating the criticism, and modifying it with more appropraite evaluations or instructions.

Implications for Practice

Many persons suffering from excessive self-criticism do not identify it as a major problem nor actively seek help for it; nonetheless, self-criticsm may interfere with other problem-solving efforts. Intervention should be used and evaluated across diverse settings and with a variety of male and female clients.

Findings suggested that women who found the treatment rationale most compatible with their own experience were more conscientious in completing assignments and tended to accrue more benefits. Not surprisingly, intervention did not have much of an impact on persons not self-critical. In some cases intervention worked well with women who were quite depressed; in others it did not. In these latter cases, detracting factors seemed to be disrespect for other group members and perception of the extreme complexity of personal problems. Since the most promising candidates for intervention are not easily identified, the main criterion must remain the individual's perception of a self-criticism problem. Practitioners using intervention must evaluate effects so empirically based outcomes with different populations can be accumulated.

Individuals may not have resources to mount a major evaluation project; however, clinicians are responsible for documenting the intervention's outcome with each client. In addition to providing information useful in planning and refining ongoing intervention, single-case evaluations yield predictive data to help identify appropriate clients. Practitioners interested in evaluating intervention should consider the Self-Monitoring Check List as one measure of outcome. Measures should always include consumer satisfaction ratings, as on the estimate of outcome scale, and from instruments like the Index of Self-Esteem (Hudson, 1977).

FUTURE RESEARCH

Future work could clarify and extend present findings. The extent to which persons continue to employ self-criticism modification techniques needs to be determined. Since behavior patterns are learned over long periods, the ultimate benefits of intervention may not be manifest until six months or a year after termination. Long-term follow-up data are necessary. The relative contribution of each intervention component should be isolated. This information is especially important in light of the finding that self-monitoring itself provided a powerful agent for intervention.

Finally, knowledge about the damaging effects of unrealistic perfectionism should be made available to parents, teachers, and others influential in forming children's behavior patterns. Mothers participating in the present study frequently observed that their increased ability to cope with mistakes and evaluate themselves in a compassionate, friendly way impressed their children. Similar adjunctive benefits were reported by client-parents who were better able to cope with childrens' problems, disappointments, and imperfections. In these ways, social workers employing behavioral methods to treat self-criticism and related cognitive problems can affect short-term changes, longitudinal maintenance of behavior change, and the primary prevention of future problems among adults and emerging adults. The full-service cycle of dealing first with immediate crisis without neglecting long-term improvements. Then operationalizes protessional objectives as well as those associated with behavior modification.

9

Assertiveness Training for Women

Cheryl A. Richey

HELPING WOMEN ACQUIRE ASSERTIVE SKILLS

As is the treatment of women's self-criticism discussed in the previous chapter, assertiveness training for women is an exciting outgrowth of the feminist movement (Baer, 1976; Osborn & Harris, 1975; Phelps & Austin, 1975) and cognate assertiveness training paradigms (Rose & Schinke, 1978). The described program for group assertiveness training, originally developed for women, was subsequently used with both sexes. Detailed are assessment, intervention, and evalution procedures used by many group leaders and with a variety of clients. These procedures reflect extensive development, testing, and refinement of each assertiveness training phase. Supporting data are drawn from clinical experiences at the Women's Institute (WI), a private, nonprofit counseling agency, and represent scores of assertiveness training groups conducted with hundreds of women during a seven year period. The chapter concludes with practice guidelines for other social workers wishing to replicate this group assertiveness training approach.

ASSESSMENT

Assessment procedures attempt to identify the nature and magnitude of difficulties in self-assertion. Relevant questions are: Do clients possess assertiveness skills? If so, in what situations are these more likely to be observed? Is interpersonal anxiety inhibiting assertiveness skills? Is aggressiveness a problem? To answer these questions, the Gambrill-Richey Assertion Inventory (1975) is generally completed and returned before training begins. The Assertion Inventory is a forty-item self-report measure of interpersonal discomfort and response probability. Each situation is rated first on degree of discomfort on a five-point scale (1 = none, 5 = very much). Clients then complete the Inventory a second time, indicating on a five point scale (1 = always, 5 = never) the probability of displaying the behavior if actually presented with the situation. Respondents also circle those items they would like to handle more assertively. The Assertion Inventory has shown good test-retest reliability over time, and has made valid distinctions between clinical and normal populations (Gambrill & Richey, 1975; Richey, 1975).

Assertion Inventory scores are summarized to determine degree of nonassertiveness and to pinpoint common topics or themes for training. Each person's total discomfort and total probability scores are obtained so that pretraining means can be computed and compared with post-training scores. Such information is also useful in determining training pace (higher scores suggest a more nonassertive person, a slower training pace), and in evaluating training outcome. An extremely high individual discomfort score (160+) may be a clue that group training would be too anxiety provoking for a particular client. Further assessment of this individual (via observation and an interview) may be necessary to determine whether a group training format or individual counseling is advisable.

Based on Assertion Inventory scores and clinical observation, most women involved in assertiveness training at WI are nonassertive; a small percentage might be labeled aggressive—loud, interruptive, argumentative, and attempting to monopolize group discussions. More often than not, Assertion Inventory scores of such people show a "super-assertive" person, with low anxiety and probability scores. Aggressive clients generally indicate they would feel no discomfort in any situation and would always react. Although highly speculative, this clinical observation needs to be researched if the Assertion Inventory and similar instruments are to be useful in assessing aggressiveness (DeGiovanni & Epstein, 1978).

In addition to being used to determine group means and profiles, Assertion Inventory scores also guide training content. After group participants circle situations they would like to handle more assertively, the trainer totals the number of circles for each item, selecting items circled by half or more of the members. Other sources of assessment information determine particular strengths and problems of group members. If leaders have time before training, clients can individually respond to role-play simulations while being audio- or video-taped.

Responses are analyzed using various verbal and nonverbal measures—duration of eye contact, latency of response, loudness and fluency of speech, posture, number of "I" statements, and general assertive content (Eisler, Hersen, & Miller, 1973). If pretraining assessment is not feasible, ongoing observation in the group develops a more thorough picture of client deficits and abilities.

Asked to monitor daily assertions, clients record the date, type of situation, nature of assertive response, other person's reaction (positive, neutral, negative), degree of anxiety (on a 1-5 scale), and number of "points" they awarded themselves as a satisfaction rating. Clients monitor their assertions after the first session and every subsequent training week. They list situations they failed to handle assertively, and practice these during group sessions. Responses from weekly data sheets can determine beginning skill levels and the effect of training upon performance. Are anxiety ratings going up or down? Are clients getting more positive reactions from others? Are they indicating more self-satisfaction?

INTERVENTION

Once assessment has identified beginning skill levels and group themes, training begins. An important variable is group size: groups at WI ranging from eight to sixteen members, average twelve. Fewer than eight reduces group interaction and practice opportunities; more than sixteen limits individual attention and feedback. More attrition takes place with groups over twelve; perhaps members of larger groups feel their absence will not be missed. With smaller groups, members become more quickly acquainted and each person holds an important position.

Duration and training site are also considered. Sessions are generally two and a half hours in length to allow for group sharing, practice, and casual interaction during a break. Facilities are informal and comfortable: many clients comment that the rug, floor pillows, and soft lighting help reduce anxiety, facilitating an atmosphere of intimacy and cohesiveness. At the very least, the training environment should be comfortable and allow clients movement for small group role plays and leader demonstrations.

Initial Session

The leader begins the first group session of a typical five-week program by providing clear definitions of assertiveness, non-assertiveness, and aggressiveness.

Assertiveness is defined as nonverbal and verbal behavior enabling people to act in their best interests, to stand up for themselves, and to express opinions, feelings, and attitudes honestly without undue anxiety (Alberti & Emmons, 1974). Assertive people exercise rights without denying or violating others' rights and feelings. Being assertive is self-enhancing and increases self-esteem because personal preferences are stated in ways generally acceptable to others (MacDonald, 1974). Assertiveness does not guarantee "winning"; it does facilitate self-expression, increasing the likelihood that satisfactory resolutions occur with the obtaining of personal goals.

In contrast, nonassertive people exhibit self-denying, restrained, and inhibited behavior. Submissive in social situations, they often experience high interpersonal anxiety. Generally avoiding confrontation situations, nonassertive persons do not express preferences, but allow others to make decisions for them and, as a result, often feel helpless, controlled, and bitter. Feelings of self-hatred and resentment towards others are not uncommon.

Compared to assertive or nonassertive responses, aggression includes hostile words or actions which coerce others. Interested in "winning," aggressive people attempt to achieve this goal by putting others down, hurting or humiliating them. Although aggressive persons may not feel anxious and frequently achieve their goals, the price for "winning" can be high. Reactions of others generally include dislike, hostility, and counteraggression. Aggressive persons may find others avoiding them and reacting in terse, sarcastic, or openly hostile ways.

To help allay concern that the outcome of training will be increased aggressiveness, trainers demonstrate differences among the responses by role playing a situation with a group member—first nonassertively, then aggressively, and finally, assertively.

After definitions and examples have been discussed, the leader describes training procedures. Behavior rehearsal, modeling, guidelines, feedback and coaching, reinforcement, and homework assignments are mentioned. Also presented are group norms and attendance expectations. Encouraged to discuss present issues and to not dwell on the past, members are expected to be supportive of each other's attempts, to praise accomplishments rather than point out shortcomings. Assertion training is not an encounter group experience. Members are expected to practice what they have learned in class and monitor their assertiveness during the week.

Group members then interview each other in dyads and introduce the partner to the rest of the group. Wrist counters are distributed and the importance of self-reinforcement procedures is discussed. Wrist counters, usually commercially available golf-stroke counters, help members acknowledge assertiveness attempts and successes. Members are also shown how to give themselves overt compliments for responses. Overt self-reinforcement is encouraged because it reduces people's reluctance regarding self-praise, anxiety is lessened since everyone is doing it, members get to hear what others say to themselves, members can be reminded to self-praise if they "forget," and the pairing of overt self-reinforcement with point-giving helps give points value.

Providing the foundation for all other assertive responses, basic conversational skills is the first training topic with concentration on specific skills such as expressing elaborated opinion statements, breaking into ongoing conversations, and resisting unwarranted interruptions. Elaborated opinion statements begin with a personal pronoun ("I", "me", or "my") and should contain a compound sentence. After the leader demonstrates elaborated opinions, members are handed a discussion topic, divided into small groups of three or four and though not prepared for discussion, asked to express an opinion on topics general enough to allow for open discussion that are stimulating and offer the opportunity for differences of opinion. Each person expresses one elaborated opinion, praises herself outloud, and gives herself wrist counter points. Members are reminded to omit any self-critical evaluations. The small groups are then ready to tackle more realistic conversational challenges: entering an ongoing conversation without aggressively cutting someone off, for example. Each member participates breaking into group conversation by leaving the group and then attempting to join the discussion. Other members engross themselves in conversation and ignore the target person until she attempts to enter. Her task is to join the conversation by making a meaningful verbal contribution without interrupting. Some "Helpful Hints" that have been employed follow. Members are encouraged to compliment the target person for what she did well, to point out the specific strategies she utilized, and to offer suggestions for improvement. If the target person was overly anxious and cut someone off, she tries the exercise again using more constraint and additional techniques. This exercise highlights individual difficulties, encourages participation from all members, and has immediate payoff for the target person.

The initial session ends with group members being assigned tasks using conversational skills, wrist counters and data-taking sheets during the intervening week. Participants are reminded to bring their data with them to share at the next group session.

Subsequent Sessions

Each of the remaining four group sessions starts with group testimonials. Participants are asked to tell about at least one assertiveness success accomplished during the week. They refer to their data sheets for details—the person and situation involved; what was said; how the other person reacted; degree of discomfort before, during, and after the assertion; and number of self-administered points. One ground rule for testimonials is that only successes are shared. Failures are not ignored, but are worked on in a problem-solving manner during role plays later in the session.

Another rule for the testimonials is brevity; the assertive situation should be reported without a summary of its historical aspects. And, members are urged to give each other attention and praise throughout testimonials.

Testimonials completed, the group leader uses Assertion Inventory priorities to identify and demonstrate a nonassertive, aggressive, and assertive response to a specific social situation. The group discusses the demonstration and how the various responses appeared. Members are then ready for individual practice on their own. If a member cannot think of a situation to practice, or feels that a real example would be too difficult, she can select from a prepared list of scripts. Practice takes approximately fifteen minutes per person, with leaders circulating among small groups, giving feedback and praise, making suggestions, and modeling alternative responses.

Before the session ends, all members are brought back together to discuss the exercise and share experiences and progress, with one or two members demonstrating their situations for feedback and reinforcement. Members then turn in data sheets, take a blank sheet, and are assigned the task of using their practiced assertive behavior in an actual situation.

The final group session includes testimonials covering what each member learned and deficits she needs to work on. Toward the end, members complete anonymous workshop evaluations on their satisfaction with their achievement of objectives, the amount of work, each training activity, and their new assertive skills.

EVALUATION

Assertion Inventories

A data sample was obtained from sixty-eight women who participated in thirteen different assertion training groups led by one of three WI staff counselors. Each of these women completed an Assertion Inventory before group training, one month after training ended, and approximately eight months later. Shown in Figure One, these scores are contrasted with normative data from 313 untrained female and male college students (cf. Gambrill & Richey, 1975). Before training, the clinical group had higher mean discomfort and probability scores than did the normative sample. After they were given training, clients reported much lower scores on the two Assertion Inventory subscales. Positive posttraining trends were maintained and became greater over time.

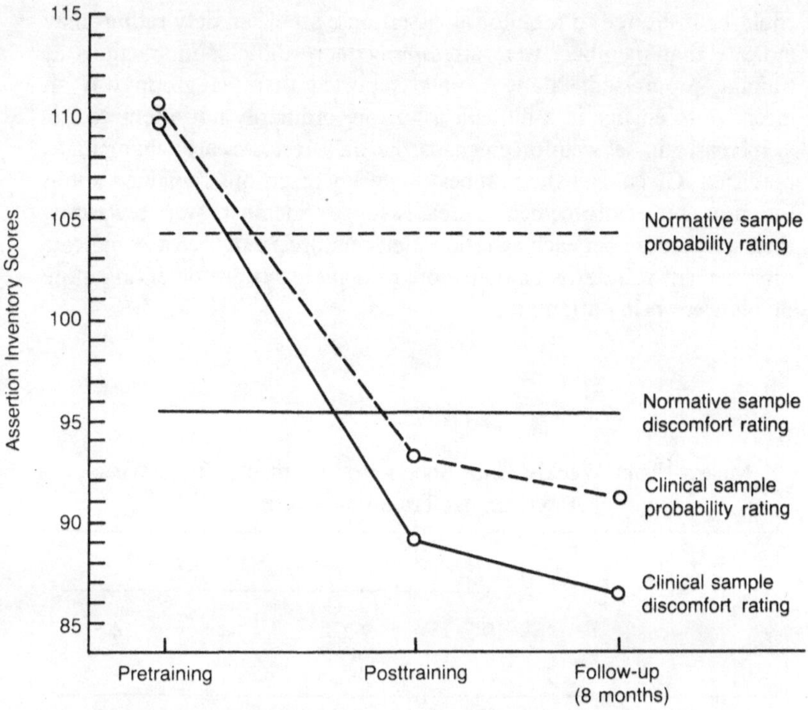

FIGURE 1. Pre-, posttraining, and follow-up means of discomfort and response probability ratings on the Gambrill-Richey Assertion Inventory for a clinical sample (N=68) and a normative college sample (N=313). Lower scores signify greater assertiveness.

Weekly Monitoring

Another source of evaluation data is results of clients' weekly monitoring of progress. Specifically, clients kept track of assertive responses, feelings of anxiety during these responses, and their awarding of self-reinforcement points after the assertive response. Data from a representative subset of women participating in assertion training at WI are shown in Table One. Over time, the women reported slight declines in their assertiveness attempts, rather stable anxiety ratings, and substantial increase in self-administered reinforcement points.

The slight decreases in reported assertions may mean members were no longer counting assertions now included in their repertoires. Some women commented that they would not list a particular interaction or behavior because "I do that all the time now and don't bother reporting it as a success." A decrease in reported number of assertions may reflect higher standards. If this is the case, alternative data-collection methods could be instituted to monitor all assertions. Stable anxiety ratings may indicate that members were attempting more difficult interactions as training progressed. Many women reported that the group was an incentive to engage in a difficult assertion, ordinarily not attempted.

Increases in self-reinforcement is the only result clearly changing as predicted. Given that the number of weekly assertions remained about the same, self-reinforcement increases suggest members were rewarding themselves more per each assertion. Self-reinforcement increases indicate more lenient standards or that more difficult assertions deserving more points were being attempted.

Table 1

Means From Weekly Data Sheets For Women In Five-Week Assertiveness Training Groups

	Weeks			
	1-2	2-3	3-4	4-5
Assertions	8.72	7.54	7.30	7.36
Anxiety rating per assertion†	2.78	2.42	2.78	2.68
Number of points per assertion	3.84	3.82	5.80	7.02

† Anxiety was rated on a 1 to 5 scale with 1 indicating no anxiety and 5 indicating high anxiety.

Consumer Feedback Ratings

Based on final evaluation forms of a large cohort of women trained at WI, a mean rating of 6.1 (on a seven point scale with seven being most positive) was assigned to overall satisfaction with the workshop. Achievement of objectives was rated at 5.3. Forty-one said the required work was "about right", four said "too little." Another section of the evaluation form asked how much each training activity contributed to overall learning. Rank-ordered in Table Two the means for eight training activities show overall positive ratings with some variation between perceptions immediately following training and at the eight-month follow-up.

Table 2

Ranks and Means of Training Activities
Evaluated at Post Training and Follow-Up

Activity	Post-Training		Follow-Up	
	Rank	Mean†	Rank	Mean†
Contributions from the leader	1	4.29	1	3.90
Group reinforcement	2	4.08	3	3.69
Testimonials	3	4.06	5	3.28
Role playing real situations	4	4.02	2	3.86
Homework assignments	5	3.50	6	3.02
Self-reinforcement	6	3.20	4	3.35
Weekly data sheets	7	3.18	8	2.70
Standard role playing scripts	8	2.88	7	3.00
Overall means:		3.65		3.35

† All items evaluated on a 5 point scale, with 5 as most positive.

Follow-up

To assess maintenance of change, generalization of training to new situations, and impact of increased assertiveness on other areas, a follow-up questionnaire and the Assertion Inventory was mailed to 144 cleints whose training concluded one to seventeen (an average of eight) months earlier. Seventy-six women, 55%, responded.

Respondents indicated on a five-point scale how effective training was in enabling them to be more assertive in current situations. With a 3.7 mean, responses to this question approached the 4.2 mean derived immediately after training. Other questions and resulting mean (M) response scores were: 1. How often do you praise or compliment yourself for an assertion (M = 3.5)? 2. What has happened to your overall level of assertiveness since training (M = 4.2)? 3. How has training affected your general self-image, self-esteem, or self-confidence (M = 4.3)? 4. What has happened to your general level of self-praise since training? (M = 4.0) 5. Has assertiveness training had any noticeable impact on other areas such as interpersonal relationships with female acquaintances and co-workers, close male friends and family, job and/or career development? (M = 3.9) 6. How did training affect any moods of depression, low self-estimation, or sense of inferiority? (M = 3.8) 7. How often do you assert yourself in situations not practiced during the training, i.e. what is the carry-over of assertiveness to "new" situations? (M = 3.6) Combined, these ratings indicated that training effects were maintained over time and had positive ramifications on self-evaluation and relationships with others.

Trainer Follow-up

Over 130 professionals have been trained in the intervention described here. A recent follow-up survey solicited feedback from these persons on training effectiveness, whether evaluation activities were carried out, and changes in the model to enhance its applicability to different clientele. Although only forty-three professionals returned the questionnaire, their responses help document training efficacy and suggest guidelines for subsequent improvements.

Assessment

In terms of assessment and evaluation, 90% of forty-two trainers who answered this question indicated they utilized some pretraining assessment procedures to determine difficulties in assertiveness. Table Three illustrates the various assessment techniques used. Of the trainers, 95%, forty-one of forty-three, reported using an evaluation procedure; however, Table Three shows relatively few administering post-training questionnaires to determine outcome. The Gambrill-Richey Assertion Inventory or another questionnaire was used before training by 88%, but only 44% reported having members complete the same assessment questionnaires after training. Most leaders used workshop evaluation forms to assess client satisfaction (81%) and observations of success via client reports (70%). Moreover, thirty of forty-three trainers used two or three evaluation procedures to determine success (seven used one technique only, four used all procedures listed). Unfortunately, all evaluation procedures were used at posttraining only; no trainer reported follow-up efforts.

Logistics

Regarding duration and scheduling, most trainers, twenty-six out of forty-three, or 61%) indicated that sessions lasted one and one half to two hours and met once weekly. Nine trainers (21%) held two and one half to three hour-sessions per week; three (7%) conducted three hour-sessions twice a week; three ran all-day workshops; and two (5%) held weekly four-hour sessions. The total number of training hours per group ranged from two to thirty with a mean of 13.6. Though showing wide variation in number and duration of sessions, these data were comparable with the 12.5 hours of training offered at WI.

Table 3

Assessment and Evaluation Methods Used

By Community Trainers

Method	Ethically Mixed Groups†	Primarily Non-White Groups	All
Pretraining Assessment			
Gambrill-Richey Assertion Inventory	83% (10)	67% (20)	71% (30)
Other questionnaire	8% (1)	20% (6)	17% (7)
Other means of assessment (interviews, group discussion, case records)	33% (4)	30% (9)	31% (13)
None	0	13% (4)	10% (4)
Post-training Evaluation			
Readminister pretraining assessment questionnaire	38% (5)	47% (14)	44% (19)
Members complete a workshop evaluation form	77% (10)	83% (25)	81% (35)
Leader listens to testimonials and success stories	54% (7)	77% (23)	70% (30)
Other procedures (individual interviews, group role plays, feedback from others)	15% (2)	33% (10)	28% (12)
None	0	7% (2)	5% (2)

Note. Number of respondents are given in parentheses.

† 10% or more ethnic minority members.

Procedures

Using a five-point scale (five as most positive), trainers indicated how much various procedures contributed to the overall effectiveness of their programs. Specific procedures and their mean ratings follow: role playing real situations (M = 4.37); group reinforcement (M = 4.15); leader's contribution (M = 3.87); testimonials (M = 3.85); self-praise (M = 3.41); homework assignments (M = 3.41); standard role-play scripts (M = 3.28); weekly data sheets (M = 3.05); and self-administration of points on wrist counters (M = 2.25). Relatively low rankings on the wrist counter technique illustrates the importance of separating this more mechanical self-reinforcement from the overt and covert self-praise strategies that receive higher rankings. Interestingly, further data comparisons evidenced trainers of mixed-sex groups rating self-praise and use of wrist counters lower than trainers of groups that were primarily or exclusively women. Trainers of women may view self-reinforcement as more important, or women clients may be more responsive than men to this technique.

Format

Asked to scale from one (no change) to five (extensive change) how much they had modified the original training format, 50% of the trainers indicated "few changes," 29% reported "a fair amount of changes," 17% said "much change," and 5% reported "extensive changes." No differences were shown between means for racially mixed groups (M = 2.67) and primarily white groups (M = 2.77); however, trainers of groups containing more men indicated slightly more alterations (exclusively women, M = 2.57; primarily women, M = 2.71; half women and half men, M = 2.94).

Effectiveness

Trainers rated how effective they viewed training in helping clients be more assertive. On a five-point scale (five as very effective), trainers of minority groups gave higher ratings (M = 3.73) than did trainers of primarily nonminority groups (M = 3.18). Trainers working with women primarily or exclusively gave slightly higher ratings (M = 3.69 and M = 3.64) than did those working with male/female groups (M = 3.50). Mean rating for the entire sample was 3.64, comparable to 3.74 for WI clients at follow-up.

Problems

Problems with implementing assertiveness training were solicited. Twenty-six of forty-three respondents (60%) reported at least one difficulty. Resistance from other staff—physicians, supervisors, personnel managers, and co-workers—was encountered by twelve trainers. Problems included reluctance of a personnel manager to give employees time off for training, "conflict with agency policies," the training's non-correspondence with business priorities, jealousy among co-workers, and lack of referrals even though appropriate clients seemed available.

Client resistance interfering with training implementation was reported by thirteen surveyed trainers. Problems included clients not viewing assertiveness training as relevant to their presenting complaint, lack of sophistication, resistance to mandatory training say, in a prison setting, value conflicts (AT seen as anti-Christian, or a women's lib plot), absenteeism, and attrition. All trainers who encountered problems said they handled them without much trouble. Staff resistance was dealt with by discussing training goals, format, and expected outcome and inviting staff to training sessions. Client resistance was reduced by trainers sharing their values, spending more time on definitions, using simpler vocabulary and role plays, and emphasizing commitment to the group and consistent attendance.

GUIDELINES FOR PRACTICE

To aid others in developing, implementing, and evaluating group assertiveness training, the following sections outline guidelines for preparation, intervention tailoring, interdependence, member self-reinforcement, monitoring, and work with minority groups.

Preparation

Practitioners leading assertiveness training groups must have knowledge of basic behavioral principles and procedures. Important among these are the concepts of anxiety as an inhibitor and techniques of shaping, reinforcement, extinction, modeling, and practice. Leaders must understand group dynamics, and be able to intervene with group problems of unequal participation, competition for leadership, and client resistance. Some have suggested that group leaders have at least ten hours of assertiveness training themselves before enrolling in trainers' workshops (Alberti 1977, p. 369). Although not a qualification for entry into trainers' workshops at WI, experience with assertiveness training is an important prerequisite. Many trainers associated with me have been in assertiveness training groups or have read extensively in the area before enrolling in trainers' workshops. Because several future leaders viewed training as an opportunity to work on their own problems, workshop descriptions for trainers make explicit the professional rather than personal emphasis. Leaders must get feedback from an experienced assertiveness trainer regarding leadership abilities and style. Trainers' workshops offered at WI include feedback from members, the leader, and videotapes on how the trainees handle typical group situations. If potential leaders are unable to locate a trainers' workshop, a professional leader can be asked to offer a class or allow a trainee to observe or co-lead a group. Practitioners can also work with each other using videotaped feedback and supervisory input. Written material alone does not provide necessary skills for conducting an assertiveness training group; practice and feedback are as important for trainers as for clients.

Intervention Tailoring

Social workers engage diverse clients in a variety of settings. Specific themes, ordering of themes, and training pace, therefore, are tailored to each assertiveness training group. Referring to earlier findings, trainers of mixed-sex groups may have rated training as less effective than did trainers of primarily or exclusively women's groups because training formats did not sufficiently address male issues. Several trainers did report that areas of difficulty chosen by men were different from those chosen by women. For instance, more men than women had problems with "expressing personal limitations" such as admitting confusion or asking someone for a favor.

Interdependence

Successful trainers help group members rely on each other more than on the leader for reinforcement and support. Leaders are facilitators, not focal points of training activities. Initially, members do rely more heavily on leaders for direction and acknowledgement; skillful leaders, however, quickly share responsibility by encouraging others to respond with suggestions, modeling, and praise. Support for assertiveness is leader instigated during the first weeks, assumed by group members from the middle to the end of training, and continued by clients through self-reinforcement after training.

Self-Reinforcement

Because explaining and practicing self-reinforcement takes considerable time and energy, leaders are tempted to omit it and rely solely on social reinforcement. When training ends, however, clients dependent on reinforcement from others may experience decreased assertiveness. Incorporating frequent self-reinforcement early and stressing its role throughout training are worthwhile investments.

Monitoring

Monitoring change and client satisfaction can significantly assist leaders in upgrading their skills and their later training endeavors. The efforts required of clients and leaders by posttraining evaluation activities is time well spent. Questionnaires yield invaluable feedback on individual goal attainment, client satisfaction, and suggestions for future groups. Having clients monitor overall weekly assertiveness also generates feedback on assertive behavior outside the group. As described previously, many monitoring procedures are available for monitoring training efficacy. Leaders taking advantage of at least some demonstrate professional accountability to clients, colleagues, and themselves.

Working with Minority Groups

Even though almost one third of surveyed clinicians successfully trained groups with 10% or more ethnic-minority clients, it seems premature to suggest that the program can be implemented with culturally diverse populations without modifications. A growing body of literature on cross-cultural assertiveness training exists (Cheek, 1977; Grodner, 1977; Hwang, 1977; Landau & Paulson in Alberti, 1977); however, relevant issues must be examined before complete confidence in the model's generalizability can be assured. Moreover, research on assertiveness training with low-income individuals is rare (Galinsky, Schopler, Safier, & Gambrill, 1978). Prejudice and discrimination may be similar whether based on income, age, color, or sex. The import of each variable on training demands systematic inquiry.

Aggression

Although most women requesting assertiveness training are nonassertive, aggressive members can present special difficulties for trainers. Indeed, ten out of forty-three trainers (23%) said they wanted to handle aggression better. One promising strategy for dealing with in-group aggression uses tokens to help members discriminate among assertive, nonassertive, and aggressive responses. For example, others report giving white tokens contingent on assertive responses, blue tokens for nonassertive statements, and red tokens for aggressive behavior.

CONCLUSION

The group approach to assertiveness training for women described in this chapter has been widely implemented. Direct-service applications at the Women's Institute have trained nearly 400 women. Other social workers in a variety of settings have applied the intervention approach with groups of women and men throughout diverse training formats. A survey from a sample of community trainers, representing 43 of 136 professionals so trained, shows over 3,330 clients participating in assertiveness training. Training outcomes and long-term follow-up provide evidence of successful experiences for both trainers and clients. Future work should build upon these data and outlined procedures for delivering and improving the assertiveness training approach, so that social work practitioners can thereby enhance their professional skills repertoires, expand the knowledge base, and help clients learn new ways to cope with personal and social distress.

10

Sexual Dysfunctions and Cognitions

Wayne D. Duehn
and
Nazneen Sada Mayadas

Direct intervention with sexual dysfunctions has been the focus of intensive research and clinical efforts following the pioneer work of Masters and Johnson (1966, 1970). Subsequent years have witnessed adoption and proliferation of sexual therapy as an established mode of social work intervention. Although its efficacy is well documented (LoPiccolo & LoPiccolo, 1978; Fischer & Gochros, 1977; Masters & Johnson, 1970), many professionals have begun to question the effectiveness of extant therapeutic procedures in meeting an extended range of sexual dysfunctions (Higginbotham & Farkas, 1977; Schumacher & Lloyd, 1976). Masters, Johnson, and Kolodny (1977) offer a partial explanation for apparent decreases in therapeutic effectiveness by attributing trends to transitory placebo effects—not unlike those accompanying newly introduced pharmaceutical agents—or to residual sexual dysfunctions insulary to intervention.

Regardless of cause, many recognize the limitations of current sexual therapy procedures. It now seems obvious that clinicians need to account more adequately for the role of other variables—especially cognitive processes—in understanding sexual functioning. Thus, cognitive and behavioral skills must be incorporated into intervention to resolve seemingly unamenable and unyielding sexual dysfunctions. This chapter outlines one such set of cognitive procedures: self-management techniques for ameliorating sexual dysfunctions. Procedures of role induction, baselining, cognitive modeling, directed mediational training, self-reinforcement, evaluation, and maintenance are defined and explicated within a single-case research design.

All self-management intervention techniques are derived from the authors' work at Marriage and Family Counselors Associates, Arlington, Texas, with individuals not responding to traditional approaches with sexual dysfunction. Presenting problems successfully remediated have included ejaculatory and erectile failure, primary and secondary orgasmic dysfunciton, vaginismus, and inadequate sexual response patterns.

SELF-MANAGEMENT

Self-management occurs when individuals systematically apply learning principles to themselves (Mahoney & Thoresen, 1974; Meichenbaum & Cameron, 1974; Goldiamond, 1965). Conceptualizations of self-management and supportive empirical research are recent developments in behavior therapy. Initial work in this area focused on methods of stimulus control, subsequently expanded to include covert control, imagery training, flooding, thought stopping, and thought management (Goldiamond, 1965).

Cautela (1969) has since identified four subcategories of self-management: 1) stimulus control: the arranging of environmental cues eliciting undesirable responses and establishing cues evoking desired responses; 2) self-monitoring: the recording of data about one's self to supply relevant and measurable information on rates of behavioral and cognitive occurrences, eliciting cues, and subsequent consequences; 3) self-reinforcement: the identifying of rewards, the specifying of contingencies under which rewards will be given, and the administering of rewards; and 4) self-punishment: the administering of aversive procedures designed to decrease behavior or cognitions.

Such self-management components are consistent with Mahoney and Thoresen's (1974) basic elements of behavioral self-control: self-observation, environmental planning, and behavioral programming. Regardless of semantics, the foundation of self-management procedures resides with behavioral specification, identification of behavioral antecedents and consequences, and intervention strategies altering these contingencies.

Permeating conceptualizations and research supporting self-management is an emphasis on covert actions. Bandura (1971a), for example, suggests that the way people perceive, anticipate, and evaluate events dictates external environmental influences. Within this context, covert responses are amenable to change much as are overt responses. The veracity of this assertion is well documented by empirical investigations and case studies substantiating the importance of cognitions in self-regulatory behavior (Meichenbaum, 1977; Mahoney, 1974; and Meichenbaum & Cameron, 1974).

That complex cognitive processes mediate and influence sexual response patterns (Geer & Fuhr, 1977; McCarthy, 1977; Masters & Johnson, 1966) suggests the necessity of applying self-management procedures to internal events and to overt sexual behavior. Certainly, most investigators in the area of sexual counseling have long recognized relationships between cognitive processes and sexual functioning. Masters and Johnson (1970), for example, declare cognitions to be a primary factor in sexual dysfunciton: "It should be restated that fear of inadequacy is the greatest known deterrant to effective sexual functioning, simply because it so completely distracts the fearful individual from his or her natural responsiveness by blocking reception of sexual stimuli, either created by or reflected from the sexual partner" (12-13). This clinical research team repeatedly emphasizes negative effects of self-administered cognitions related to particular stimuli, faulty monitoring processes, and perceived adverse consequences. Labels—such as "performance fears," "spectatoring," "anxiety" "sensate blockage," and "goal orientation," and various sexual myths, misconceptions, and prejudices—have been assigned to such self-administered internal states and their negative effects documented (Masters & Johnson, 1970). For Hartman and Fithian (1974) the import of cognitions is limited to effects of negative body image on sexual expression. Combining cognitive restructuring procedures with imagery exercises to change body concepts, these experts also advise post-hypnotic suggestion for managing performance anxiety. Kaplan (1974), however, recognizing the importance of cognitive processes in sexual dysfunctioning, emphasizes only need for counselors to employ analytic strategies to bring unconscious material into cognitive awareness.

Although discussion of cognitive processes has begun to appear in recent clinical literature (Zilbergeld, 1978; Heiman, LoPiccolo, & LoPiccolo, 1976; Lobitz & LoPiccolo, 1972), far more specific procedural guidelines are provided for self-management of overt sexual behavior than of internal states. For example, detailed instructions such as sensate focus exercises, the squeeze technique, and body positioning, have all been suggested for altering sexual responses. Addressing cognitive components of sexual dysfunction, Masters and Johnson (1970) suggest that thorough explanations of the spectator role, performance anxiety, and goal orientations are in themselves sufficient to modify accompanying negative cognitions, and attention will be diverted from self-evaluative cognitions to the immediacy of interaction simply by engaging in prescribed behavioral processes. Similarly, Kaplan (1974) assumes that sexually problematic behaviors are functional because they manifest unresolved and unrecognized inner conflicts. Sexual dysfunctions are then to be alleviated either by relying on behavioral prescriptions bypassing internal processes or by ego-analytic strategies to uncover repressed impulses and unresolved conflicts. Procedural guidelines for the latter action are left unspecified and assumed in each worker's clinical repertoire.

Even though the published literature emphasizes the interplay between overt behavior and covert cognitions in sexual functioning, clinical procedures have been targeted primarily to the former; thus, the intervention reported here was developed and tested to redress these deficiencies. The case study presented below is illustrative of the assessment, data collection, intervention, and evaluation of covert cognitions in sexual treatment.

CASE STUDY

Clients

Mr. and Mrs. L—aged thirty-nine and thirty-five, married for twelve years with two sons—were referred to the agency by their physician because of Mr. L's erectile failure and Mrs. L's increasing inability to reach orgasm. From the beginning of their marriage, the L's sexual relationship had been less than satisfactory. Mrs. L experienced orgasms infrequently through husband's manual manipulations due to his increasing difficulties in obtaining and maintaining an erection. Mr. L was becoming more insistent that his wife become orgasmic with each sexual encounter. Mr. L stated that it was highly arousing for him to "give his wife an orgasm," and that if such did not occur he felt inadequate, guilty, and usually lost his erection. The couple had previously sought remediation through two other clinical programs. The first focused on marital communication; although helpful, the program did not specifically address the L's sexual problems. The second consisted of ten sessions apparently based on Masters and Johnson's (1970) therapeutic procedures. It is of interest that the couple—Mr. L particularly—seemed well versed in concepts of distractibility, performance anxiety, and spectatoring; however, they continued experiencing sexual distress.

Intervention

Intervention was delivered in four phases by a male social worker with extensive clinical and research experience in human sexuality. For descriptive purposes, these phases are presented sequentially; in practice, intervention is rarely so systematic. A flexible stance must be maintained to apply varying combinations of each phase, consistent with immediate and dynamic practice needs. Intervention also involved a research design with repeated measures. Such procedures were adapted from Meichenbaum's (1977) format of systematic data collection, cognitive modeling, graduated tasks, directed mediational training, and self-reinforcement for cognitive self-management. Each procedure is defined and described in the context of four intervention phases: I. Role Induction; II. Baseline; III. Intervention; and, IV. Maintenance and Follow-Up.

PHASE I: ROLE INDUCTION (One session, Mr. and Mrs. L interviewed jointly.) Often overlooked, role induction is crucial in preparing clients for active involvement in change. Because clients experiencing sexual distress have undoubtedly engaged in a number of negative mediating processes (thoughts), they may enter sexual counseling with self-defeating ideas. Generally, clients fall into two categories: those recognizing that uncontrolled thoughts are themselves sources of sexual dysfunction; and those aware of thoughts impeding performance and enjoyment, but feeling helpless to manage cognitions. The objective of role induction is to arrive at a mutual conceptualization of problems linking negative mediating processes to specific sexual dysfunctions. This objective can be accomplished either through a didactic educational approach relying heavily on worker status and expertise (Masters & Johnson, 1970), or more indirectly, by client and worker conjointly arriving at an inclusive definition of the problem. We prefer the latter approach, characterized by a non-authoritarian worker style, increased specificity and full exploration of cognitive processes (Meichenbaum, 1976), active client participation in data collection and assessment procedures, and cognitive and behavioral assignments both in-session and at home. The following dialogue illustrates role induction procedures with the L's.

Mrs. L: In answer to your question, I guess I don't feel as aroused as I used to...I just don't get turned on and if I do, it seems I have to work so hard. When we are having sex or when I masturbate I don't understand what is happening to me.

Worker: It's understandable that you are fearful and confused—as you must be, Ed. Sexual arousal or "turning on," involves physical and emotional tension exciting in themselves and essential for orgasm. Arousal is not simply vaginal lubrication, nor is it other physical processes, pulse rate, muscle tension, wet palms, tingling sensation throughout the body. These physical signs are influenced by feelings and thoughts, either of the situation, the circumstances, your partner or yourself.

Mrs. L: I still think there is something wrong with me. Nothing has really changed in my life and it didn't use to be so hard or so important.

Mr. L (to worker): I agree with you. Sometimes I think it's all in here (pointing to his head). I know my thoughts are my worst enemy. I keep thinking, will I get a hard on, how long will it take, and if I do can I keep it? What is Shirley thinking now? Why can't I give her what she wants or is it only what I want?

Worker (nodding agreement to Ed, then turning to Shirley): Previously, Shirley, you managed to become aroused most of the time, but now if you don't get aroused when you or Ed thinks you should, do you start thinking you are frigid or inadequate?

Mrs. L: Well, Yes! Wouldn't anyone who experiences this?

Worker: I wonder if it is these fears—that many people have at one time or another—that are making you two lose confidence in your own sexuality and putting you at the mercy of forces or thoughts you don't think you control?

Mrs. L: Well, I know I am reluctant to get involved in sex or show any emotion because I am scared it won't work. Even now, since we failed before, I'm not the one pushing for counseling again.

Worker: Let's stop right here. Your last comment in itself is a real sexual turn off. We all know that certain thoughts may be highly arousing. Is the thought "I'm scared it won't work" a turn on for you?

Mrs. L: Of course not!

Worker: Is the statement you give yourself "I wonder what Shirley is thinking now, when I'm working so hard to get an erection," arousing to you Ed?

Mr. L (shrugs and sighs): I've known all along it is in my head! But knowing doesn't help much—in fact, it may be making the problem worse.

Worker: I wonder if these are the only negative thoughts getting in the way of your sexual enjoyment. A first step in solving this problem is to find out how many, what kind of, under what circumstances, and how often such thoughts get in your way. As we go along, I will be giving you a number of assignments—some completed here, some at home—designed to help you understand what sexual activities, thoughts, feelings, and circumstances contribute to the current situation. These assignments will also give us information on how you can best accomplish what you want.

Mrs. L: I think I understand; but getting back to what you said first, are you saying that thoughts I have are preventing me from enjoying sex and getting an orgasm?

Worker: Precisely; and in our sessions together, you, Ed, and I will be working on managing the thoughts that prevent you from enjoying each other.

Here, the L's begin to meet Phase I's objectives by verbally acknowledging mediating processes in sexual functioning. Throughout intervention, practitioners need to reconfirm clients' acceptance of cognitive components in sexual activity.

Other procedures in Phase I include readings and in-session and home assignments. In-session assignments involve clients generating lists of sexually arousing thoughts—sexual fantasies, forbidden sexual pleasures, and practices. Lists are then compared with negative self-statements noted by worker and client.

Attributes of arousal and the extent to which nonarousing thoughts control behavior are explained and modeled during Phase I. Modeling may take the form of worker self-disclosure and sharing the negative statements of others who have experienced sexual distress. Home assignments are given to further help client acceptance of the import of cognitions on sexual activity.

Client in-session verbalizations supporting effects of self-statements on sexual behavior are monitored. A second indicator of self-statement effects on sexual behavior is derived from Cognitive Behavior (CBR) Forms. Figure One presents data on Mrs. L's in-session verbalizations of thoughts affecting sexual behavior. Showing an increase in self-statements, data indicated Mrs. L's continued acceptance of the importance of self-statements. Substantial increases followed sessions two and three when the worker explained cognitive processes, and again across three through nine when intervention focused on cognitive self-management procedures.

Compliance in record keeping is an index of task orientation and the extent to which clients self-manage behavior and cognitions. Increased compliance with record keeping and homework assignments is achieved through an explicit contractual agreement involving forfeiture of monetary deposit for noncompliance (Welch, 1979). Clinical data suggest low frequency of verbal statements and disparities between behavioral and cognitive components in daily log-keeping may indicate cognitions are being excluded from the definition of sexual distress.

PHASE II: BASELINE (Mr. and Mrs. L seen individually for two hourly sessions.) In baselining, worker and clients collect data for behavioral and cognitive functional assessment. The latter aspect is in the tradition of the former but includes sequential ordering of the clients' thought processes preceding, accompanying, and following behavioral performance. Clients' thoughts or self-statements are crucial in developing cognitive and behavioral skills regarding sexual interaction. In short, assessment focuses on the why, how, and what of behavior; according to Meichenbaum (1977), assessment is an inventory of cognitive strategies.

Throughout the interview, the worker models and provides discrimination training for clients to identify incompatible, self-depreciating, distracting, anxiety-producing, and inhibiting cognitive processes in sexual activities. Questions elicit specific behavioral

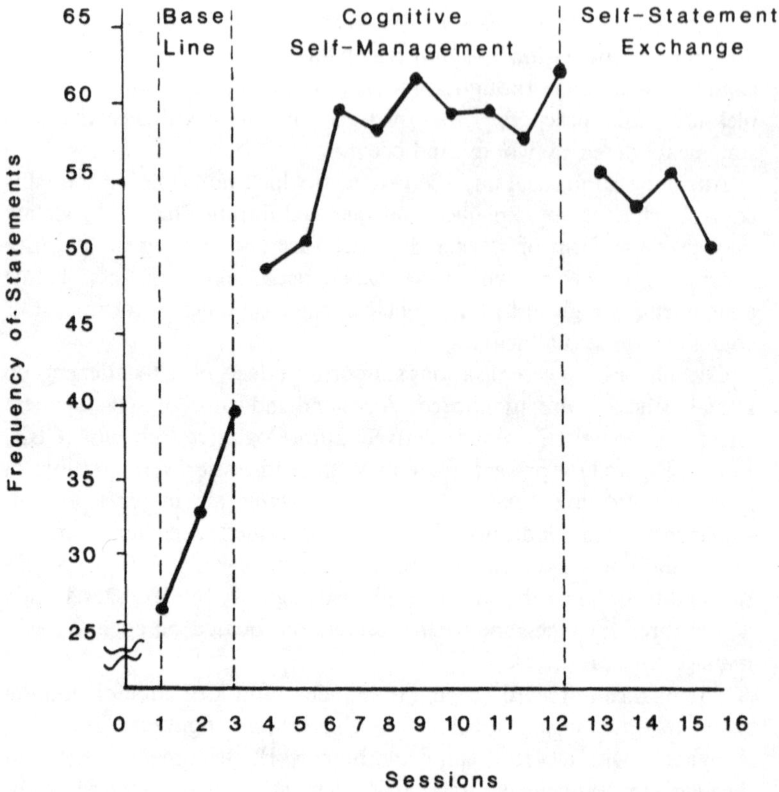

FIGURE 1. Frequency of Mrs. L's In-Session Statements Affecting Sexual Behavior.

information, and clients are taught to attend to self-statements intervening between sexual stimulation and behavior. On days when sexual activity occurs, clients are asked to note the activity, identify the range of related cognitions, give a numerical rating for pleasure derived from the activity, and determine whether accompanying self-statements contribute to or distract from arousal.

Attempting to quantify self-observations of covert behavior has raised questions related to reactivity, observer characteristics, reliability, and validity (Lipinski, Black, Nelson, & Ciminero, 1975; Jeffrey, 1974; Mahoney, 1972). A crucial issue is whether internal behavior can be accurately and repeatedly measured without being affected by the measurement procedures or instruments. Since individuals are not usually the most accurate observers of their own behavior, they are trained in discrimination and systematic data collection. Objectivity is enhanced by modeling, immediate feedback, and reinforcement for accuracy (Thoresen & Mahoney, 1974). Such techniques and use of the Reliability Enhancement Package (Bornstein, Hamilton, Carmody, Rychtarik, & Veraldi, 1977) help increase client self-report veracity.

Specific techniques include asking clients to close their eyes, reconstruct a recent sexual behavior sequence, and verbalize accompanying self-statements. For clients having difficulty, the Sexual Self-Statement Inventory (Duehn & Mayadas, 1978) is either formally administered or used as stimulus material. The SSSI is designed to identify negative and positive self-statements and the frequency of their occurrence. Below are negative examples from the 100-item inventory. 1. I'm supposed to engage in this sexual behavior which I don't really like. 2. My breasts are mishaped, I don't want him to look at them. 3. I am aware of his/her unpleasant body odor. 4. I hope I can hold my erection. 5. If this movement continues, I know I'll come too soon. 6. I wonder what s/he is thinking right now. 7. Is s/he pretending to be enjoying this?

Homework assignments are also given and serve as additional resources for behavioral-cognitive analysis, underscoring the import of self-statements in sexual dysfunctions. Using CBR forms, clients note duration, degree of satisfaction (on a 1 to 7 scale), accompanying self-statements, and arousal value of self-statements (+ or -) for each sexual activity. CBR data are maintained by clients throughout intervention, providing ongoing feedback on various techniques. Clients are instructed to complete CBR forms at their convenience, relying largely on recall. Figure Two shows a typical CBR form for Mrs. L during an early stage of therapy.

Additional assessment includes administering the Sexual Interaction Inventory (LoPiccolo & Steger, 1974). Quantifying a range of heterosexual interactions, the SII elicits responses on frequency, preference, and pleasure ratings for seventeen sexual activities. Each dimension is then summed across the seventeen activities and graphically displayed. Through in-session instruction, audiotapes, and home assignments, clients also initiate Bernstein and Borkovec's (1973) relaxation training.

PHASE III: INTERVENTION A (Separate weekly appointments for Mr. and Mrs. L; Mrs. L, nine sessions, Mr. L, eight sessions.) This phase helps develop alternative arousing self-statements likely to initiate desired sexual behaviors. Formulating alternative self-statements is a joint client-worker undertaking. Initially, workers model self-statement construction and provide major input on content. In home assignments, clients generate additional self-statements to accompany each existing or desired sexual behavior. Baseline information is helpful in constructing

Excerpts from Mrs. L's Cognitive-Behavioral Record (CBR) Form

Sexual Activity	Duration	Degree of Satisfaction 1234567	Self-Statements	Non-Arousing (-) Arousing (=)
Touches my ears, arms, neck, thighs, and breasts in living room while watching TV. I have arms around Ed and nestle close.	30 min.	3	This feels good.	+
			I haven't had a chance to relax all day.	+
			Ed really knows me very well.	+
			I wish we could always feel so close.	+
			I like my arms touched.	+
			I hope Ed likes it when I hold him.	-
			He's touching my legs, I wonder what's next?	-
			Here we go again, I knew it, he's touching my breasts.	-
			Too many commercials on TV. I really shouldn't be spending time here, with laundry to be done.	-
			His touch seems matter of fact—he's not into it.	-
(In bed) Ed holds me and caresses my clitoris.	10 min. Too long!	2	I'm floating.	+
			This feels so good	+
			He's going too fast.	-
			This is becoming irritating.	-
			Should I tell him?	-
			Now that I've told him he looks hurt—I feel guilty.	-
			I'm taking too much time.	-
			Why can't I come?	-
			He must be disgusted with me.	-
			It used to be so easy.	-
			It hurts.	-
			Now this is better.	+
			Sometimes, I don't think Ed listens or cares. He's doing exactly what I told him not to do!	-
			How can I tell him again?	-

FIGURE 2

alternative self-statements, but direct conversion of each statement to its opposite form may be an over-simplification and therapeutically misdirected. Thus, consistent with Bandura's (1971b) and Marston's (1964) contention that clients' internal dialogues are frequently polarized—i.e. viewing self as totally sexually inadequate, and then constructing alternative self-statements of unattainable and idealized sexual performance—workers provide numerous examples of positive and realistic self-statements. When at least twenty alternative self-statements have been generated by each partner, self-management procedures begin.

Following Meichenbaum's (1977) guidelines and empirical evidence supporting self-instruction training (Sarason, 1973; Tori & Worell, 1973; Bem, 1967), self-statement management emphasizes cognitive modeling, graduated tasks and directed mediational training, and self-reinforcement. Operationally, these procedures occur as follows:

Cognitive modeling: Conjointly with progressive relaxation exercisees, clients visualize a sexual activity while worker reads newly constructed alternative self-statements.

Graduated tasks and directed mediational training: Subsequent to cognitive modeling, clients instruct themselves aloud while visualizing a sexual activity. This procedure is repeated with clients whispering, and then silently thinking self-statements.

Self-reinforcement: Workers model self-reinforcement, rewarding client efforts for positive self-evaluation.

Client involvement in these procedures has a number of benefits. Active participation provides detailed scripts for initiating and engaging in self-statements congruent with sexual activities. By focusing on discrete sexual activities and managing self-statements, a process-oriented cognitive model is developed. Involvement further helps clients construct reliably based self-statements. Finally, clients increase sources and frequency of self-reinforcement and reinforcement from partners.

Once clients master self-management procedures, they practice them separately or in combination with selected sexual activities. Clients are taught to handle persistent negative self-statements with thought stopping—covert instruction stopping incompatible self-statements—or with coping self-statements constructed for particular sexual activities.

PHASE III: INTERVENTION B (Four conjoint, weekly appointments with Mr. and Mrs. L.) When CBR data indicate an increase in performance self-statements and arousal levels, joint appointments are scheduled. This decision is based on experience indicating that individuals derive maximum benefit from conjoint exchanges after learning self-management.

In the first session, workers again review the impact of self-statements on sexual functioning. This provides a rationale for verbal exchange of sexually arousing self-statements. In explaining the rationale, workers sanction and model the range of mental activities, imageries, self-statements, and fantasies that are as significant in sexual response as is cardiovascular functioning. Covert activities are acceptable and normal components of sexual functioning. Just as sexual behavior is selective and situation specific, so are cognitive and affective activities. In practice, couples exchange only self-statements contributing to mutual sexual satisfaction.

Within the session, partners read aloud and discuss self-statements reflecting positive evaluations of their own and their partner's sexual contribution. At home, couples read aloud CBR forms, give feedback on self-statements eliciting positive reactions, and provide corrective information on self-depreciating statements. Individuals are reinforced for positive self-statements and learn to recognize these as erotic stimuli. During sexual activity, statements become part of the sexual behavioral repertoire. The procedure also allows for feedback when the partner's positive evaluation of sexual contribution is at variance with persisting negative self-statements. Workers continue to monitor results of these exchanges throughout counseling.

To keep emphasis on client self-management, the final intervention sessions are directed toward maintenance. Workers assist couples in evaluating and planning the behavioral and cognitive self-management program. Clients become their own therapists. They plan homework assignments, list behavior and self-statements contributing to positive interactions, identify behavioral and cognitive changes, and outline intervention procedures for coping with possible problem recurrence.

PHASE IV: MAINTENANCE AND FOLLOW-UP (Conjoint appointments with Mr. and Mrs. L. at one, three, and six month intervals following Phase III.) Couples are seen periodically for ongoing monitoring of change maintenance and evaluation. They bring completed CBR forms to each session. They also return to self-statement management procedures should a sexual concern recur. The Sexual Interaction Inventory (LoPiccolo & Steger, 1974) is administered at each follow-up session.

Satisfaction ratings of sexual activities and percentage of positive self-statements for Mr. and Mrs. L are presented in Figure Three. Each data point represents the mean of all sexual activities recorded during a particular day for satisfaction ratings and positive self-statements. The percentage of positive self-statements was calculated from CBR forms by dividing total negative and positive self-statements by the number of positive statements and multiplying by 100.

Data collected by Mr. and Mrs. L during baseline indicate surprisingly

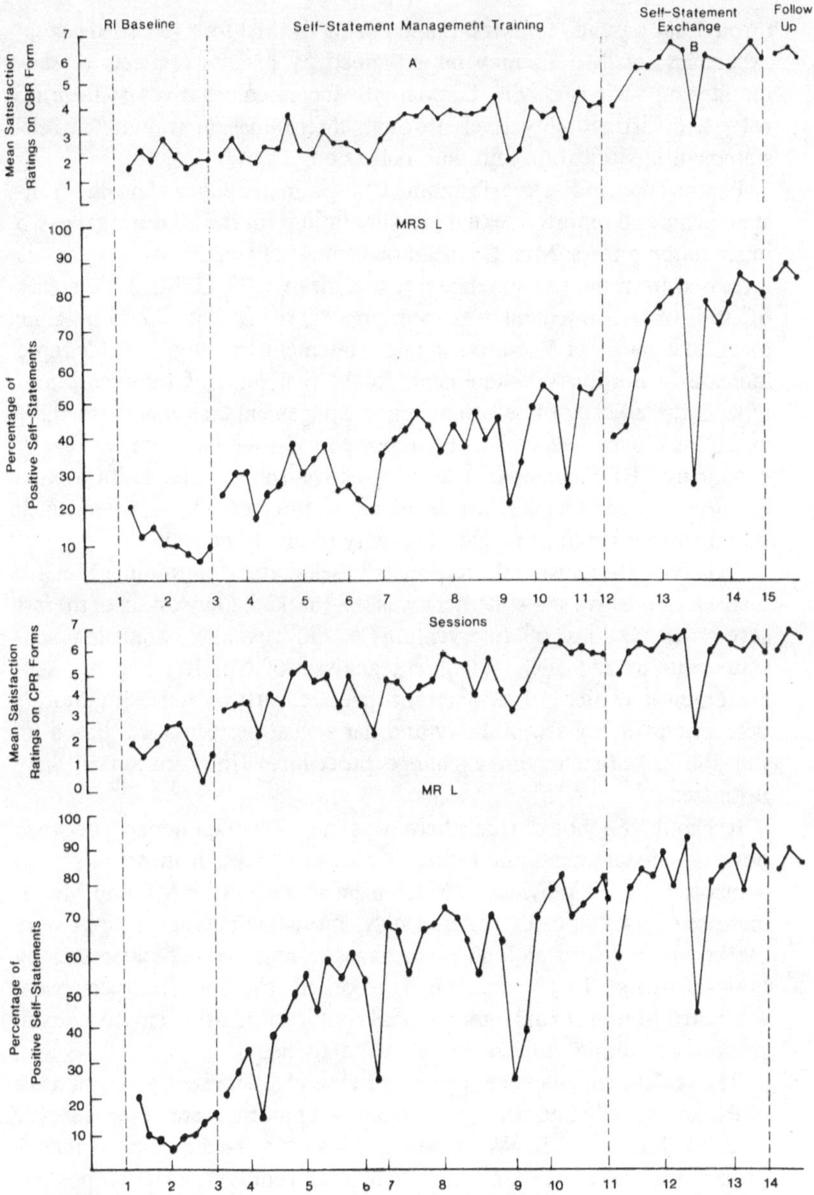

FIGURE 3. Percentage of Positive Self-Statement and Mean Satisfaction Ratings for Mr. and Mrs. L.

similar low pleasure ratings of sexual activities (Mr. L, M = 2.0; Mrs. L, M = 1.9) and low percentage of positive self-statements (Mr. L, M = 12.45; Mrs. L, M = 12.40). These data represent recorded self-statements of sexual activities for eight days over a two-week baseline period. Percentage decrease in positive self-statements, consistently occurring throughout baseline for Mrs. L and during the first four recorded sexual exchanges for Mr. L, may be explained by reactivity effects of self-monitoring—Mr. and Mrs. L apparently increased negative spectatoring roles and distractibility levels through discrimination training in self-statement identification and data collection.

Figure Three indicates substantial changes in frequency of positive self-statements and reported sexual pleasure ratings for the L's during the two intervention phases: Mrs. L's mean percentage of positive self-statements increased from the 12.4 baseline rate to a mean of 38.43; Mr. L's increase of positive self-statement was even greater, rising from 12.45 baseline mean to a mean of 57.54, during self-statement training. Mr. L's rapid increase in positive self-statements in the first third of Intervention A reflects the efficacy of self-statement management training. With three exceptions, over half of Mr. L's reported self-statements were sexually enhancing. His increased use of positive self-statements in sexual activities is seen in the last segment of Intervention A where such statements occurred at a rate of seventy to eighty percent.

Relative to her husband's responses to self-statement training, Mrs. L's increase of positive self-statement was less marked. Only on six of the last seven observations of Intervention A did sexually enhancing self-statements exceed 50%. A content analysis of Mrs. L's negative self-statements indicated consistent preoccupation with husband's perceptions of her acceptability and her sexual performance. Based on the above, self-statement exchange procedures (Intervention B) were instigated.

It should be noted that there was high correspondence between positive self-statements and ratings of pleasure derived from actual sexual activities for both individuals. Mean pleasure ratings for Mr. and Mrs. L increased to 4.8 and 3.1. Interestingly, most low pleasure ratings were marked by a return of high percentages of negative self-statements by both partners. Low percentages recorded by both partners were attributed to non-sexual interpersonal conflicts and other environmental pressures resulting in decreased sexual activities.

The self-statement exchange procedure is characterized by an increase of enhancing self-statement ($M = 70.38$) and reported rate of pleasure ($M = 5.80$) for Mrs. L. With instigation of self-statement exchange procedures there was an immediate and rapid increase in positive enhancing self-statements. In this period, Mrs. L more than doubled her rate of self-administered enhancing cognitions.

Gains occurring in Intervention B may be attributed to husband's shared self-statements serving as corrective feedback on Mrs. L's negative self-statements, interpersonal modeling for constructing arousing self-statements, and positive reinforcement of Mrs. L's sexual behavior. Whereas Mr. L's increases were made during the self-statement training phase, his reported percentage of enhancing self-statements (*M* = 8.13) and pleasure ratings (*M* = 6.07), with one exception, remained at a high level. Follow-up interviews at one, three, and six months indicated that the couple maintained high percentages of desired self-statements and reported pleasure ratings.

Sexual Interaction Inventory (SII) profile scores at preintervention, postintervention, and six-month follow-up are presented in Figure Four. SII scores changed in the desired direction and in some cases improved by more than three standard deviations. Combined for both partners, preintervention profiles indicate a considerable degree of sexual dissatisfaction, particularly on frequency and range of sexual behavior (scales one and two), self-acceptance (scales three and four), and pleasure derived from the sexual activity (scales five and six). The high degree of rated displeasure for both Mr. and Mrs. L (scales five and six) is consistent with low self-reported pleasure ratings on CBR forms. Each partner perceived self as having little knowledge of the other's sexual preference (scales seven and eight). Only in areas of acceptance of partner's sexuality, did Mr. and Mrs. L's preintervention scores fall within one standard deviation of sexually undistressed couples. Postintervention and six-month follow-up scores on the SII indicated increased sexual satisfaction on all scales, clustering along standard mean scores of fifty.

Results presented thus far have focused on the successful management of self-statements and thoughts; but, such findings would have little value if not associated with gains in sexual behavior. Thus, behavioral data were collected before, during, and after intervention. Presented in Table One, these data showed positive changes throughout intervention and follow-up.

DISCUSSION

The case material presented in this chapter illustrates cognitive management of sexual dysfunction. The rationale for managing self-statements was based on assessment data indicating that distracting and other negative spectatoring processes rather than behavioral deficits were primary sources of sexual distress. Managing self-statements and self-statement exchange were effective in increasing cognitions compatible with successful sexual activity. This approach systematically identified, measured, and altered cognitive targets during intervention. Within the field there is agreement that sexual problems are a function of individual cognitions (negative sex attitudes, lack of information, unrealistic expectations, performance anxieties, misinformation, preoccupations, and irrational fears) and communication failures. Unfortunately, self-statement management and interpersonal exchange of self-statements have received little clinical or research attention. As a result the literature

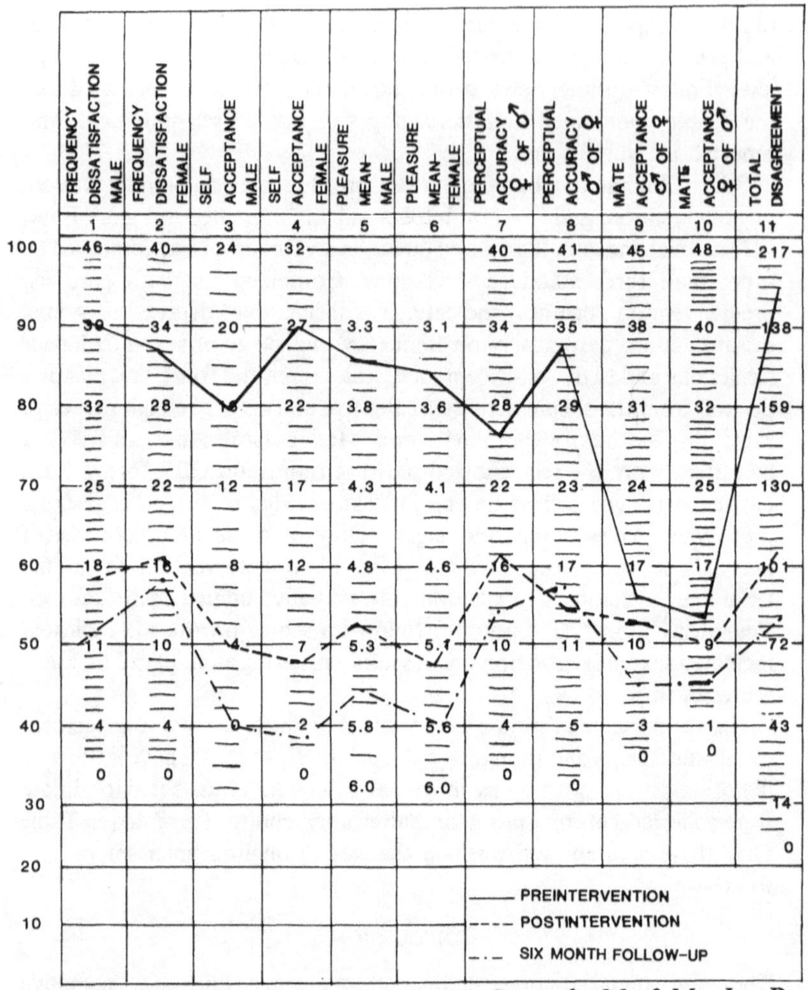

FIGURE 4. Sexual Interaction Inventory Scores for Mr. & Mrs. L at Pre and Postintervention and six month Follow Up.

has emphasized technologies directed primarily toward behavioral intervention.

Cognitive self-management is not intended to be applied apart from the more traditional behavioral approaches or unilaterally to all individuals. Instead, we advocate highly individualized, problem-specific intervention, leaving choices open and contingent on assessment of presenting problems and ongoing feedback of intervention efficacy. Workers are thus cautioned against applying the monolithic intervention packages as outlined by Masters and Johnson (1970), Kaplan (1974), or the present chapter. In short, empirically based practice stresses

Table 1
Preintervention, Postintervention and Follow-Up Sexual Behavior Data on Mr. and Mrs. L

	Pre-Intervention	**Post-Intervention**	**Six Month Follow-Up**
Frequency of Intercourse	Twice Monthly	3-4 Times Weekly	3 Times Weekly
Frequency of Sexual Activities (Excluding Intercourse and Self-Stimulation)	0	Twice Weekly	Twice Weekly
Reported Percentage of Female Orgasm Through Genital Self-Stimulation	20	100	100
Reported Percentage of Female Orgasm Through Partner Non-Coital Stimulation	20	80	100
Reported Percentage of Female Orgasm in Coitus		50	75
Reported Percentage of Erection Sufficient for Sustaining Coitus		80	90

sequencing of objectives in the continuing process of assessment, modification, and evaluation.

Past literature has focused on negative effects of selected cognitions related to sexual functioning. Particularly, spectatoring has come to have negative connotations with deleterious effects. Case study findings reported here indicate that spectatoring need not have adverse consequences; indeed, content analysis of CBR forms showed spectatoring as arousing, with potentially positive and enhancing effects. Research needs to examine the extent to which such arousing and positive cognitions are present in sexually well functioning individuals. Work by the present investigators (Duehn & Mayadas, 1978) suggests that spectatoring may be inherent in sexual activities and only when cognitions take on a negative evaluation component are they dysfunctional. Further, self-statements' exchanges procedures provide a structured format for additional sources of sexually enhancing stimuli, corrective feedback, cognitive models for self-disclosure and reinforcement.

Benefits result from clients recording their own sexual activities. Self-observation gives clients repeated opportunities to redefine problems in manageable terms. Clients recognize that thought sequences have antecedents, follow predictable patterns and have consequences. Clients are active in the intervention process, eventually becoming their own assessors, data collectors, and intervention planners. They also grow less dependent on their workers, accepting responsibility for intervention outcome and continued maintenance of change. Clients self-observations provide valuable feedback on motivation and continued cooperation. Finally, content from recorded self-observations serves as assessment data. In-depth content analysis helps identify negative evaluation themes and suggests directions for intervention. For example, if client self-statements reflect a negative body image, behavioral procedures altering body concepts may be indicated (Barbach, 1975; Graber-Kline & Graber, 1975; Hartman & Fithian, 1974).

Self-observation and self-statement monitoring are not without limitations. Inherent definitional problems are involved in self-recorded data on covert events. Self-statements are continuous; distinctions between where one self-statement ends and another begins are arbitrary and dependent upon subjective judgment. Because clients are not reliable observers of their own behavior (Jeffrey, 1974; Kanfer & Karoly, 1974; Kazdin, 1974d), they need specific instructions in objective data collection. Self-observation requires recalling recent overt and covert behavior—frequently filtered and distorted. Accuracy checks are made through repeated completion of CBR forms. Initially, clients may resist self-observation recording, stating that it inhibits sexual activity and requires too much time and energy; as negative self-statements are supplanted by sexually enhancing ones, however, this assignment becomes reinforcing—particularly when associated with increased arousal and sexual performance.

Despite promising outcomes of self-statement management, specific effects need to be isolated and tested. Although the clinical steps of self-management were highlighted here, differential intervention effects, progressive relaxation, worker behavior, client and worker characteristics, were not controlled. Practice dictates that self-statement management procedures be combined with other techniques. Current research is underway to examine separate components of our program.

Introducing self-management procedures into social work practice stresses the import of cognitions in cuing, altering, acquiring, and maintaining behavior. Since self-management is individual and requires clinical expertise in delivery, it challenges stereotypic notions that behavioral intervention is simplistic and mechanistic. In summary, the scope of behavioral intervention is being expanded to address internal cognitive events and external environments—a promising direction compatible with competent social work.

11
Control of Addictions

Betty J. Blythe

Despite extensive and increasingly well documented risks, millions of Americans persist in jeopardizing their lives by smoking cigarettes, abusing alcohol, and maintaining excess weight. For example, fifty-four million men and women smoked 615 billion cigarettes in 1978 (Department of Health, Education, and Welfare, U.S. Public Health Service 1979). In addition to damaging their own health (Department of Health, Education, and Welfare, U.S. Public Health Service 1972, 1973, 1979), smokers harm unborn (Greenwood 1979; Quigley, Sheehan, Wilkes, & Yen, 1979) and living children (Lebowitz & Burrows 1976), and nonsmokers, especially those suffering chronic cardiovascular and pulmonary disease (Department of Health, Education, and Welfare, U.S. Public Health Service 1979). Moreover, smoking's impact on society is registered in other ways. Smoking-related medical care, accidents, absenteeism, and lost work cost this country an estimated seventeen billion dollars each year. Overall, more than ten percent of all hospital and medical expenses are tobacco-related, thereby raising the price of health insurance and taxpayer-supported health programs (Department of Health, Educaiton, and Welfare, U.S. Public Health Service 1977).

Estimates of alcohol abuse are equally arresting. Although the National Institute on Alcohol Abuse and Alcoholism estimates that ten million U.S. problem drinkers manifest alcohol-related disabilities, another fifteen million men and women report that they drink too much (Noble 1978). Certainly, heavy alcohol use causes severe physical and psychological problems; moderate intake is hazardous when combined with other drugs and can lead to alcohol dependence (Noble 1978). Even slight alcohol consumption during pregnancy can cause birth defects, developmental disability, and mental retardation (Clarren & Smith 1978). Social, economic, and emotional problems for drinkers, their families, friends, employers, and others are considerable (Byles 1978; Noble 1978). Further, authorities estimate fifty to seventy-five percent of all automobile accident deaths and injuries are associated with alcohol (Knowles 1977). As a final indication of the extent of its toll, the seventh leading cause of death in the U.S. is cirrhosis of the liver, a disease resulting from excessive intake of alcohol (Thomas 1977).

Along with cigarette smoking and alcohol abuse, obesity is a major health problem. Gaining an average one to two pounds a year from ages twenty to fifty, Americans are heavier than citizens of any other major country (Farquhar 1978). Approximately eighty million Americans are sufficiently overweight (twenty or more pounds) to reduce life expectancy (Knowles 1977). In 1975 alone, 1,109 persons in every 100,000 in the U.S. population died prematurely because of obesity (Thomas 1977). Hull (1979) reports data estimating the average loss of life expectancy at 337 days for overweight males and 470 days for overweight females. Specific disabilities experienced by the overweight include hypertension, diabetes mellitus, heart and gall bladder diseases, emotional maladjustment, loneliness, social problems, and job-related discrimination (Mayer 1968; Rimm & White 1977).

Obesity is more prevalent than cigarette smoking and alcohol abuse, perhaps because harmful habits are formed at an early age and reinforced throughout childhood and adolescence. Thus, parents encourage infants and youths to eat more than necessary, advertisements promote fattening foods, and our life-styles become increasingly sedentary. At present, the odds against an overweight adolescent becoming an average weight adult are estimated at twenty-eight to one (Coates & Thoresen 1978).

Although few people wish to damage their health by excessive smoking, drinking, or eating, self-directed attempts to control addictive behavior are not often successful. Some people turn to the medical profession for help; but doctors are ill prepared to assist patients in changing habits. Others consult social workers, counselors, and psychologists; unfortunately, human services professionals have had to rely on ineffective, traditional therapies (Lovibond 1977; Schinke, Blythe, & Doueck 1978; Stevenson 1978).

Recently, behavioral interventions derived from social-learning theory have shown promising results. This chapter reviews current behavioral methods for assessing and treating addictive behaviors. A description of a clinically evaluated, smoking-reduction group provides a case example. Issues of special concern to practitioners conclude the chapter.

ASSESSMENT STRATEGIES

The first step in helping clients control addictive behavior involves selecting appropriate assessment strategies, which must serve the following functions: 1) determining whether the client actually has a smoking, drinking, or eating problem; 2) measuring the extent of the problem; 3) selecting the appropriate intervention; and 4) evaluating the outcome of intervention. Tools for assessing addictive behavior encompass self-report, physiological, and behavioral measures. The following discussion describes each measure as it relates to problems of smoking, drinking, and eating.

Self-Report Measures

Self-report measures require that clients record their smoking, drinking, or eating patterns. In addition to revealing how much the client engages in addictive behavior, self-report data collected prior to intervention provide both therapist and client valuable information about environmental stimuli and rewards controlling the behavior. This is crucial in planning effective intervention. Figure One depicts a form smokers can wrap around their cigarette packs to collect data about each smoking incident. Producing more extentive information, Marlatt's nineteen-page Drinking Profile (1975) renders a behavioral outline of drinking preferences, rates, patterns, settings, and reinforcers. The instrument provides relevant pretreatment information and may be administered to assess treatment outcome. Stuart and Davis's Daily Eating Record (1972) helps dieters identify where, what, with whom, and when they eat.

Although addictive behavior interventions often rely on self-report data (Beneke & Paulsen 1979; Bowman, Stein, & Newton 1975; Hay, Hay, & Nelson 1977), self-reports of smoking, drinking, or eating patterns may be somewhat inaccurate. Some clients may not take the time to record data precisely; others may exaggerate their progress to please therapists or to keep pace with group members. Nevertheless, several studies support the reliability and validity of self-reports (Cautela & Upper 1976; Katz, Heiman, & Gordon 1977; Sobell, Maisto, Sobell, & Cooper, 1979). Moreover, self-report records are economical and provide clients with immediate feedback. Corroborative reports from family, friends, or other professionals who have contact with the client can frequently enhance self-report data (Miller 1977), although client consent should be obtained before seeking such reports (Schinke in press a).

Physiological Measures

Physiological measures vary widely in cost, intrusiveness, ease of access,

Form for Recording Self-Reported Cigarette Smoking

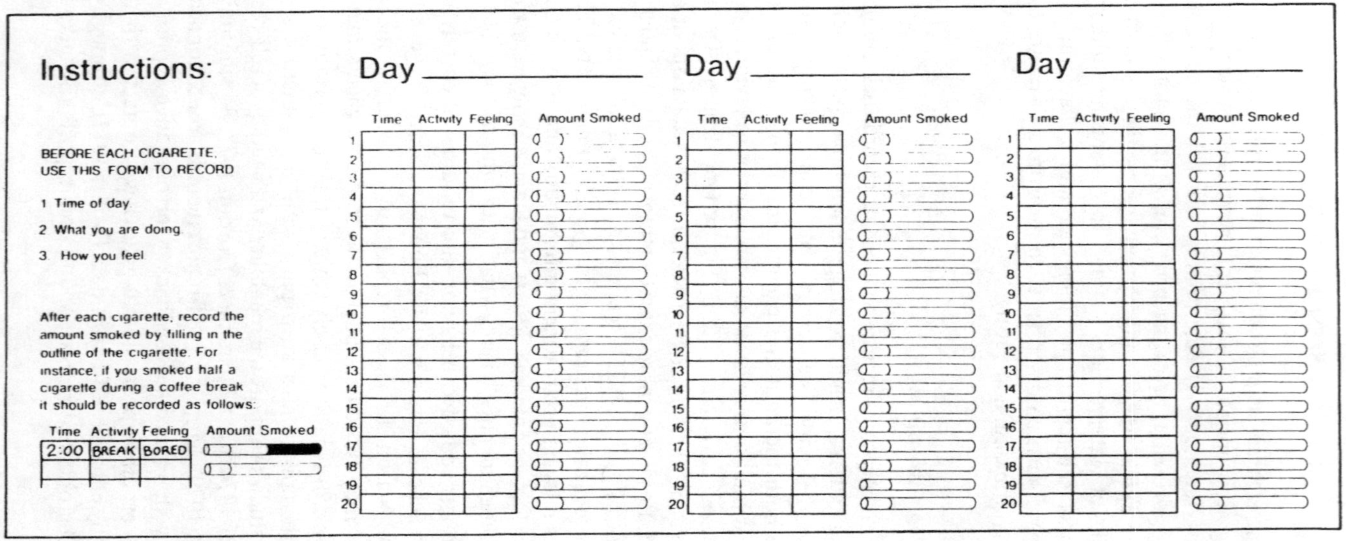

FIGURE 1.

technology required, and reliability. In work with smokers, measurements of carbon monoxide, nicotine, and thiocyanate have been tested. Carbon monoxide concentrations can be measured in breath samples or blood samples. The former are easier and less traumatic to obtain than the latter. Either method, however, requires expensive equipment and both are sensitive to time lapse following smoking, prior use of alcohol, and ambient cigarette smoke (Hughes, Frederiksen, & Frazier 1978). Analysis of nicotine concentration in urine or saliva is a second, though expensive and complicated, measure of smoking. Although easier to collect, samples must be taken soon after a smoking episode. These tests are also sensitive to ambient smoke (Horning, Horning, Carroll, Stillwell, & Dzidic, 1973; Russell & Feyerabend 1975). Finally, thiocyanate levels can be assessed in urine and saliva samples. Saliva samples are probably less intrusive and easier to obtain; collection vials and inexpensive laboratory analysis are the only costs in either case. Time lapse following smoking is less critical with the thiocyanate test, but results are affected by diet and ambient smoke (Brockway 1978).

One physiological measure of drinking behavior is the breathalyzer test which analyzes breath samples for blood alcohol concentration. Gas chromatography instruments costing several thousand dollars provide the most accurate analysis. An inexpensive portable test, the mobile breath-alcohol test, is adequate for evaluating success of intervention (Sobell & Sobell 1975). Lovibond (1977) suggests sample points be based on a knowledge of the individual's drinking patterns rather than a random schedule.

Body weight and skinfold thickness are two common physiological measures of obesity. Because it fails to assess excessive body fat directly (Franks & Wilson 1978), body weight is not always an accurate measure of obesity. For instance, different activity histories may cause two persons of equal weight to be unequally fat (LeBow 1977). Another weakness of the body weight measure stems from the Metropolitan Life Insurance Tables used as normative weight charts. Based on a nonrandom sample population, these tables fail to provide standardized criteria for estimating individuals' frame size. LeBow (1977) recommends measuring skinfold thickness, although he and others (Johnson & Stalonas 1977) note difficulties in obtaining reliable measures. Skinfold readings can vary according to site selected, method of pinching subcutaneous fat, and application of measurement instrument.

Social workers may encounter difficulty using physiological measures, especially those requiring costly equipment or laboratory analysis. Medical facilities and universities, however, often contract to collect or analyze such data. Or social workers can use "bogus pipeline" procedures, in which physiological data are collected but not analyzed, to increase the validity of self-reports. Since individuals are more likely to provide accurate self-report data if they believe their reports will be verified (Evans, Hansen, & Mittelmark 1977), thiocyanate analysis might be simulated with smokers, for example. The process of measuring thiocyanate in saliva would be fully explained to clients. Saliva specimens would be collected, but later discarded, and smoking activity questionnaires completed. Bogus pipeline procedures are also applicable to eating and drinking behavior.

Behavioral Measures

Although they have only been used to assess drinking, behavioral measures represent a novel approach and deserve further attention. This set of measures focuses on objective behaviors associated with drinking rather than solely on the actual amount of alcohol consumed. Marlatt (1978) has developed a simulated bar which approximates a typical drinking environment. While various beverages are ordered and consumed, observers record amount and type of drinks and frequency of sips. Rankin, Hodgson, and Stockwell (1980) suggest that these simulated conditions can be used to differentiate the degree of dependence on alcohol. This measure can only be employed with persons aiming to control, rather than abstain from, drinking.

More accessible to social workers than Marlatt's simulated bar is Sobell and Sobell's (1976;1978) behavioral measure comprised of multiple dependent variables. Here clients and collateral information sources are contacted every three to four weeks. Appropriate for nondrinking or controlled drinking interventions, the variables include occupational circumstances, residential arrangement and stability, driver's license status, marital situation, and physical health. Alcohol consumption is coded into one of five mutually exclusive categories: 1) drunk day; 2) controlled drinking day; 3) abstinent day; 4) incarcerated day, jail; and 5) incarcerated day, hospital. This unique measure, evaluating functioning in several areas, allows a broad view of outcome.

Follow-Up

Follow-up data are essential for evaluating long-term effects of therapy. A comparison of relapse rates for smokers, drinkers, and heroin addicts reveals that about two-thirds of all relapses occur within the first ninety days following intervention (Hunt, Barnett, & Branch 1971). Thus, three- and six-month follow-up reports are standard. Follow-up reports should be collected over longer periods of time, as interventions become more sophisticated and include skills for handling and preventing relapse (Cooke & Meyers 1980; Marlatt & Gordon 1979). Recalling events over the past six to twelve months is difficult; as Nathan and Lansky (1978) suggest, more frequent follow-up checks are appropriate.

Several means of defining and assessing outcome must be considered, since, in many instances, a single assessment measure is not enough. Corroborating information from significant others or physiological measures provide validity checks on self-report data. As suggested above, simply collecting (but not always analyzing) physiological data can improve the accuracy of self-report information. Outcome goals must be carefully specified before appropriate assessment measures can be selected. Finally, practicality and precision need to be balanced: certain kinds of data collection can be extremely costly (Sobell & Sobell 1975).

INTERVENTION METHODS

Based on a social-learning model, behavioral interventions for addictive behaviors typically have one of three objectives: 1) to *modify the antecedents* associated with addictive behavior; 2) *to teach new behaviors* incompatible with harmful use of the addictive substance, or 3) to arrange the environment to *manipulate the consequences* of engaging in addictive behavior. Various procedures to accomplish these objectives have been designed and evaluated.

Modifying Antecedents

The first objective of behavioral treatment methods concerns antecedent events (the stimulus) which call forth addictive behavior (the response). A candy store may cue eating for the overeater; a drinking buddy may stimulate the alcoholic to drink; a smoker may associate a cup of coffee with a cigarette.

STIMULUS CONTROL The most common procedure for modifying cues to addictive behavior is stimulus control. Although this procedure has been used in the treatment of drinking and smoking behavior (Blittner, Goldberg, & Merbaum 1978; Edinger, Nelson, Davidson, & Wallace, 1978; Lovibond 1977), its widest application has been to eating problems.

Studies in the laboratory and the field indicate obese individuals are influenced to eat by the sight, taste, and smell of food (Schachter 1971) and by environmental cues suggesting mealtime (Schachter & Gross 1968). Innovative treatment efforts by Ferster, Nurnberger, and Levitt (1962) included suggesting that clients store food only in the kitchen and that they eat more slowly and only in the dining area. Since then, increasingly sophisticated stimulus control techniques have been developed concerning food purchase, storage, preparation, and eating. Bellack (1977) provides a helpful table containing over a score of procedures to reduce stimulus control of eating.

Baseline data on eating habits, collected on a form similar to Figure One, identify stimulus situations that control eating behavior. Appropriate stimulus control procedures can then be selected to associate eating with fewer and less frequently occurring stimuli. Ultimately, the only operating stimulus should be hunger.

Evaluations of stimulus control procedures applied to overeating are positive. In most studies, however, stimulus control is only one part of a multicomponent intervention package; other techniques such as financial contingencies (Castro & Rachlin 1980) and self-monitoring (Katell, Callahan, Fremouw, & Zitter, 1979) have been included in the package. Bellack (1977) suggests stimulus control procedures are only effective as one segment of a complex treatment program.

Youdin and Hemmes (1978) combined stimulus control and cognitive strategies to help five women lose weight. The stimulus control intervention involved four rules: 1) always eat in the same location; 2) eat small pieces of food and chew thoroughly; 3) drink a glass of water when craving a snack; and 4) never eat when engaged in another activity. During intervention, the women lost a mean of 26.6 pounds or 34.6 percent of their total excess weight. Mean weight loss had increased to 40.2 pounds at the one-year follow-up.

THOUGHT STOPPING The technique of thought stopping assumes that ruminations about the addictive behavior or "urges" provide the stimulus. The client is instructed to imagine a situation likely to cue the addictive behavior and then to emit a subvocal "stop," thereby interrupting the thought. Thought stopping can be used inconspicuously whenever an urge is experienced.

Evaluations of thought stopping for treating addictive behaviors tend to be limited to smoking. Lamontagne, Gagnon, Trudel, and Boisvert (1978) compared thought stopping to other techniques aimed at helping male hospital workers to reduce their smoking. In the thought-stopping intervention, tape-recorded messages instructed workers to close their eyes and imagine a situation in which they were likely to smoke. Following a brief period of silence, a voice shouted "stop" simultaneously with a loud handclap. The procedure was repreated twenty times in each half-hour session. In succeeding sessions, the workers themselves shouted and then whispered "stop," until it became subvocal in Sessions Nine and Ten. They were encouraged to practice thought stopping for twenty minutes daily and when they encountered temptations to smoke. At the end of treatment, workers exposed to thought stopping had made significantly greater reductions in smoking than workers receiving the other interventions. Subsequent follow-up data, although positive, failed to confirm the superiority of thought stopping. Flaxman (1979) cautions that thought stopping is most helpful in overcoming the habit component in smoking.

Training New Behaviors

The objective of the second group of interventions focuses on the behavior itself. The underlying assumption is that individuals have a limited repertoire of nonsmoking, nondrinking, or noneating skills (Miller 1978). The solution is to teach new behaviors that are incompatible with indulging in the addiction. Representative of this approach are substitution, relaxation training, and social skills training. A new alternative in treating alcohol abuse is teaching moderate drinking skills.

SUBSTITUTION Substitution is straightforward and simple to teach. It requires that clients substitute some other behavior for smoking, drinking, or eating. For example, overeaters and smokers learn to leave the table and take a walk or do dishes rather than have a dessert or a cigarette after dinner. Drinkers learn to call a friend or practice relaxation when craving alcohol. The addition of self-reinforcement strengthens substitution behavior.

RELAXATION Stress is a frequent precipitant of abusive drinking, eating, or smoking (Miller, Hersen, Eisler, & Hilsman, 1974; Tompkins 1968; Wollersheim 1977); relaxation training provides an alternative coping response to anxious and stressful situations. Jacobson's (1978) deep muscle relaxation paradigm has detailed instructions for reducing tension in seventeen identified body regions. Clients learn to recognize tenseness and cultivate relaxation, working on one region at a time.

Behavior therapists often incorporate relaxation training in intervention packages for addictions (Edinger, Nelson, Davidson, & Wallace, 1978; Schinke, Blythe, & Doueck 1979; Wollersheim 1977). Several studies support its inclusion. Blake (1967) found a higher abstinence rate in alcoholics exposed to relaxation training and aversion therapy than in those exposed only to aversion therapy. Similarly, Sutherland, Amit, Golden, and Rosenberger (1975) reported that smokers receiving a smoking aversion treatment plus relaxation training were more successful in reducing smoking than those receiving only the aversion treatment. Flaxman (1979) suggests relaxation training, like thought stopping, is important in combating the habit component of smoking.

SOCIAL SKILLS TRAINING Social skills training also provides alternatives to addictive behavior (Marlatt & Donovan, in press). Various techniques at improving interpersonal, assertive, and marital skills, have been studied. Such training is most frequently applied to drinking behavior, although smokers and overeaters have been given assertive training to refuse offers of cigarettes or food (Brockway, Kleinmann, Edleson, & Gruenewald, 1977; McMillan 1977).

Social skills training provides alcoholics with more effective responses to environmental demands so they are less likely to turn to alcohol. O'Leary, O'Leary, and Donovan (1976) cite several studies that indicate inadequate social skills in prealcoholic male adolescents and nonsober alcoholic adults. Miller, Hersen, Eisler, and Hilsman (1974) report chronic alcoholics increased their alcohol consumption but social drinkers did not when confronted by stressful interpersonal situations requiring assertive responses. In two case studies, assertive training was given to two alcoholic subjects who reported difficulty responding to social pressure to drink (Foy, Miller, Eisler, & O'Toole, 1976). Modeling, focused instructions, role play, and verbal feedback on their performance helped them acquire more effective responses. Three months following intervention, both had maintained their new, assertive behaviors and both reported increased self-confidence after they had successfully refused drinks.

Although marital problems related to alcohol have received considerable attention, few studies on marital skills training for alcoholic famlies have been conducted. A male alcoholic whose drinking was triggered by marital conflicts (Eisler, Miller, Hersen, & Alford, 1974) was the client in a case study. Skills training with a surrogate wife modified several target behaviors and improved his ability to express his opinions. Further, weekly blood alcohol levels taken six weeks following training showed a significant decrease when compared with weekly blood alcohol levels taken six weeks prior to training.

Marital skills training, like relaxation, is rarely the sole treatment method for addictive behaviors. In a well controlled study, Hedberg and Campbell (1974) investigated the effectiveness of marital skills training as the only intervention for fifteen chronic alcoholics. Couples rehearsed use of feedback, positive reinforcement, assertiveness, and contracting. Treatment goals were complete abstinence or moderate, controlled drinking; seventy-four percent of the clients had achieved their goal at one-year follow-up.

CONTROLLED DRINKING SKILLS Certain investigators have suggested that efforts be directed toward controlling rather than eliminating intake of the addictive substance (Polich, Armour, & Braiker, 1980; Lichtenstine 1977; Miller & Joyce 1979; Sobell & Sobell 1978). Obviously, complete abstinence is not an acceptable goal for obese persons; until the 1970's, it was the only acceptable goal for smokers and drinkers. This issue is highly controversial, especially in the alcoholism field (Larkin 1979), although alcohol abuse is the only addiction in which specific skills have been developed to teach controlled use (Sobell & Sobell 1978; Vogler, Weissbach, Compton, & Martin, 1977). Controlled drinking interventions typically include: 1) blood alcohol discrimination training;

and 2) drinking instructions and behavior rehearsal.

An early contribution to research on controlled drinking came from Australia (Lovibond & Caddy 1970). Two phases of blood alcohol discrimination training were delivered on an outpatient basis. In the discrimination training phase, behavioral effects of different blood alcohol concentrations were explained. Clients then drank alcohol mixed with fruit juice and estimated their blood alcohol levels every fifteen to twenty minutes for a two-hour period. Breathalyzer readings provided immediate feedback. In the conditioning phase, clients received shocks when their blood alcohol levels reached a predetermined level. Shocks were delivered on a schedule designed to maximize uncertainty and increase the likelihood of generalization. Intervention included one discrimination session and between six and twelve conditioning sessions. Clients who participated in the training program were drinking significantly less alcohol than another group of clients randomly assigned to receive no intervention at posttreatment follow-up.

Further investigations refined and extended the findings of Lovibond and Caddy's Australian study (1970). Huber, Karlin, and Nathan (1976) determined that social drinkers can acquire and maintain accurate blood alcohol discriminations using only such internal cues as subjective mood and bodily sensations. An attempt to replicate Lovibond and Caddy's study found the most important factor influencing alcoholics' ability to make accurate discriminations was continuous feedback on blood alcohol level. When this feedback was removed, control of drinking decreased significantly (Silverstein, Nathan, & Taylor 1974).

Based on observations of external components of drinking behavior, Miller, Becker, Foy, and Wooten (1976) taught three in-patient alcoholics controlled drinking skills. Clients rehearsed taking smaller sips, increasing the time between sips, and drinking less alcohol while receiving drinking instructions from another room. All three were able to bring drinking components under instructional control. Unhappily, "negative reactivity" was observed in two clients: positive changes in one component were paired with negative changes in another component (e.g., as they took smaller sips, they drank more rapidly). Refinement and further assessment of this procedure are needed.

Manipulating the Consequences

The focus of the last category of intervention methods is on the consequences of engaging in addictive behavior. Positive reinforcement is given for avoiding the behavior; indulging in the behavior is punished. Reinforcement, covert sensitization, and aversion are used to accomplish this objective. Aversion therapies are perhaps the best known behavioral treatments for addictions. In addition to manipulating the consequences of addictive behavior, aversion therapies may be used to modify cues associated with smoking, drinking, or eating. Although they rarely use aversive techniques, social workers must be able to answer questions and help clients decide whether or not to seek this kind of therapy.

REINFORCEMENT Reinforcement can be delivered by therapist, significant other, or client. Most therapists implicitly or explicitly give social reinforcement (Jeffrey 1976), but such tangible reinforcers as money, enriched environments, or tokens can also be employed (Bigelow, Cohen, Liebson, & Faillace, 1972; Cohen, Liebson, Faillace, & Allen, 1971). Often a written contract formalizes and strengthens reinforcement procedures, extending the therapist's impact to the client's environment. In reviewing studies of therapist reinforcement for weight control, Abramson (1977) concluded that the technique can be effective in a therapist-controlled environment, such as a hospital. Unfortunately, when clients leave the setting and reinforcement is withdrawn, maintenance becomes a problem.

Persons important to the client are also good sources of reinforcement. Israel and Saccone (1979) documented that reinforcement by a significant other produced more persistent weight loss three and twelve months following intervention than reinforcement by a therapist. The significant others (usually spouses) attended one training session where they learned basic contingency management and behavior moinitoring techniques. The researchers speculate the significant other's presence continues to remind the client of new eating habits after program termination. Self-help manuals often suggest enlisting the support and reinforcement of friends and family (Farquhar 1978; Jordan, Levitz, & Kimbrall, 1976; Stuart & Davis, 1972).

Because they must eventually monitor and maintain their own behavior, clients should be taught to self-reinforce positive changes. Reinforcers might be a covert self-statement or such tangibles as money or a phone call to a friend. Jeffrey and Christensen (1972) had clients read daily a list of positive consequences of behavior change. Bellack (1976) found the rate and amount of weight loss for self-reinforcing subjects similar to results of more elaborate and intensive programs. He suggests directly instructing clients in self-reinforcement procedures to ensure their using them contingently.

COVERT SENSITIZATION One form of aversion therapy, covert sensitization, requires clients to associate thoughts of drinking, eating, or smoking with thoughts of unpleasant experiences (e.g., nausea, vomiting, unpleasant odors). Working with two clients, Cautela (1966) researched the treatment of alcoholism and obesity with covert sensitization. Subsequent work questions the utility of this technique with overweight clients (Abramson 1977). Successful outcomes have been reported with alcoholics (Ashem & Donner 1968; Miller & Hersen, 1972) and smokers

(Hynd, Stratton, & Severson 1978). For example, Edinger, Nelson, Davidson, and Wallace (1978) showed male prison inmates a film depicting smoking hazards and chest surgery for lung cancer. The men then smoked cigarettes while imagining scenes from the film that were especially aversive. They were instructed to practice this covert sensitization procedure daily. Significant reductions in smoking were reported at termination of intervention and at a thirteen-week follow-up.

CHEMICAL AVERSION Chemical aversion therapy is used primarily in treating alcoholism. Drugs inducing nausea and paralysis have been associated with the sight, smell, or taste of alcohol (Farrar, Powell, & Martin 1968; Raymond 1964). Although some empirical support exists for inducing nausea, none exists for inducing paralysis. Wilson and Davison (1969) speculate that nausea-inducing drugs are more "biologically appropriate" aversive stimuli.

In a few instances, chemical aversion therapy has been applied to smoking. A nicotine substitute, Lobeline, was determined no more effective than an appropriate placebo in one study (Davison & Rosen 1972). Cigarette consumption was successfully reduced, however, by an antismoking chewing gum which produced an unpleasant taste if cigarettes were subsequently smoked (Rosenberg 1977).

Unusual aversive stimuli have been paired with eating. Thus, a noxious odor, butyric acid, was associated with the aroma of foods preferred by one overweight client (Kennedy & Foreyt 1968). Unfortunately, well controlled studies of this technique are lacking. Associating cigarette smoke with the act of eating was effective in another weight-reduction study (Morganstern, 1974).

ELECTRICAL AVERSION Electrical aversion has been widely used in the treatment of all three addictions under discussion with varying success rates. In a classic conditioning paradigm, electric shock was paired with the taste, smell, or sight of alcohol (Voegtlin 1940). Blake (1965; 1967) tested an escape-conditioning technique in which clients terminated the shock by spitting out alcohol they had been instructed to sip but not swallow. Because it was not carefully controlled, the study's positive results are questionable. In another study, shock was contingent on presentation of alcohol-related visual stimuli (Hedberg & Campbell 1974); only one of four alcoholic clients showed improvement at the six-month follow-up. In view of inadequate supporting evidence, Wilson (1978) calls for terminating use of electrical shock for alcholics. Doleys, Ciminero, Wallach, and Davidson (1977) discuss related ethical issues.

In obesity studies, electric shock paired with movement toward or discussion of favorite foods has yielded disappointing findings (Meyer & Crisp 1964; Stollack 1967). Likewise, shock failed to produce positive, long-term results in smoking studies (Conway 1977; Steffy, Meichenbaum, & Best 1970). A successful case study suggests shocking imagined urges rather than shocking actual smoking is more effective (Berecz 1976).

SMOKING AVERSION Other aversive procedures for smoking reduction or cessation have been evaluated, including warm, smoky air (Schmahl, Lichtenstein, & Harris 1972) satiation (Dericco, Brigham, & Garlington 1977), and rapid smoking (Lichtenstein, Harris, Birchler, Wahl, & Schmahl, 1973). Only results from satiation have been unencouraging. Since the warm, smoky air requires complicated procedures, it has been abandoned in favor of the equally effective rapid smoking, which typically requires individuals to inhale smoke from their usual cigarettes every six seconds until they feel unable to continue. Two additional trials are completed following three- to five-minute rest periods. Hauser (1974) voiced concern over possible hazards of rapid smoking. Subsequent investigations of cardiopulmonary risks of increased nicotine and carbon monoxide exposure resulted in some precautionary recommendations such as medical screening prior to participation (Hall, Sachs, & Hall 1979; Russell, Raw, Taylor, Feyerbend, & Saloojee, 1978). When used cautiously, rapid smoking can be effective. Recent outcome studies suggest better results are obtained when rapid smoking is combined with other treatment methods (Best, Bass, & Owen 1977; Best, Owen, & Trentadue 1978).

Several of the techniques discussed above may be combined to form an intervention package. These "broad spectrum" interventions have several advantages. Social workers may find that certain individual methods are not appropriate for their client population or setting, or that required equipment is inaccessible. Taking into account the changing needs as clients modify their eating, drinking, or smoking behavior and the unique needs of individual clients (Lando 1977; Nathan 1978), broad spectrum packages strengthen intervention and improve service to a wide range of clients. The following case example evaluated a broad-spectrum interventive packaged designed to help clients reduce cigarette smoking.

CASE EXAMPLE

Two social workers conducted a smoking-reduction group at the request of faculty at a local community college. Newspaper advertisements and posted announcements recruited seventeen student and nonstudent members of the community interested in reducing or eliminating cigarette smoking and offered them a noncredit evening class.

Participants were assigned randomly to an intervention condition or to a waiting-list control condition. Geographic location changes and schedule conflicts reduced the intervention and control conditions to six and two members respectively. Ages ranged from sixteen years to fifty-one years, with a mean (M) of 34.16 and standard deviation (SD) of 9.88.

Participants had been smoking for one to twenty-nine years ($M = 18.29$, $SD = 10.30$).

Assessment

Self-reported smoking behavior assessed the extent of each participant's smoking at baseline and following treatment. The date, time, number of cigarettes smoked, and activity and mood associated with the smoking incident were recorded on a monitoring sheet similar to Figure One. Data were collected for each of the eight weeks of intervention. Experimental participants submitted their data at weekly group meetings; control participants mailed their data. Because of known high relapse rates, follow-up data were gathered at one, three, and six months and at three years after intervention.

Intervention

During the first session, two social work group leaders discussed smoking within the framework of antecedents, behaviors, and consequences. Group participants were encouraged to apply social-learning principles to their own smoking experiences. An overview of the intervention package emphasized its grounding in social-learning theory.

To address problems of antecedent control, group members practiced stimulus control and thought-stopping procedures. Using baseline information from monitoring sheets to identify environmental stimuli facilitating smoking, each member planned his or her own individually tailored stimulus control interventions. These plans were reviewed in the group, with leaders and participants providing additional suggestions. Thus, because she often smoked while drinking coffee or alcohol, one group member temporarily replaced these beverages with herbal teas, soft drinks, and bottled water. She also removed all cigarettes, lighters, and ash trays from her environment and socialized with nonsmoking friends during the initial weeks of treatment. Thought stopping helped participants control urges to smoke, a frequent stimulus condition. After group leaders modeled thought stopping, members practiced stopping cigarette-related thoughts.

Substitution, relaxation, and assertion training provided new behaviors incompatible with smoking. Regarding substitution, group members studied a list of alternative behaviors and selected activities suitable to their life styles. Suggested incompatible behaviors included talking a walk, chewing flavored toothpicks, rubbing a "worry stone," or whittling.

Beginning with the third session, participants practiced deep-muscle relaxation (Jacobson 1978) during each meeting. After one group leader modeled the use of relaxation as an alternative coping behavior, members rehearsed the response. Leaders coached and gave feedback, stressing the importance of frequent practice to achieve deep relaxation.

Next, group participants identified and described interpersonal and social situations in which it was difficult not to smoke. Following procedures described by Schinke and Rose (1976), the two leaders demonstrated new assertive behaviors. Members practiced refusing offered cigarettes, asking people not to smoke in public areas, and negotiating with smokers in their environment. Other participants and leaders provided coaching, feedback, and reinforcement following behavior rehearsals.

Completing the intervention package, reinforcement, contracting, covert sensitization, and rapid smoking altered the consequences of smoking and nonsmoking behavior. Based on their monitoring sheets, group members reported smoking-reduction progress and use of treatment techniques. Group leaders and participants provided verbal and nonverbal reinforcement (praise, applause, a pat on the shoulder) for positive reports. A group norm requiring at least three participants reinforce the reporting member ensured consistent reinforcement. Members were also instructed to self-reinforce their nonsmoking behavior outside the group and their practice of treatment methods such as thought stopping and assertiveness.

Participants wrote weekly contracts with themselves agreeing to use

Table 1.
Daily Mean of Cigarettes Smoked
for Intervention and Control-condition Participants

Monitoring Period	Interventive[a] *M*	Control[b] *M*
Week 1 (Baseline)	35.91	33.46
Week 2	27.10	33.42
Week 3	21.32	33.89
Week 4	10.88	34.43
Week 5	6.21	33.94
Week 6	5.90	33.74
Week 7	4.54	35.61
Week 8 (Postintervention)	5.13	33.87
Follow-up		
1 Month	12.53	36.15
3 Months	13.64	36.73
6 Months	15.08	37.14
36 Months	20.33	38.51

Note. Means were computed on 7-day monitoring periods.

[a] $n = 6$ [b] $n = 2$

specific smoking-reducting techniques. Contracts were read aloud, adding an element of public commitment.

Depending on their physical health and personal wishes, group members practiced covert sensitization or rapid smoking. In the covert sensitization treatment, participants followed a paradigm outlined by Dawley and Dillenkoffer (1975). Group members smoked and inhaled at their regular rates while handling the litter of approximately twenty spent cigarettes. Simultaneously, they imagined the harmful and undesirable consequences of cigarette smoking (e.g. heart and lung damage, monetary expense, lingering unpleasant odors). Participants selecting rapid smoking read a description of associated risks and signed informed-consent statements. Under the direction of a group leader, members practiced rapid smoking according to standard procedures. All members were instructed to use covert sensitization or rapid smoking if they smoked cigarettes outside the group.

Daily means of cigarettes smoked by intervention and control condition participants during the eight weeks of intervention, and at four follow-up periods, are presented in Table One. Baseline smoking levels were comparable. Beginning with the second week of intervention, however, differences between conditions were evident. Participants in the smoking-reduction group smoked fewer cigarettes than did control-condition participants.

The data indicate this broad-spectrum intervention package successfully reduced group participants' smoking. Especially impressive are the long-term smoking levels when compared with previously reported follow-up rates for smoking-reduction programs (Best 1975; Danaher 1977; West, Graham, Swanson, & Wilkinson, 1977).

In short, social workers frequently work with clients addicted to cigarettes, alcohol, or food. The present case illustrates an evaluation of a behavioral approach to controlling smoking with a straightforward, economical, valid, and easily collected measure assessed outcome. The intervention package was composed of techniques found effective by previous researchers; these techniques were easily learned and quickly applied. Positive long-term findings support continued use of the interventive package.

CLINICAL ISSUES

A discussion of behavioral approaches to treating addictive behaviors is incomplete without considering related clinical issues social workers may encounter. Choice of assessment and intervention strategies is very important. Equally important is the particular way the strategies are employed. Whether intervention is delivered individually or in groups, certain clinical considerations emerge.

Clients frequently ask what personal experience, if any, the practitioner has with smoking, drinking, or eating problems. The social worker should explore with the client why this is of concern. Some clients believe that practitioners who have themselves struggled with problems of addiction will be more understanding and less judgmental. Although practitioners may find it helpful to disclose their own experiences, the primary focus should be on client needs and concerns.

A case has been made for broad-spectrum intervention packages. Presenting all the techniques simultaneously, however, confuses and overwhelms clients. Techniques should be introduced individually and when clients most need them. In the case study, rapid smoking and covert sensitization helped group members initially reduce their overall smoking. Assertion training procedures later provided skills to deal with less frequently occurring interpersonal situations in which nonsmoking was difficult. Adequate time for practice and shaping increases the likelihood that techniques will be correctly and consistently applied.

Unlike many problems treated by social workers, addictive behavior often extends over a long period of time. Lifelong habits are best changed on the basis of plans, with particular attention to maintenance. Marlatt and Gordon (1979) have developed a unique skills training model to prevent relapse. Based on research with smoking, drinking, and heroin addictions, they classified relapse episodes according to interpersonal and intrapersonal/environmental determinants. Specific coping skills are suggested for handling high-risk situations where relapse is likely to occur. Further testing of this model is certainly warranted.

Social workers serve a critical function in helping clients control their addictive behavior. Often individuals have made several futile attempts to gain control prior to seeking professional help. During the initial phase of intervention, the practitioner may be the primary source of reinforcement for behavior change. These facts, coupled with the extended time required to change these behaviors, call for careful fading of the social worker's role. Structuring intervention so that clients are gradually provided skills for handling difficult situations is helpful. Clients should be allowed to experiment with new, independent coping skills while still maintaining practitioner contact and support. They also should be encouraged to self-reinforce positive behavior change. Gradually reducing contact helps clients make the transition to independently maintained intervention gains.

Addiction to cigarettes, alcohol, and food presents grave problems for individuals, families, and society as a whole. Promising interventions for controlling addictive behaviors have been developed; more work remains. Under-represented in past efforts, social workers are well qualified to continue these endeavors. Social workers have skills that are particularly suited to designing and conducting programs in the community—exactly where remedies are most needed.

12

Helping Mentally Retarded Persons Get Jobs

Richard M. Grinnell, Jr.
and
Alice Lieberman

For whatever reasons, unemployment among mentally retarded persons is disproportionately high. Current literature in the field of vocational rehabilitation expresses a deep and abiding concern with this inequity and implores the helping professional to look beyond general economic conditions for alternative explanations for the scarcity of retarded people in the job market (Eagle, 1967; Tobias, 1970). Although one of the prime objectives of educational and rehabilitative efforts with mentally retarded persons is to prepare them for successful employment, little attention is devoted to this area. Clearly, job interviews are an initial step in a sequence leading to their employment.

Training retarded persons for job interviews has received little attention because they were usually assisted by advocates often present during job interviews to mediate communication difficulties. Trends toward community living mean social workers must help retarded people learn appropriate interview skills so they may eventually act without advocates, a process likely to increase self-reliance and self-esteem and provide a sense of accomplishment, as well as employment, for thousands of retarded adults not in the work force.

Recent research shows that retarded persons possess low self-concepts, limited ranges of life experiences, and little confidence in their ability to succeed (Brolin & Kokaska, 1974). Each of these variables, in conjunction with a lack of experience, may impede the development of the skills necessary to interview successfully. Previous studies indicate that sound interviewing behavior is critical to the employment of retarded people. Most studies, however, have neither specified the structure nor the result of training with retarded people in helping them prepare for job interviews. To provide concrete assistance, this chapter presents a training approach in which some of the necessary interviewing skills were successfully taught through the microcounseling model of communication. A total of seven skill areas were utilized with the assumption that, if these skill areas were modeled to the clients and subsequently mastered by them, chances of employment would significantly increase.

Because of its repeated successes with similar populations, microcounseling, a model widely used to train a variety of students, clients, and professionals was chosen (Boyd, 1973; Saltmarsh & Hubele, 1974; Ivey, 1973; Haase & DiMattia, 1970). When adapted to fit the specific needs of diverse populations, it achieves well documented success. The first section discusses the setting where this project was initiated and executed; the second section subsequently describes the clients who participated in the project, continuing to describe the training model utilized. After a detailed discussion of what procedures were used to implement the training model and presenting the findings from the research, the last sections discuss possible implications of the results to social work practice.

METHOD

Setting

This project was initiated and executed in one of the largest Goodwill Industries facilities in the country, located in western Dallas, Texas and surrounded by a moderate amount of industry. The agency provides permanent sheltered employment and also serves as a vocational training center for the handicapped. Approximately 540 people with disabilities restricting them to sheltered employment are permanent employees. An additional seventy people are clients of the Texas Rehabilitation Commission (TRC), an agency whose primary aim is the preparation of clients for successful employment with professional teachers available on a part-time basis to help clients acquire the General Equivalency Degree.

Other professional staff include a social worker, a vocational rehabilitation counselor, a psychologist, a psychometrician, and a vocational placement advisor.

This exceptionally large facility has a sheltered workshop area, a lunchroom, two large classrooms, a chapel, seven large staff meeting rooms, and equipment storage areas. The workshop area includes many sections. One section, for example, is responsible for the pickup of discarded goods. These items are returned to the Goodwill facility for cleaning, repair, and pricing before being dispatched to the outlet stores for resale.

Clients

Clients for the job-interviewing training project were selected through a classification system in which each active case in the agency could be categorized into a problem typology in which seven problem categories comprise the entire array of problems for which a person may need social work services (Grinnell & Kyte, 1975). Screening consisted of first classifying each of the 537 active cases on file into the problem categories, with the most heavily populated category comprising the potential clients from which the sample would be drawn. Mental retardation, mental illness, physical handicaps, or some combination of these problems were present in most cases with varying degrees of severity, so the range of problems, with respect to rehabilitation potential, was wide. The largest number of clients, fifty-four, was placed into the problem category of "individual maladjustments."

Each file contained the following information: demographic data, such as name, age, race, address, and phone number; the nature of the person's handicap; previous job experience, if any, and reasons for employment termination; scores on pencil and paper tests assessing fine and gross motor skills, such as the Wide Range Achievement Test and the Purdue Pegboard Test; bi-weekly progress reports from the area supervisor on the client's rates of skill acquisition; and "incident reports," consisting of narrative recordings of rule infringements.

Prior to securing access to the files of clients selected for project participation, permission was obtained from each parent or guardian for observation and videotaping. Fortunately, few objections were raised; none could not be overcome. Requests most frequently met with positive responses, with several parents or guardians requesting information on the researchers' credentials. Only one parent expressed concern that the observation of videotapes by the "wrong people" might hamper her son in his work. After she was informed that the videotapes would be viewed only by professional researchers and not by any staff at Goodwill, she consented.

A revised Beta Examination (Lindner & Gurvitz, 1946) was administered in groups of six to the fifty-four potential clients to determine the extent of mental retardation, because previous research has demonstrated that groups of between six to eight members accomplish tasks more effectively. To ensure an adequate number of clients for the study, lower and upper limits of fifty-four and seventy-four were established. Within these parameters, fourteen clients scored too high and three scored too low on the examination for project inclusion. An additional five had left the facility, their vocational training completed. Thus, thirty-two clients were theoretically eligible for participation in the project; four groups with six clients in each comprised the training sample, fourteen females and ten males with an average age of twenty-three. Eight clients were Caucasian and sixteen were of other ethnic origins. The average IQ score on the Revised Beta Examination was sixty-five, indicating "moderate" retardation.

Two problems common in applied research appeared in subject selection procedures. First, since only one worker participated in the content analysis and classification process, the implementation of the classification system used may have poor reliability. If more than one person had classified these cases into problem categories, there may well have been differences of opinion. Second, because the IQ limits used included both moderate and mild levels of retardation, the inclusion of these two levels may have obscured different ability levels. These two potential flaws seemed justified, since the goal of the study was clinical relevance as well as research rigor (Azrin, 1977; Thomas, 1975).

Training Model

The microcounseling model of communication training relies on imitation to teach particular skills. The model is a scaled-down interviewing situation in which a beginning counselor and a volunteer talk about a problem while focusing attention on a single specific behavior (Ivey, 1974); generally, the paradigm proceeds as follows:

1. The behavior to be learned—eye contact, body posture, other attending skills, etc.—is *modeled* by the instructor.
2. The trainee *practices* that skill.
3. At this point, a videotaped recording may be made of the trainee role playing a counseling situation.
4. The videotaped recording is played back to the trainee with *feedback* given regarding performance on the *behavior in question only*. In this manner, trainees observe their own performance and repeat videotaped trials until they are satisfied that they are observing themselves performing correctly. In short, microcounseling focuses on specific skills and behaviors that can be defined,

> observed, practiced, and evaluated. Rather than confuse the interviewing trainee with an overwhelming amount of data, the component skills approach divides interviewing into workable and observable dimensions.

The model includes eleven general skills ranging from extremely simple ones, requiring no conceptual ability, to very complex skills demanding great ability in conceptualization. It was decided that the seventh skill on the continuum, reflection of content, would be the last skill the clients could master. Beyond that point, imitative skills cease to be the major factor in learning, and it becomes necessary to possess conceptual skill. Thus, the study concentrated on these seven skills rather than on the entire model.

Eye contact, the easiest skill to master, was modeled first; reflection of content, the hardest skill area, was modeled last. A conscious effort was made to demonstrate the skill areas to the clients in a continuum from easy to difficult over six modeling sessions. Skills concentrated on during the training were:

A. *Attending Behavior—four components:*

A.1 Eye Contact: To look at the partner comfortably without a fixed stare.

A.2 Body Posture: To be physically relaxed and seated without slouching or fidgeting.

A.3 Minimal Encourage: Verbal cues of understanding, e.g. "um-hum," "yeah," "really," "then?"

A.4 Verbal Follow: Repetition of one or two key words from the partner's immediately preceding verbalization.

B. *Questioning Skills—two components*

B.5 Open-end question: Provide limited categorization so that the partner cannot answer question in only one or two words.

B.6 Close-ended question: Greater categorization is imposed such that the partner has to answer with a "yes," or "no."

C. *Reflection Skill—one component:*

C.7 Reflection of content: To paraphrase or summarize the partner's verbalization.

Procedure

Clients were randomly assigned to one of three training groups or to a control group. Each group was composed of six clients; group content differed only in videotaped playback presentation. The training groups met twice a week for three continuous weeks during which skill areas were taught.

TRAINING GROUP ONE received a detailed skill training package: each Tuesday and Thursday, clients were excused from work areas for an hour to an hour and a half to participate in training. The first session was devoted only to eye contact and body posture. A social work graduate student gave a didactic presentation on these two skills, using large drawings to emphasize these skills in a job interview. With one of the participants, she also demonstrated a job-interview situation in which both poor and good eye contact and body posture were present. Thus, didactic information, pictorial aids, and modeling were the primary means of presenting the skills.

Following this presentation, each client was given two opportunities to demonstrate the ability to execute each skill in a videotaped trial interview situation one and one half minutes to two minutes long with a fellow trainee. The tape was stopped by either the worker or a member of the group each time a target skill-behavior was observed. A nickel was given along with positive social reinforcement (e.g. "you really maintained good eye contact," "you did that very well," etc.), the skill behavior commented upon, and the tape playback resumed. All other sessions in training group one were conducted similarly, using the following schedule: the second session, minimal encourage and verbal follow; the third session, open-ended questions; the fourth session, close-ended questions; and the fifth and sixth sessions, reflection of content. At each session, previously focused skills were reviewed to enhance cumulative learning.

TRAINING GROUP TWO received the same skill training package as did training group one, but clients did not view videotaped trial performances. Although the equipment was present during each session, the monitor was never activated. A nickel and positive social reinforcement were given at the close of the viewing in response to each skill behavior exhibited by clients.

TRAINING GROUP THREE received the same skill training package as groups one and two, but clients did not view videotaped performances. Although the equipment was present during each session, the monitor was never activated. A nickel and positive social reinforcement were given at the close of the session for each skill behavior exhibited by the client.

CONTROL GROUP clients recieved no skill training package and were told only that they would participate in pretest and posttest.

Objective Evaluation

Clients were given both pre- and posttests to assess training effects. For both testing periods, clients were randomly paired and were seated in a large room under the following conditions. Two schooldesk chairs were seated next to each other. Facing them was a tripod with a portable videotape camera atop it. A microphone was placed between the two desks equidistant between clients. After seating themselves, each pair was given two and a half minutes to respond on videotape to three stimulus presentations.

At pretest, clients were told: "Thanksgiving is only one week off and each of you has a five-day vacation. Discuss with your partner what you plan to do over Thanksgiving. Or what you would do and where you would go if you could do anything or go anywhere." The clients were then asked to respond to the visual stimulus—a print of a painting by Chagall. The instructions were: "This picture looks like many different things when different people look at it. Examine the picture, turn it upside down or sideways. Then, discuss with your partner what you think the picture is, and what you like or don't like about it." The third set of instructions asked clients respond to the following dilemma: "You have been accidentally locked in a department store for the night and surrounded by toys, games, clothes, televisions, stereos, and furniture. You haven't been able to find a phone, so you decide to make the best of the situation. How would you spend the night?"

Posttest assessment was administered on the day following the last training session. Similar to pretest, the first vignette requested a general discussion of Christmas—"What would you like to get for Christmas if you could have anything you wanted?" "What are you giving other members of your family?" "Does Christmas have other meanings for you?" The second vignette required responses to a visual stimulus, administered identical to its pretest counterpart. The third vignette asked each client pair to discuss plans for the coming year, goals, or New Year's resolutions. "Do you look forward to leaving this training?" "What pleased you most about the training received at Goodwill?" Tapes from pretest and posttest were rated by five second-year graduate social work students. Raters, unfamiliar with clients and experimental conditions, were asked to independently measure the quality or quantity of each target behavior using the following components.

EYE CONTACT Clients were rated on this variable by the way they maintained an attentive look at their partner. This meant looking without staring for sustained periods of time. Since the most common problem in teaching eye contact was overcoming tendencies to look at the floor, eye contact was an accurate measure of attentiveness. Raters measured the quality of eye contact for each vignette using a four-point scale: one represented "very poor;" four represented "very good."

BODY POSTURE Measured on the same four-point scale as eye contact, body posture ratings determined whether or not clients were sitting comfortably or slouching, leaning slightly forward to indicate attentiveness, and whether or not they fidgeted excessively.

MINIMAL ENCOURAGES, VERBAL FOLLOW, OPEN- AND CLOSE-ENDED QUESTIONS, AND REFLECTION OF CONTENT The remaining five skills were measured on a quantity basis only. For each client, rater scores were averaged for each skill area across each vignette. A total score, consisting of each skill behavior average for the three vignettes, was then computed.

Subjective Evaluation

Pre- and posttest assessment of job interview readiness was also measured subjectively. Each client completed a five-minute interview consisting of three open-ended questions, four close-ended questions, and an opportunity to question the two TRC counselors/interviewers, at the end of each interview. Counselors then independently rated clients in response to the question, "To what extent is this person ready to interview for a competitive employment position?" Based on a six-point scale where one represented "not ready at all" and six represented "ready right now," ratings were averaged to form a mutual single score.

FINDINGS AND DISCUSSION

Data were first analyzed to determine if any significant difference existed between pre- and posttest scores in the seven skill areas across the four groups. Summarized in Tables 1 and 2, significant differences were found for all three training groups on eye contact and body posture. As expected, the control group showed no significant differences for these two skill areas. Moreover, there were no significant pre- to posttest differences for any of the four groups on the last five skill areas.

As stated previously, the seven skill areas were taught in ascending order from simple to complex. Since eye contact and body posture are descriptive in nature, failure to master these two skill areas may predict unsuccessful learning of the last five skill areas. Data showing clients who mastered training for the first two skill areas much more effective with the remaining five support this proposition. Further, this finding suggests that mentally retarded persons can master skills entirely physical in nature, regardless of the presence of videotape feedback. Because the relative effectiveness of videotape as a primary teaching tool has been reported in work with another populations (Gutride, Goldstein, & Hunter, 1973), additional investigation is needed regarding who can benefit most from self-observation via videotape.

Data collected at each modeling session helped identify the first session in which significant improvement over pretest scores would occur,

Table 1

Distribution of Mean Scores by Training Group for Eye Contact

	Mean Pretest Score	**Mean Posttest Score**	**Mean Gain Score**	t	p*
Training group 1	1.9	3.0	+1.1	6.0	.01
Training group 2	2.7	3.5	+0.8	3.4	.01
Training group 3	2.4	3.2	+0.8	4.6	.01
Control group	3.2	3.3	+0.1	0.5	.33

*one-tailed test

Table 2

Distribution of Mean Scores by Training Group for Body Posture

	Mean Pretest Score	**Mean Posttest Score**	**Mean Gain Score**	t	p*
Experimental group 1	2.0	3.3	+1.3	7.3	.01
Experimental group 2	1.5	2.7	+1.2	6.1	.01
Experimental group 3	1.8	2.8	+1.0	12.1	.01
Control group	2.7	3.1	+0.4	1.4	.12

*one-tailed test

revealing that after modeling session two, eye contact and body posture improved and subsequently remained significant throughout the duration of the project. Suggesting that clients retained what they learned, this finding may have resulted from clients seeing the two skills demonstrated on the videotape monitor and viewing them in live vignettes rather than simply hearing skills containing certain words or phases via audio equipment. The training group that never viewed themselves on the monitor also showed and retained significant improvements after modeling session two, so modeling is probably an important variable explaining mastery of eye contact and body posture (Doster & Brooks, 1974).

The constant review and practice of these two skill areas after the initial learning sessions is helpful. Certainly, the importance of constant repetition to achieve mastery of these skills is well documented (Doubros, 1966). Since results showed skills taught later in training not incorporated into clients' repertoires—perhaps because of lack of sufficient practice combined with the skills' increasing complexity—its seems likely that training expanded over a longer period of time may be successful in helping clients gain mastery over the last five skill areas.

A second level of data analysis determined if any significant differences existed among the groups themselves for each skill area. Analysis of variance on difference scores revealed no such differences in each training group showing a higher difference score than the control group in each skill area. The three training groups' difference scores were then averaged and compared to the control group's difference score. The training groups' average difference score for each skill area was greater than the difference score for the control group.

Next, data were analyzed to see if the average difference score for each group decreased as videotaped feedback was delayed. For each skill area, it was hypothesized that training group one would have a higher difference score than training group two, training group two would have a higher difference score than training group three, and training group three would have a higher difference score than the control group. Pre- to posttest change scores were calculated to determine the average difference score for each group for each skill area. Correlation coefficients revealed no meaningful coefficients (*r V .2)* in all skill areas. However, it appeared that videotape feedback with immediate social and monetary reinforcement was more effective than videotape feedback with delayed social and monetary reinforcement, which in turn was more effective than no videotape feedback with social and monetary reinforcement: each was more effective than no training.

Results of subjective interviews indicate significant pre- to post-test improvements for training groups one and two; the other two groups showed no such improvements. Difference scores for each training group, however, decreased in the delay of videotape feedback. Consistent with objective measures, subjective assessment results support the impact of training.

IMPLICATIONS

Experiences in using the skill training microcounseling model in a mentally retarded population have yielded several guidelines for future work. First, data suggest that the three training programs might have produced stronger results if expanded over time: six sessions may have been too few for participants to master the last five skill areas. Increasing the number of sessions to ten or twelve might be better. Second, participants appeared motivated primarily by two aspects of the program: the opportunity to view themselves on "television;" and monetary and social reinforcement. Thus, future studies may wish to examine both for differential effects. Finally, this project demonstrates that intensive training with mentally retarded clients can be acomplished inexpensively. Even with videotape equipment and monetary reinforcement, the microcounseling program was administered very inexpensively. For under $500 others could operate similar programs by maximizing professional staff involvement.

Unintended Consequences

In retrospect, it seems that this project may have been more efficiently conducted if the major goals of Goodwill Industries were considered more carefully: providing sheltered employment and rehabilitation services for appropriate clients, retrieving, refurbishing and selling household items. Unfortunately, the two goals create an inherent paradox: when trained, people leaving Goodwill to take competitive employment weaken the agency workforce. Thus, the study posed a potential threat to agency staff valuing efficient production and not wanting to lose trained clients because of newly acquired job interview skills. Although initially unaware of this dilemma, the project personnel became cognizant of its ramifications as the study progressed. Supervisors began to complain that the hours clients spent in the training program and away from their tasks were hampering production. Often, it was necessary to discuss the importance of a client's attendance at training sessions with the supervisor. Not an uncommon phenomenon in applied research, such resistance may doom one's best efforts to failure (Glaser & Taylor, 1973). If project personnel had not met with administrative and line staff prior to the project, had not invited their suggestions, and had not explained in detail study goals, the project may have not been so successful.

Serendipitous Findings

Conducting training sessions with the present clients, project personnel observed a by-product of the microcounseling model not usually evident when working in non-retarded groups: as clients became more skilled in eye contact and body posture, they grew more assertive. In retrospect, this seems logical, since eye contact and body posture are two physical components of assertive behavior; however, although student trainees may exhibit these qualities regardless of training, assertive behavior is often absent among retarded persons—due perhaps to low self-esteem. But, learning to exhibit physical qualities evidencing high self-esteem, client behavior appeared positively influenced. This new behavior was further reinforced as skills increased by initiating conversation and questions. Despite the lack of provision to assess videotape content, raters noticed a more positive and forceful tone in posttraining taped dialogues.

Practice Guidelines

Without question, applied research with clinical populations should be a major part of social work. Such research affirms accountability of practice and provides other social workers with knowledge to improve their practice. As an aid to others conducting applied social research, several guidelines revealed by the present project follow:

1. The clients selected must be sufficiently motivated toward behavior change. An oversight in the present project was failure to consider that some clients clearly preferred the security and friendship of working at Goodwill; thus, they were not sufficiently motivated to acquire skills that would facilitate leaving the agency.
2. Advanced planning is essential to avoid potential problems. Rooms for assessment and training must be reserved. Any technical equipment—video monitors and recorders, audio tape recorders, films, etc.—should be checked thoroughly the day before they are needed.
3. Clients' informed consent, even if not required by the agency, should be obtained from all study participants with a copy kept in the client's file. Certainly, all questions must be dealt with honestly; when appropriate, clients should be informed that intervention is untried and experimental.
4. If the project team does not work for the agency, all effective agency personnel should be fully knowledgeable about study goals and process. Comments and suggestions often must be actively solicited; moreover, staff are generally more positive when reminded of how potentially beneficial the project may be to subsequent agency operations.

5. Where possible, research staff should avoid other roles while conducting the project. Conflicting roles that may confuse clients and staff may have potentially contaminating effects, jeopardizing study results.

SUMMARY

This study represents a pioneering effort to evaluate the use of videotape and microcounseling in job-interview training for mentally retarded adults. Seven skill areas were modeled with three training groups, each employing videotape in a different capacity. Data revealed that microcounseling is most effective with eye contact and body posture, regardless of videotape use. Significant improvement occurred in both skill areas after two modeling sessions and remained improved thoughout the study. Thus, only two modeling sessions may be needed to give mentally retarded persons basic skills in these two areas.

It appeared that two modeling sessions produced positive results which, in turn, can help clients prepare for job interviews. Many clients, mentally retarded or not, have difficulty obtaining jobs because they lack adequate interview skills. This project demonstrated that in only two sessions a counselor could create significant positive changes in body posture and eye contact. The use of videotape playback allowed clear and precise performance feedback.

It also provided clients with opportunities for self-observation; as a teaching tool, however, it was an adjunct to the skill training package. Vocational training facilities without video equipment need not rule out the microcounseling model as a job-interview-skill teaching method.

Some employers have a negative bias toward mentally retarded persons. The literature reveals that these biases may play a more important role in a dyadic interchange such as a job interview than does objective assessment. It therefore becomes extremely important for retarded persons to present themselves as potentially competent employees by exhibiting behavioral traits more likely seen in a non-retarded population. Since nonverbal communication is a very important ingredient in total communication (Kadushin, 1972; Gorden, 1975), mastery of the two areas will help achieve this goal. If mentally retarded persons can improve their eye contact and body posture, they would have a better chance for future employment. Any interviewee would have difficulty obtaining a job when s/he never looks at the interviewer, slouches or excessively moves around during the initial interview. All of the skill areas modeled in this study are desirable for any interviewee in any interview; if interviewees lack eye contact and proper body posture, they may not favorably impress the interviewer, resulting in a negative overall evaluation of his/her total capacity and future employment potential.

13

Social Interactions in Nursing Homes

Raymond M. Berger

In 1970 almost one million persons sixty-five years of age or older lived in institutional settings. Although it is estimated that four to five percent of the elderly population are institutionalized at any one time, Kastenbaum and Candy (1973) have presented evidence to buttress the argument that the chances of an older person entering a long-term care facility of some type are nearly one in four. With projected increases in the relative proportion of older persons in the total population and the high incidence of chronic disease and disability in this group, the phenomenon of the institutionalized older person is here to stay.

All too often the nursing home is perceived by older persons, their relatives and by professionals as a final waiting station before death. This attitude has led to a neglect of services for the institutionalized elderly. Under Medicare and Medicaid, extended care facilities have been required (with somewaht inconsistent results) to maintain basic standards in their physical plant, its maintenance, and the provision of medical services. However, scarcely any attention has been paid to the development of psychosocial programs for the institutionalized older person (Gottesman, 1970). It is ironic that the helping professions have devoted so little attention to the two events which are among the most difficult social and emotional adjustments in the life cycle—the process of growing old and moving to an institution.

The adjustment of the older person is made difficult by a number of role changes associated with aging. The wholesale retirement of individuals at the age of sixty-five leaves many unprepared for the accompanying change in status and re-orientation to a new life-style. (Butler, 1975).

Social expectations demand that the older person relinquish the assertive style of earlier years (Havighurst, Neugarten, & Tobin, 1968): the older worker is expected to "step aside" to make room for younger workers. Often the older person is perceived by others to be unproductive. Whereas in earlier years the older person played the role of provider, now he or she is perceived as someone who must be "cared for." There is a sudden increase in leisure time for which the older person is often unprepared because of earlier devotion to career.

With retirement, work associates are left behind and kinship ties assume greater importance (Cumming, 1964). However, the older person's role in the family may change dramatically. Decision-making within the family often shifts to the younger members. Important decisions regarding finances and other personal matters are increasingly made without the approval or input of the older person.

As the discrepancy between male and female life span increases, extended widowhood has become a regular feature of growing old (Butler, 1975). Women who previously relied on husbands for financial security, emotional support and daily chores are abruptly deprived of a familiar resource. A new set of individuals must be relied upon: children, friends, relatives or providers of services, such as the delivery person and the visiting nurse.

Along with these changes many older persons must cope with serious illness, and physical disability. Reduced mobility eliminates many opportunities for social interaction. Impaired hearing makes it difficult to communicate freely with others. The use of a crutch or prosthesis may be embarassing for the older person.

With such changes it is not surprising that the level of social interaction decreases with age (Bellin, 1961; Cumming & Henry, 1961; Phillips, 1957), though this increasing social isolation may not be desired (Havighurst, Neugarten, & Tobin, 1968).

Particularly for the institutionalized older person role changes may be dramatic. Often these changes are abrupt, allowing little time to develop the skills necessary to cope with a new or altered environment. For instance, many older persons are institutionalized as the result of a crisis such as the death of a spouse or a serious illness, and made suddenly dependent on institutional staff for daily maintenance needs and on other residents for fulfillment of social and emotional needs. Novel, problematic situations may arise. How does the resident get staff to schedule bath times that will not interfere with a relative's visit? How does the resident ask for a change of medication? or assistance in getting to a recreational activity? How does the resident ask for a change in diet or additional items added to the dinner menu? How does the resident approach other residents for a card game or a session of friendly reminiscing? What does the resident do about the disappearance of valuable items from his dresser? What does the resident say to a confused resident who repeatedly wanders into his or her room uninvited?

The growth of our elderly population and the accompanying proliferation of geriatric long-term care facilities has led in turn to the recruitment of a large number of service workers to care for the institutionalized elderly. Unfortunately, care for the elderly has assumed a position of low status in our culture (Bennet & Eisdorfer, 1975). This is reflected in the low wages, poor education and high turnover of non-professional nursing home staff. The routine nature of maintenance tasks and lack of career opportunities result in the recruitment of inexperienced persons who may be unsuited for work with the elderly. High rates of turnover for professional staff result from much the same reasons.

In addition, problems of communication among levels of authority and staff differences concerning treatment of residents may adversely effect the resident: (Stanton and Schwartz (1954) reported this to be the case in mental hospitals. Gubrium (1975) for example, found that ward attendants effectively sabotaged innovative procedures and treatment programs designed by professional staff. Ineffective ways of interacting with residents and poor awareness of the special needs of the elderly may also lead to a nontherapeutic environment.

SETTING

The research program discussed in this chapter was carried out within two long-term care institutions for the elderly. The Dane County Home is located in Verona, Wisconsin, a small town several miles from the capital, Madison. Oakwood Village is a voluntary nursing home under the auspices of Lutheran Social Service and is located in Madison. Both homes are skilled nursing care facilities. Both are above average in terms of the general quality of care and physical facilities. The residents of Oakwood Village tend to be of somewhat higher socio-economic status. Residents at Oakwood are more likely to be "private-pay" patients than their counterparts at the County home.

Residents' perceptions of their own roles give some clue as to the different orientation of the two homes. In response to our questioning we found that Oakwood Village occupants prefer to be called "residents," while County home occupants insist on being called "patients." This was true even though the subjects who participated in our program at the two homes were of comparable mental and physical status and health. Oakwood Village is part of a complex of several buildings which vary in level of care from skilled nursing to semi-independent living within an "apartment-complex" setting. There is an emphasis on preserving the resident's independence and discouraging the effects of institutionalization and the patient role. Although there are several hundred elderly in the entire complex, there are only sixty to seventy-five residents in Oakwood Village.

The Dane County home, in appearance and philosophy, is more typically an "institution." Wards are painted in drab hospital colors unlike the bright orange and blue walls at Oakwood Village. There is no semi-independent living facility associated with the home and there is a larger proportion of severely ill patients among the 160 occupants.

Both homes were very receptive to the presence of our research project. The Dane County home had previously served as a field placement agency for social work students, so staff were used to the sight of students interacting with patients. Staff at both homes were very cooperative with our research staff and regularly assisted in tasks ranging from finding a missing patient to interpreting medical records. Most staff, professional as well as nonprofessional, seemed genuinely committed to the welfare of the patients. At the Dane County home this was reflected in an unusually low turnover rate for all staff. Many of the nurses and aides had been with the home for over ten years.

SOCIAL SKILLS TRAINING FOR RESIDENTS

The theoretical background for the present program is a social-skills learning model consisting of a set of principles and procedures derived from social learning theory. In this model both assessment and treatment are focused on readily observable behavior, and the subject is provided with direct instruction and practice in a range of interpersonal situations. Unlike traditional treatment models which seek to eliminate inner psychological conflicts, the social skills model teaches the subject skills in which he or she is deficient.

Some models of the aging process assume that behavioral deficits of the elderly are products of irreversible biological deterioration, but a social learning theory approach assumes that behavioral deficits may be lessened or overcome through environmental modficiation (Hoyer, 1973; Hoyer, Kafer, Simpson, & Hoyer, 1974; Mueller & Atlas, 1972). Lindsley (1964) first suggested the use of environmental manipulation to overcome behavioral deficits among the elderly. Environmental deficits may be seen as contributing substantially to reduced competence, and "pathological" behaviors may be a result of the patient's setting (Gottesman & Brody, 1975). For instance, social withdrawal behaviors (e.g. reduced verbalizations, fewer interactions with others) may be shaped and maintained by the reinforcement of nursing home staff because "quiet" patients are perceived by staff as more easily managed. From a social learning perspective such behaviors may be modified by providing programs to train patients in interactive skills and by instructing staff to reinforce appropriate patient behaviors.

Gerontology was a late comer to the field of behavioral intervention. The present author found only three reports of behavioral intervention with the elderly prior to 1968. Since that time nearly forty studies have appeared in the literature—(a good review of studies prior to 1975 is provided by Hoyer, Mishara & Riebel, 1975)—by and large dealing with simple operant behaviors. Mueller and Atlas (1972), for instance, successfully used cigarettes, candy and token reinforcement to increase appropriate interactions among members of a group of five elderly men in a nursing home. Hoyer, Kafer, Simpson, and Hoyer (1974) increased appropriate verbalizations among elderly male residents on an old-age ward of a state mental hospital. Linsk, Howe and Pinkston (1975) modified member behaviors in three ongoing group activities in a nursing home for the elderly. They utilized stimulus prompting (i.e. leader question-asking) to increase a number of group behaviors. Blackman, Howe, and Pinkston (1976) used prompting and reinforcement to increase pro-social behaviors of handicapped elderly women in a nursing home.

Intervention Paradigm

The research reported in this chapter goes beyond the modification of simple operant behaviors. The skill training programs described here are designed to develop the complex social behaviors that determine an individual's competence in social situations. A comprehensive model for behavioral assessment developed by Goldfried and D'Zurilla (1969) serves as the basis for the programs.

The central theoretical concept of Goldfried and D'Zurilla's Behavioral Analytic Model for Assessing Competence is competent behavior. *Competence* is defined as the "effectiveness or adequacy with which an individual is capable of responding to the various problematic situations which confront him" (p. 161). A problematic situation is one "which requires a solution to a problem or some decision for appropriate action" (p. 159). The basic "unit" of personality is the *effective response.* Effective behavior is defined as "a response or pattern of responses to a problematic situation which alters the situation so that it is no longer problematical, and at the same time produces a maximum of other positive consequences and a minimum of negative ones" (p. 158). The greater the range and number of situations to which the individual can respond effectively, the greater is that individual's competence.

Goldfried and D'Zurilla describe five steps that can be applied to develop an assessment procedure and training program for any client population: 1) situational analysis, 2) enumeration of the response 3) evaluation of the response, 4) development of measurement format, and 5) evaluation of the measure.

The purpose of situational analysis is to obtain a comprehensive list of the relevant situations with which the individual must cope. Each situation must be described with sufficient specificity so that effective response(s) can be enumerated. Situations should be relatively problematic for members of the population under assessment. For example, at least some members of the population should have some difficulty in responding to some of the situations. An individual who is effective in a large number of these situations, however, is a "competent" individual. Goldfried and D'Zurilla suggest a number of methods by which the situational analysis could be conducted: direct naturalistic observation, interviews with individuals who experience the problematic situations, and self-observation and recording of these situations as they occur.

The response enumeration phase provides a collection of possible responses for each problematic situation. According to the model the effectiveness of a response varies on a continuum from superior to inferior. Therefore, different responses may vary in their effectiveness. Some situations may elicit a wide variety of responses while others may elicit few responses. The optimum method for response enumeration involves direct observation of individuals responding in real life situations. A more practicial method is to create a simulated situation such as a role play. The situation may also be simulated through verbal or written descriptions to which the subject responds orally or in writing. Where the subject's responses are described rather than enacted, the response description must be sufficiently detailed so it is clear exactly what the subject did and how he did it.

The purpose of the response evaluation phase is to determine the relative effectiveness of each of the responses enumerated in the previous step. Goldfried and D'Zurilla suggest that this determination be based on the judgment of "significant others." These should be influential individuals who "a) have frequent contact with the people to whom the assessment technique will be applied, b) have an important role in labeling or judging behavior as effective or ineffective...., and c) whose opinions are likely to be respected by others" (p. 166). Once these judgments of effectiveness are obtained it should be possible to get some consensus regarding which responses are effective or ineffective.

The end result of this procedure is to have established both the *content* for an assessment measure (the list of situations) as well as the *criteria* by which this measure can be scored (ratings of response effectiveness).

Development of the Program

Our skill training program followed the steps of the Goldfried and D'Zurilla model. Intensive situational analysis interviews were conducted with twenty-two residents. In the interview, residents were asked to think about situations over the past few weeks in which they interacted with one or more other persons—residents, staff, or visitors. Then they were asked to identify any situations in which they felt they could have acted more effectively than they actually did. We were also interested in situations in which the residents perceived they had acted in the best possible way but were less than satisfied with the way they *felt* afterwards. Examples were provided of the types of situations desired. The interviewer guided residents to discussion of a particular occurrence of the situation. Residents were asked to describe the situation in as much detail as possible, including: 1) what led up to the situation, 2) the purpose of the interaction, 3) the characteristics of the other person or persons, 4) the physical location, and 5) who said what to whom. These details were recorded in writing by the interviewer.

It was found that approximately fifteen to twenty interviews were sufficient to identify the core of problematic social situations in the first nursing home in which we conducted the program. (Only minor modifications were necessary when the program was expanded to include the second nursing home). The situations could be divided into four categories: 1) making a request, 2) responding to a request, 3) starting or continuing a conversation, and 4) responding to an annoying statement or action. Situations that were substantially similar were combined and reworded for clarity to produce a final list of thirty-four situations.

Having identified a core of common problematic social situations our next step was to determine how we might instruct residents to respond to these situations (response enumeration). Each situation was presented one at a time to a staff member who was asked to act out a verbal response that would be effective for a resident. (These sometimes included nonverbal components, such as getting up and changing the TV channel.) We interviewed a total of sixteen staff members (professional and nonprofessional) who had extensive experiences in nursing home settings. (To reduce the length of the interview, half of the staff respondents received one set of situations and half received the other.) The end result of this step was a series of eight potentially effective responses to each of the identified social situations.

The next step was response evaluation. The rationale behind this step was that there exists within a social environment, consensual validation as to what constitutes an effective response to a social situation. In other words, the most effective behaviors are those defined by those in the social setting as being the "best" way to handle the situation. For our purposes ten individuals were selected who had "expert" knowledge of the nursing home environment. These included professional and non-professional staff from one of our nursing homes as well as others with extensive nursing home experience. The experts were asked to rate each response to each situation on a five-point scale from "one = very ineffective" to "five = very effective" and to explain their reasons for each rating.

The expert ratings were summarized and used to identify those responses to each situation considered to be effective. An effective response was defined as one which was rated as "effective" or "very effective" by four out of five experts. By this criterion, all situations had at least one effective response.

The reasons provided by the experts for their ratings were carefully examined. These rationales provided us with basic principles of responding later used in the training program. Principles applicable to a number of similar situations were termed General Criteria. Principles unique to a specific situation were termed Specific Criteria. Thus, each situation had a set of both General and Specific Criteria for an effective response.

Figure One provides an example of a problematic social situation, criteria for responding effectively, and an effective response.

Example of Problematic Social Situation, Criteria for Responding, and an Effective Response.

Situation: Let's suppose that you do not like uninvited residents to come into your room. Sometimes a resident will wander into your room and look at and touch your things. You find this very annoying.

You are returning to your room after lunch. As you enter your room you notice that one of the residents from down the hall is standing in your room.

Criteria

General

1. Tell the other person specifically that his(her) behavior is annoying to you.
2. Suggest an alternative behavior that would be less annoying.
3. Do *not* "name-call."

Specific

1. Offer to assist resident to his(her) own room.
2. Do *not* make an accusation or give an order e.g. "stay out of my room unless asked to be there!"
3. Do *not* use swear words.

FIGURE 1

An Effective Response

"I wish you wouldn't come in here when I'm not here. You know it's not nice to be in my room when you are uninvited. I'll help you to your room if you would like."

Training Program

The identified situations, responses and principles of responding form the basis of the training program. The program assumes that the best way to learn new effective behavior is to practice that behavior in a non-threatening simulated situation. The more similar the situation to situations which are actually encountered, the more effective the training will be. In addition, the resident must be given specific instructions and examples of effective responding.

There are five key elements in the training program.

1) *Coaching.* The General and Specific Principles are presented for each situation. Index cards may be useful to help the resident retain this information.

2) *Modeling.* The resident observes effective responses which are provided by a trainer, another resident or a tape-recorded model.

3) *Rehearsal.* The resident practices the response as if the situation were actually occurring.

4) *Feedback.* After rehearsal the resident is told specifically how her response did or did not meet the criteria for an effective response. Alternating rehearsal and feedback may occur if necessary.

5) *Gradual response building.* One principle or set of principles is presented at a time. The resident is given adequate opportunity to practice part of a response before the entire response is taught. Presentation of new material then, is tied to the resident's ability to rehearse appropriately.

In the first year's study residents were trained individually following the training sequence summarized in Figure Two. In the second year's study residents were trained in pairs so that a "buddy" would be available to enhance feedback and discussion and to provide support for practice of new responses. An example of a typical training sequence for a session with two residents is provided in Figure Three.

Several points should be noted in this example:

1) Three types of index cards provided to each resident served as prompts and memory aids. The General Principles card listed all the General Principles for one type of situation. In this case, the situation was of the type involving a response to an annoying statement or action. After the resident received training in each type of situation s/he was given a personal copy of the General Principles card to refer to between sessions. Notice in the example in Figure Three that the trainer reviewed the

General Principles at the beginning. The Specific Principles cards were presented during coaching steps. At each point in the training sequence the trainer presented a Specific Principles card which listed only those principles covered so far. Modeling cards are particularly useful for residents who are forgetful or hard of hearing.

2) A response building procedure was followed with the general and specific principles presented in a cumulative fashion.

3) The training sequence made maximal use of pairs of residents. Each partner alternates self rehearsal and feedback on the other's rehearsal. In order to keep feedback specific, residents were asked to refer to the General and Specific Principles cards when giving feedback. The partners were also encouraged to continue discussion and feedback of everyday situations between training sessions.

Training Sequence Utilizing One Resident

1. Situation presentation
2. Coaching
3. Modeling
4. Coaching
5. Discussion
6. Situation Re-presentation
7. Rehearsal
8. Feedback
9. Discussion
10. Steps 6, 7 and 8 are repeated until resident has adequately learned response or three minutes have elapsed, whichever comes first.

FIGURE 2

Training Sequence Utilizing Two Residents

1. *Situation presentation:* Let's suppose that you do not like uninvited residents to come into your room. Sometimes a resident will wander into your room and look at and touch your things. You find this very annoying.

You are returning to your room after lunch. As you enter your room you notice that one of the residents from down the hall is standing in your room.

2. *Coaching:* This is a situation in which you need to *respond to an annoying situation.* Let's first look at your list of general principles for this type of situation. (Refer residents to their General Principle card for responding to an annoying action or statement.)

Card: RESPONDING TO AN ANNOYING ACTION OR STATEMENT

You tell the other person in a polite way *specifically* the behavior that is annoying to you.

Suggest an alternative behavior that would be less annoying.

Do *not* name call.

In *this* situation, you want to let the resident know that it annoys you to have her/him in your room. You want him/her to know that you do not like to have people come in uninvited. You do not say it as an order or use swear words.

Let's listen to an example. (Refer to modeling cards.)

3. *Modeling:* I wish you wouldn't come in here when I'm not here. You know it isn't nice to be in my room when you are not invited.

4. *Coaching:* Notice that the model immediately stated what the person was doing that annoyed him. You want to let the wanderer know that it not only annoys you to see him in your room now, but that you *never* like to have people come to your room uninvited when you're not there. The statement was made in a very polite way. The speaker didn't accuse the resident, use any swear words or name call. Instead, he clearly got across his feelings about the annoying situation.

5. *Discussion with Mrs. Brock. Then repeat with Mrs. Able:* Did you see how the General Principle was used in this annoying situation? Do you feel that the other parts of the statement would help you get your point across? Can you picture yourself saying this in this situation? O.K., you want to let the resident know what annoys you. You do not order or use swear words.

6. *Situation re-presentation.* Let's suppose that you do not like uninvited residents to come into your room. Sometimes a resident will wander into your room and look at and touch your things. You find this very annoying.

You are returning to your room after lunch. As you enter your room you notice that one of the residents from down the hall is standing in your room. (Refer to Specific Principles card.)

7. *Rehearsal with Mrs. Brock:* Two successful responses required before moving on.

8. *Feedback and discussion from Trainer and Mrs. Abel.* (Refer to Specific Principles card.)

9. *Situation re-presentation:* You are returning to your room after lunch. As you enter your room you notice that one of the residents from down the hall is standing in your room. (Refer to Specific Principles card.)

10. *Rehearsal with Mrs. Able:* Two successful performances required before moving on.

11. *Discussion and feedback from Trainer and Mrs. Brock:* (refer to Specific Principles card.)

12. *Situation re-presentation:* You don't like uninvited residents to

wander into your room or touch your things. You find this very annoying. You are returning to your room after lunch. As you enter you notice that one of the residents from down the hall is standing in your room.

13. *Coaching:* You have now let the person know, in a polite way that you do not like him to come into your room uninvited. Now you can offer to assist the resident to his/her own room. This would help get the person out of your room. It would also reinforce your message that you don't want people in your room uninvited. It gives him an alternative to touching your things that would be less annoying.

Let's listen to an example. (Refer to modeling cards.)

14. *Modeling:* I wish you wouldn't come in here when I'm not here. You know it's not nice to be in my room when you are not invited. *I'll help you to your room if you would like.*

15. *Coaching:* Notice how you can suggest the resident go to his room. This is telling him to do something that would not annoy you.

16. *Discussion with Mrs. Able. Repeat with Mrs. Brock:* How did that sound to you? Can you picture yourself responding to this situation in this way? O.K. You want to let the resident know what annoys you. You don't order or use swear words. You suggest the resident do something else—something that is not annoying to you.

17. *Situation re-presentation:* You don't like uninvited residents to wander into your room or touch your things. You find this very annoying. You are returning to your room after lunch. As you enter you notice that one of the residents from down the hall is standing in your room. (Refer to Specific Principles cards.)

18. *Rehearsal with Mrs. Able:* Two successful responses required before moving on.

19. *Discussion and feedback from Trainer and Mrs. Brock.* (Refer to Specific Principles cards.)

20. *Situation re-presentation:* You are returning to your room after lunch. As you enter your room you notice that one of the residents from down the hall is standing in your room. (Refer to Specific Principles card.)

21. *Rehearsal with Mrs. Brock:* Two successful responses required before moving.

22. *Discussion and feedback from Trainer and Mrs. Able.* (Refer to Specific Principles card.)

FIGURE 3

Selection of Residents

In selecting residents for the Skill Training Program we sought to eliminate those who were too severely ill or disoriented to participate.

Thus, the training procedures described are most suitable for those who are able to interact in a coherent way with others.

The present program however, did include residents who were temporarily or partially disoriented and those with physical problems such as paralysis or impaired hearing. Selection of eligible residents was made by the Director of Nurses in each home. Ninety of 160 residents at Dane County and thirty-five of 110 residents at Oakwood Village were selected as eligible; each of these was requested to participate in some phase of the program: only those who agreed to participate were included in the program.

During the first year of the program the study was limited to the Dane County Home. Twenty-five residents participated in skill training procedures. Median age of these residents was 77.3 years (70.9 years for males and 83.9 years for females). Median length of residence at the home was 5.2 years (5.9 years for males and 2.9 years for females). Six males and four females were never married. The remaining residents were widowed or divorced. Seven males and three females had a psychiatric or psychiatric-related diagnosis indicated in their medical record such as schizophrenia or organic brain syndrome due to arteriosclerosis. All were white.

During the second year the program was conducted at both homes. Demographic data for the second year's training program are similar. Median age of these residents was 85.4 years (78.9 years for males and 86.6 years for females). Median length of residence at the home was 1.9 years (3.2 years for males and 1.9 for females). Five residents were never married, one was currently married. The others were widowed or divorced. Six residents had a psychiatric or psychiatric-related diagnosis indicated in their medical record. Again, all were white. At both homes former occupations included farmers, laborers, housewives, clerks, nurse's aids, librarians and salesmen.

Brief descriptions of several typical residents are presented below.

Ms. O. Ms. O. was seventy-two years old and had been a resident in the Home for twelve and one-half years. She was bright and articulate and had formerly worked as a medical librarian. Never married, she displayed an excellent memory and took pride in remembering the names of social work students and the dates they had visited her. Quick-witted and known by the staff for her mild sarcasm and frequent jokes, Ms. O had a partial paralysis of her legs. With the assistance of a leg brace she took regular walks along the wing by pushing a wheelchair in front of her for support. Most of the day was spent in her room where she read, embroidered or watched television. Her room was filled with many personal possessions, mostly notably various items she had embroidered or crocheted.

Ms. G. Ms. G. was a housewife whose husband had died many years earlier. Eight-four years old, she was very alert, articulate, responsive, and in touch with the present. She had been a resident of the Home for the past two years. She revealed no major physical impairments, and although she appeared somewhat fragile, she was quite mobile. Photos, embroidery work and a rocking chair of her own added a personal touch to her tiny room.

Ms. U. Ms. U. had been a housekeeper for an elderly gentleman for a major portion of her adult life. Never married, at sixty-three she was afflicted with multiple sclerosis which had slurred her speech and left her paralyzed below the waist. She had been at the home for the past six years and spent most of her time in bed or sitting up in a wheelchair in her room. Despite these limitations, Ms. U. was always alert and in touch with reality. Through extensive speech therapy she had learned to speak audibly, but slowly. Her room was decorated with many pictures and personal belongings.

Mr. J. Forty-eight years old, Mr. J. was the youngest resident in the Home. Never married, he had been a psychiatric inpatient since his early thirties. Mr. J. spent part of each day helping staff to set up recreational activities and assisting other patients by pushing their wheelchairs or relaying messages for them. He was actively involved in the preparation of a newsletter written by the patients. Mr. J. had been diagnosed as suffering from "cerebal atrophy." Although he stuttered and displayed some facial twitching, he was very alert and articulate, able to engage in intelligent conversation about sports, the weather and other common topics. Despite frequent hypochondriacal complaints he did not have any obvious physical impairments and was able to get around the Home with apparent ease. Mr. J's room had a highly personal touch, filled with many personal possessions and decorations such as a radio, clock, television, magazines, books and pictures.

Mr. K. Mr. K. was a sixty-five year old retired accountant who had been institutionalized as a result of medical problems associated with alcoholism. He had been divorced and separated from his wife some twenty years before and had been living in the Home for three years. He was well educated and intelligent, and had run a successful accounting business for many years. He displayed no apparent physical handicaps and spent most of his time in one of the lounges or outside during good weather. He talked readily about his daily walks, trips into town and visits to his children. Although Mr. K's room was somewhat stark and undecorated, there were several books, magazines, a cigarette rolling machine and tobacco, all of which were important parts of Mr. K's use of his leisure time.

Mr. N. Mr. N., a former bricklayer, was ninety-three years old. He had been widowed many years previously and had been a patient at the Home for ten years. Confined to a chair for most of the day and totally blind, he was very alert and responsive. Mr. N. frequently related amusing anecdotes and reminiscences of his earlier years. His room was devoid of personal possessions with the exception of a small radio within reach of the bed. Although his social interactions were extremely minimal due to his physical condition, he remained very responsive to human contact.

EVALUATION

Behavioral researchers have stressed the importance of multiple forms of evaluation (Mischel, 1968). In general, evaluation seeks to document a change in behavior that occurs in the resident's natural environment. Direct observation of the resident is the preferred form since it is the most accurate measure of real change. Other forms of evaluation in order from most direct to least direct are: simulated interactions, roleplays, and self-report. Each of these procedures was used to evaluate the present training program.

For the direct observation student observers were trained to monitor residents. In this procedure each observer was provided with a monitoring form, as illustrated in Figure Four. Observers worked in pairs, monitoring resident behavior simultaneously in order to provide a measure of interobserver agreement. Four to six residents were monitored at a time. (On the form each resident is indicated by a capital letter from A to F.) Monitoring followed an interval recording procedure and occurred three days prior to and again three days after intervention. During each day the paired observers made four observations or "sweeps" of the nursing home. Each sweep followed a fixed order from day room, down the wing, and so forth. Observers made their recordings independently without conversing or interacting with each other. For each observation the observer recorded the location of the resident from the list indicated at the bottom of the form. A resident may have been in the dayroom, his or her own room, or a "social hot spot." Social hot spots were identified as a number of locations in which residents regularly congregated. Each time a resident was in his/her room the observer recorded whether the room door was open.

Inter-observer agreement for these data were consistently high. Data were summarized across observation times and days and averaged across pairs of observers to yield the proportion of instances in which the resident was in the day room, his or her own room, or a social hot spot. In a similar manner, for each of these locations the researchers determined the proportion of times the resident was interacting with another person. Collapsing across locations the researchers also computed the overall

Observational Inventory Monitoring Sheet

Date _____/_____/_____ Pilot Pre Post f/u (circle one) AM PM (circle one) Observer

Residents observed A __________ B __________ C __________ D __________ E__________ F __________

Time 1 __________ Time 2 __________ Time 3 __________ Time 4 __________

Resident's name	A	B	C	D	E	F	A	B	C	D	E	F	A	B	C	D	E	F	A	B	C	D	E	F
Where was resident?*																								
Listening/talking to another person? Y=Yes N=No																								
Own room door at least half way open? Y=Yes N=No																								

* D= day room on resident's wing: 0= own room; S= social hot spot: (1) opening of wing onto main hallway (downstairs only), 2) TV room across the way from the dining room (downstairs only), 3) front lounge by main entrance (downstairs only); E= Elsewhere (indicate where); ?= could not be found.

Note: Begin observation at day room, proceed down the wing checking residents' rooms, then to social hot spots, then elsewhere. Always follow this order.

FIGURE 4

Observational Inventory:
Information from Institutional Records

Information from Chart

For period from ______________ (mo./day) to ______________ (mo./day)

1. Number of times resident visited with his/her family or friends outside the Home.
2. Number of times resident visited the doctor or dentist (include visits outside as well as inside the Home).
3. Total number of milligrams of prescription medicine administered to resident.

Information from Activity Director's Records

For period from ______________ (mo./day) to ______________ (mo./day)

1. Number of activities attended by resident.
2. Number of times resident helped Activity Director set up an activity.

FIGURE 5

proportion of times in which the resident was interacting with another resident or staff person.

Observers were also responsible for collecting relevant data from the institution's own on-going recording. This included the items listed in Figure Five.

It is not always possible to observe the target behavior as it occurs in the resident's natural environment. For instance, if we wanted to assess the resident's ability to refuse unreasonable requests we may not have the time or resources to observe continuously until the target behavior occurs. An alternative is to create as realistic as possible an interaction between the resident and one or more other persons. In the present study such a simulated "real-life" test was constructed.

For this test the assessor (who will be referred to as *E*) read the following statement to the resident:

> I would like you to imagine that I am a social worker you have never met before. I will leave the room. Then I will knock on your door. I will pretend that I am a social worker, and I will ask you if I can interview you right now. I would like you to do three things. 1. First, ask me what agency I'm from. 2. Next, get me to agree to come back tomorrow. Whatever I say, don't let me stay to talk to you now. 3. Then, get me to leave the room.

E reviewed these instructions with the resident carefully until they were understood. Then *E* left the room, paused, and knocked on the door to the resident's room. *E* entered the room and introduced himself: "Hi. My name is __________ I'm a social worker. I'd like to talk with you now." *E* was instructed to honor the resident's first request (informing the resident of the social worker's agency). However, if the resident asked *E* to return tomorrow *E* was instructed to reply: "I won't be here tomorrow. Can we talk right now?" If the resident again requested *E* to return tomorrow *E* agreed to do so. *E* left the room as soon as the resident made a direct request that he leave or three minutes had elapsed since *E*'s knock on the door.

After the roleplay *E* recorded the number of tasks successfully completed by the resident, his or her impression of the resident's effectiveness in the role play, and the duration of the role play (three minute maximum). The resident was asked to rate how she acted and felt during the role play on a four point scale ranging from 1 = "comfortable and able to handle it well" to 4 = "uncomfortable *and* unable to handle it well." *E* was instructed to spend no more than fifteen minutes on the initial instructions and the "real-life" test.

Although the simulated real-life test may be a desirable assessment instrument because of the highly realistic nature of the simulation, it does limit the range and number of situations on which the subject may be tested. First, the test consumes a great deal of time. Second, it is impossible to simulate the broad range of types of interactions which the resident is likely to encounter. A role-play test overcomes these difficulties at the expense of being an additional step removed from the real situation.

A role-play test consists of a series of imagined interpersonal situations which are presented to the resident. The resident is asked to respond to the situation as if it were really occurring, and is encouraged to answer out loud as if she were actually experiencing the situation. The test itself is usually preceded by one or two practice situations during which *E* uses coaching, feedback and verbal praise to shape a role play.

In this study the situations were read to the resident from a transcript. Presentation of tape-recorded situations did not work as well since many of the residents had difficulty hearing or understanding the tape. The role-play situations were selected from the situations developed during the situational analysis of the assessment phase (see above). The test included situations on which the resident received training as well as untrained situations. A comparison of responses to the two types of situations provided a measure of generalization of learning.

All subject responses were tape-recorded and evaluated by trained raters. The order of responses was randomized with respect to resident, time of test (pretest, posttest, and followup), experimental condition and situation. All responses were rated independently from the tapes by at least two raters, and inter-rater agreement was computed. The measure of inter-rater agreement utilized in this study was the proportion of situations which received the same rating from both raters.

In the present study all ratings were based on a Judges' Manual. The Judges' Manual consisted of a list of from one to five criteria for effective responding in each situation. These criteria were generated from the response evaluation interviews described above, and therefore represent the judgment of "significant others" in the resident's environment. These criteria are the same as those employed in training.

In the first year's study raters evaluated the resident's response to each situation by assigning a number equivalent to the number of criteria fulfilled. Resident's final scores represent the proportion of criteria satisfied, averaged across situations. The final score subjected to analysis was the average of the two raters' scores for each subject.

Although high interrater agreement was obtained across situations using this procedure, agreement on particular situations was not consistently satisfactory. Therefore, in the second year's study a simplified rating procedure was used. The following scale was used to rate responses to each situation:

1	2	3	4
Very Ineffective	Ineffective	Effective	Very Effective

In this study raters utilized a list of criteria to rate each situation. However, the criteria were divided into General Criteria (applicable to all situations of that type) and Specific Criteria. In addition, separate groups of judges either listened to the tape-recorded responses or read transcribed responses (there were no differences in the two methods). Judges then followed a set of rules for rating responses as summarized in Figure Six. As before, order was randomized with respect to resident, experimental condition, situation and time of testing. The resident's final score was his/her mean rating across all situations. Interobserver agreement was high for individual situations and overall scores.

A variety of resident self-report measures were also used. Although self-report may be less accurate than observation as an indicator of overt behavior, the resident's own perceptions and feelings are an important aspect of the program's effectiveness.

An Interpersonal Situation Inventory was constructed. It consisted of a list of all the situations derived from the situational analysis described above. (It included the situations on the roleplay test.) Each situation was read to the resident, who was asked to rate how she would personally feel and act in each situation. The response alternatives were:

1 = comfortable *and* able to handle it well
2 = uncomfortable *but* able to handle it well
3 = comfortable *but* unable to handle it well
4 = uncomfortable *and* unable to handle it well
5 = would never come up

The subject's final score was the average of her responses with irrelevant ("5") situations eliminated.

Self-report can also be combined with other forms of assessment. For the roleplay test, after the resident's response to each situation he or she was asked to rate personal satisfaction with the response:

1 = Very Dissatisfied
2 = Dissatisfied
3 = Neither Satisfied Nor Dissatisfied
4 = Satisfied
5 = Very Satisfied

The resident's final score was an average of responses to all the situations.

The resident may also be used as a source of information on behaviors and activities that could be expected to change as a result of the skill training program. In some cases self-report data can be checked with institutional records to verify the accuracy of the resident's self-report. For example, one of our nursing homes recorded the number of times a resident asked the Activity Director to purchase a personal item for the resident on one of the Activity Director's regular shopping trips. In

Rules for Rating

Behavior Roleplay Test Responses

Assign A Rating of	*If The Following Are Met*
4 = Very Effective	All but one general criteria and all specific criteria. or All but one specific criteria and all general criteria.
3 = Effective	Half or more of general criteria. *and* one or more specific criteria. or Half or more of specific criteria *and* one or more general criteria. or All specific and no general criteria. or All general and no specific criteria.
2 = Ineffective	None of the above but at least two criteria (general or specific)
1 = Very Ineffective	Zero or one criterion (general or specific).

FIGURE 6

addition, the Activity Director regularly recorded the number of recreational activities attended by each resident. At the program's request she also recorded the number of times each resident helped set up an activity in the auditorium. Residents' requests for medication and personal services are recorded in the charts.

In our program a Self-Report Inventory was administered to each subject. The subject was asked to record the number of times s/he engaged in a number of activities related to interpersonal effectiveness. The items on the Self-Report Inventory are listed in Figure Seven. Several of the items are drawn from situations included in the training program. The Inventory recorded the number of times the activity occurred over the past month. Since this is a fairly long time

Summary of Items from Self-Report Inventory

In the past month

1. Have you left the home to visit friends or family?
2. Other than visits with family or friends, have you participated in an activity outside the home?
3. Have you written and mailed letters to family or friends?
4. Have you received letters from someone outside the home?
5. Have you made phone calls to someone?
6. Have you received phone calls from someone?
7. Have you attended activities held in the auditorium?
8. Did you make any special request of the server at meals?
9. Have you helped a fellow resident push his/her wheelchair?
10. Have you helped a visitor to find a resident, room or staff person?
11. Have you helped a staff member to find a resident or get a message to a resident?
12. Have you helped a resident find another resident or staff member, or helped a resident get a message to another resident or staff member?
13. Have you helped the Activity Director set up activities by doing such things as passing things out, arranging chairs, or setting up Bingo cards?
14. Thinking over the past month, did you spend time in the day room? If yes, how much time on an average day?
15. As you know, Bill or other staff go on a weekly shopping trip to buy things for residents. In the past month have you made a request to buy something on their weekly shopping trip? If yes, how many times?

FIGURE 7

experimenters were instructed to ask the resident how many times the activity occurred in the past week and then to help the resident construct a reasonable estimate for the month.

Self-report instruments can also be used to assist in program development. After a total of thirty-four situations were developed from the situational analysis interviews with residents, it was necessary to select a subset of situations for the training program. In the first year's study the Interpersonal Situation Inventory was administered to an independent sample of residents. Situations that these residents identified as most problematic and most common were selected for inclusion in the training program. All residents received training on the same set of situations.

In the second year each resident in the training program completed a Situation Selection Checklist prior to training. The checklist asked the resident to select the situations in which s/he felt the least competent. Residents were paired for training sessions. The particular set of situations selected for training was derived by making the best possible fit between the Situation Selection Checklists of the two residents, with the proviso that all of the four types of situations would be represented.

Self-report measures can be useful in other ways as well. A major requirement of the research design is the presence of a control group so that the "placebo" effect, induced by contact with the experiment, can be ruled out as an explanation for any difference between experimental and control groups. In the present study, Discussion Control Groups were formed for this purpose. In order to ascertain that expectancy effects were indeed equivalent in the Experimental and Discussion Control Groups, an Expectancy Questionnaire was administered to both groups. The trainer read the following questions to each resident: 1) How much do you think this training will help you to handle difficult social situations in the future?" and 2) "How much do you think this training will help you in general?" The subject chose one of five response alternatives to each question: 1 = Not at All, 2 = Very Little, 3 = Somewhat, 4 = Much, 5 = Very Much.

PROGRAM EVALUATION

The research described in this chapter was conducted over a two-year period in two phases which will be referred to as Study I and Study II. Several major changes designed to improve program effectiveness were incorporated into Study II. These changes will be explained below.

Study I

Study I was conducted in the Dane County Home. Twenty-seven residents were recruited for participation in the Program Evaluation.

Residents were randomly assigned, nine each, to one of three experimental conditions: Interpersonal Skill Training, Discussion Control, and Assessment-Only Control, with the restriction that males and females be about equally distributed among conditions. Two female residents in the Assessment-Only Condition subsequently dropped from the program because of unwillingness to participate.

Seven graduate students with experience in nursing home settings served as experimenters. All treatment and assessment was conducted in individual sessions with residents. Three experimenters conducted the training sessions for Interpersonal Skill Training and Discussion Control residents. Each of these experimenters was randomly assigned to three Skill Training and three Discussion Control residents. The remaining four experimenters administered the assessment measures and were randomly assigned to residents. Each resident met with one experimenter for the two post-treatment assessment sessions and with another experimenter for the two follow-up assessment sessions. In no case was the resident trained and assessed by the same experimenter.

The nine Interpersonal Skill Training and nine Discussion Control residents received three one-hour training sessions on eight social situations developed from the situational analysis interviews described earlier. These training situations involved interactions with both other residents and staff and dealt with a range of tasks. All of these eight situations were included on the sixteen item Behavior Roleplay Test. Residents in the Interpersonal Skill Training condition received training on these eight situations according to the training sequence in Figure Two, which included situation presentation, coaching, modeling, rehearsal and feedback.

Residents in the Discussion Control Condition were told that discussing social situations makes one better able to handle these situations. The experimenter read out loud the same situations as used in the Interpersonal Skill Training sessions, in the same order. Each situation was followed by a fifteen to twenty minute discussion which focused on similar experiences which occurred to the resident, the resident's feelings in those situations, and discussion of probable causes for those feelings. Specific behavioral solutions to these situations were not presented. Residents in both the Interpersonal Skill Training and Discussion Control conditions were also asked to respond to two questions (described above) to determine their expected gains from training. Assessment-Only residents participated only in the assessment procedures.

ASSESSMENT MEASURES All residents were assessed after the completion of training (or in the case of Assessment-Only residents, at approximately the same time as Training Condition residents were assessed) and again eight weeks later.

The Interpersonal Situation Inventory (ISI) and Behavior Role-play Test (BRT), as described above, were administered at the first and second posttreatment sessions respectively. For each BRT situation enacted, the resident rated satisfaction with his response on a five-point scale from 1 = "Very Satisfied" to 5 = "Very Dissatisfied", and the experimenter recorded the patient's pulse immediately before and after the BRT. In addition, at the second posttreatment session, a Simulated "Real-Life" Test was administered to all residents (as described above).

The Interpersonal Situation Inventory and the Behavior Role-play Test were readministered to all residents in the same order, approximately eight weeks after posttreatment assessment.

To summarize, the dependent variables were (1) Interpersonal Situation Inventory (ISI) score, (2) Behavior Roleplay Test (BRT) score, (3) Behavior Roleplay Test Satisfaction rating, and (4) Simulated "Real-Life" test scores.

RESULTS In the Interpersonal Skill Training and Discussion Control Conditions residents' responses to the two questions assessing their expectation of gain were summed and subjected to a nondirectional two independent sample *t*-test. The two conditions did not differ in expectancy.

Each resident's BRT responses were scored independently by four raters according to procedures described above. Correlations between all pairs of raters on this variable were consistently above 0.8, indicating high interrater reliability.

BRT scores are summarized in Figure Eight. On this variable the Interpersonal Skill Training Condition was significantly superior to the Discussion Control Condition and to the combined Control Conditions at posttest but not at follow-up. On closer examination, it was seen that the Interpersonal Skill Training Condition was significantly superior to the Control Conditions only for those situations for which residents received training but not for untrained situations alone. For the subset of eight situations for which residents received training, Interpersonal Skill Training was significantly superior to Discussion Control, and to the combined Control Conditions, at both posttest and follow-up. None of the remaining dependent variables—Interpersonal Situation Inventory, BRT Satisfaction Rating or Simulated "Real-Life" Test Scores differentiated significantly among conditions.

Study II

A number of modifications were made in Study II. Rather than training all residents on the same set of situations, as in Study I, each resident was asked to select a number of situations from a master list. Based on data from this list, each resident was matched with another resident or "buddy" who chose the most similar set of situations.

Forty-six residents were recruited for participation in Study II, as described above. Twenty-three "buddy pairs" were assigned to an Interpersonal Training and twenty-three pairs to Discussion Control Discussion. Subsequently twenty-one residents were dropped from the program prior to the posttest because of illness, lack of interest, or death, leaving twenty-five residents who completed the training and posttest assessment.

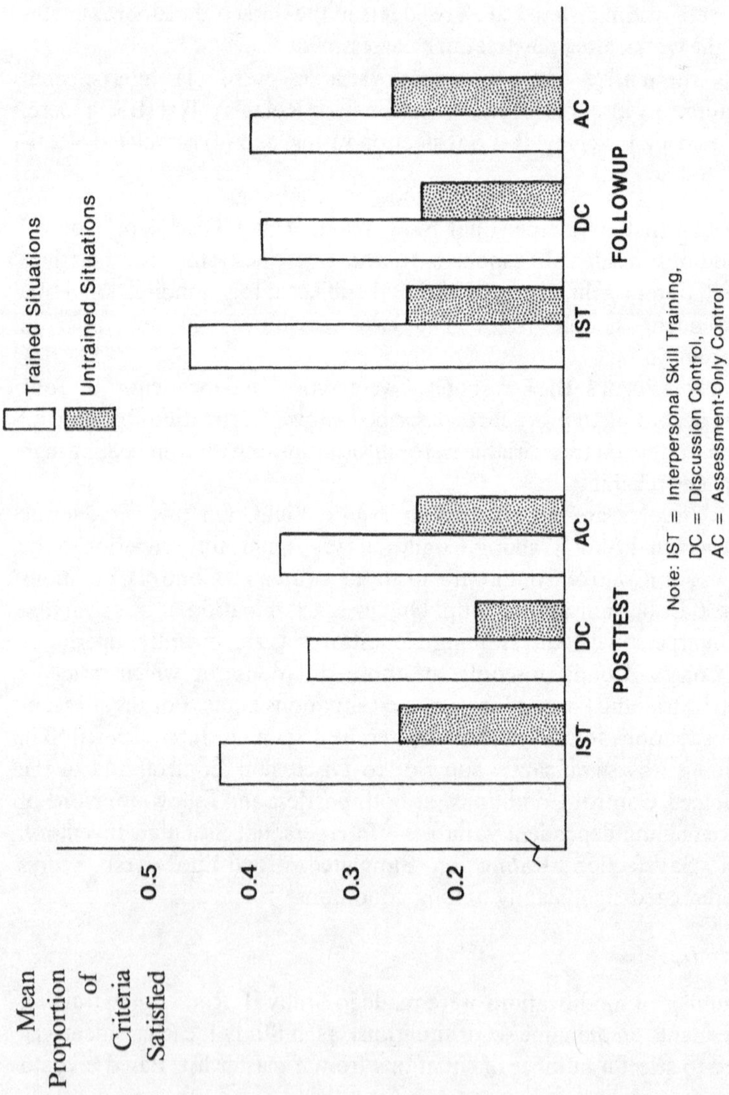

FIGURE 8. **Study I: Mean Behavior Role Play Test Scores for Experimental Conditions**

Interpersonal Skill Training pairs received five intensive training sessions on nine situations utilizing coaching, modeling, rehearsal and feedback from trainer and buddy as in the example of a typical training sequence summarized in Figure Three. Discussion Control pairs were presented with the same number of situations from each category of situations as Interpersonal Skill Training pairs: three situations which involved making a request, two situations which involved responding to an annoying action or statement, etc.

The pairs were informed that discussion of social situations has been shown to be helpful in learning how to better handle those situations. The number and length of training sessions was the same as for Interpersonal Skill Training pairs. Trainers focused the discussion around similar experiences encountered by the residents, their feelings in those situations, and speculation on the cause of those feelings.

Four trainers received extensive training in conducting the Interpersonal Skill Training and Discussion Control sessions with residents. A number of students from the School of Social Work administered the assessment instruments and judged the Behavior Roleplay Test responses.

RESULTS Scores on the Behavior Roleplay Test are summarized in Figure Nine. There were no significant differences between the Interpersonal Skill Training and Discussion Control conditions at posttest or follow-up. In addition, no differences were found between the conditions on any of the remaining variables. These variables included the number of visits outside the Home, number of grams of medication consumed, number of recreational activities attended, time spent in the dayroom and in social hot spots, and time spent interacting with other residents or staff. These analyses were computed with both univariate t tests and a multivariate T^2 test, and repeated with the single resident and the paired resident as the unit of analysis. None of these analyses revealed significant differences between residents who received Skill Training and those who did not.

DISCUSSION OF RESULTS

In Study I, on a direct behavioral measure (BRT), residents who participated in Interpersonal Skill Training were significantly more effective than control residents in responding to social situations to which effective responses had been explicitly taught. Skill Training residents retained this learning even two months after training. The results of Study I however, provide only limited evidence for the efficacy of Interpersonal Skill Training with elderly residents. On the BRT it was

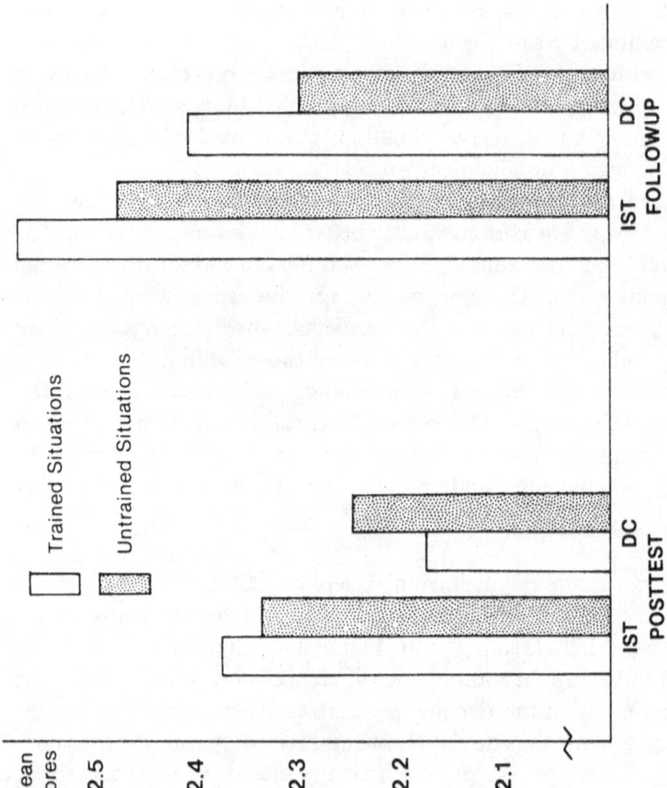

IST = Interpersonal Skill Training,
DC = Discussion Control
Scores could range from one to four.

FIGURE 9. **Study II: Mean Behavior Role Play Test Scores for Experimental Conditions**

clear that learning did not generalize to novel situations, Skill Training residents did not learn how to apply general rules of effective behavior to new situations. In addition, although these residents did increase their effectiveness, this was not reflected in the self-report measures. That is, Skill Training residents were not more satisfied with their responses and did not rate social situations as less problematic or difficult. Also, Skill Training had no effect on the resident's performance in a simulated interaction with a social worker.

It is noteworthy, however, that a treatment effect was demonstrated for the Roleplay Test. After direct observation in real situations, roleplay simulation is the most direct and hence preferred measure of behavior. (Mischel, 1968). In fact, in similar programs with other populations it is not uncommon to find a behavioral improvement on a role-play test with no accompanying change in self evaluation (e.g. Brockway, 1976;

Schinke & Rose, 1976). This phenomenon has been described as "attitudinal lag" (Goldsmith, 1973). That is, enhanced self-evaluations are considered consequences of improved performance and would be expected to lag behind performance change.

However, the treatment effect on the BRT in Study I was not replicated in the BRT in Study II. It was hoped that the modifications in the training program in Study II (greater duration of training, use of general principles, use of memory aids, and buddy pairs) would enhance the effectiveness of Interpersonal Skill Training and facilitate maintenance and generalization. This was not the case.

Study II failed to demonstrate that Interpersonal Skill Training was superior to a nonspecific discussion in training elderly nursing home residents how to be more effective in interpersonal interaction. The training program also did not affect a range of variables which might be related to interpersonal effectiveness in the institution, such as the frequency of interaction with others and the number of visits outside the institution.

One reason for the discrepancy in findings between Study I and Study II was the extended duration of training and assessment in Study II. Although more practice on a greater number of situations would seem likely to increase the program's effectiveness, in fact the extended nature of the program was objectionable to many residents. This was reflected, in part, in the high drop-out rate in Study II. Effective programs will have to limit the amount of time devoted to training and assessment or will have to make participation more attractive to residents.

The use of buddy pairs may have had an adverse effect. Some residents may have felt anxious performing in front of another resident. In almost all cases the paired residents had not interacted with each other prior to the study and this lack of familiarity may have heightened resident anxiety. Use of pairs and critical feedback between members of the pair may have created an undesirable competitive situation which interfered with learning. Use of a larger group may or may not have resolved these problems. The optimal setting (individual, pair, or group) for training is still undetermined.

There were interesting trends in the data in Study II which should be explored in future investigations. IST residents did seem to attend a greater number of recreational activities, confirming an observation of the Activity Director in response to Study I. If this treatment effect is indeed real, skilltraining programs may be useful in increasing level of interaction among residents. When data were analyzed with the single subject as the unit of analysis, a marginal treatment effect was demonstrated on the Behavioral Roleplay Test but only at follow-up. The The absence of such an effect at posttest suggests a possible "delayed" effect of treatment.

Despite the "improvements" added to Study II (use of general principles, etc.), a treatment effect was not demonstrated. Future investigations may be directed at discovering the optimal mix of training components for direct instruction with nursing home residents.

However, it may be that the most important changes could be directed at altering the interpersonal environment of the institution, rather than targeting interventions only at residents. For instance, attention should be paid to the effects of physical environment, and architectural variables on the behavior of residents (Danford, 1978).

Behaviorally oriented programs such as the one described in this chapter could be applied to volunteers and staff. Preliminary work by the present author has shown that the Goldfried and D'Zurilla model can be applied to develop an interpersonal skill training program for staff. When these procedures were carried out in the context of group-training incorporated into the regular in-service training program, they were warmly received by administrative and ward staff. Such procedures could be incorporated into requirements for nursing home staff currently required to receive in-service training. Reviews of the quality of care in nursing homes, such as the current utilization reviews required for Medicare/Medicaid programs, could include assessment of the interpersonal environment of the institution by utilizing some of the assessment procedures discussed here. The future is likely to see the application of behavioral procedures in these and other areas within the geriatric setting.

III

Professional Competence and Accountability

PROFESSIONAL COMPETENCE AND ACCOUNTABILITY

Professional competence and accountability are integral to contemporary social work. In light of growing competition from other human service disciplines and of shrinking public and private dollars for social programs, our profession is undergoing scrutiny from outside and within the field. Outsiders include a White House aide who thought the President ought to tell social workers, "Look, your social program of the 1960's isn't working, and we're going to dismantle it so you'll just have to go out and find honest labor somewhere else" (Ehrlichman quoted by Gannon, 1972, p. 1). From within the field we hear cries for a more clearly defined mission, greater professional competence, and better casework effectiveness (Schinke, 1979a, 1979b). Accordingly, the chapters included in the present section are essential to this text and our profession, and are placed at the end of our survey of applications of social work in the community to establish professional competence and accountability as final mandates for behavioral social work.

These chapters answer two questions: How can professionals acquire behavior modification techniques? What are some ways for evaluating the use of behavior modification in everyday social work? The practice-relevant answers to these questions give behavioral workers handy and sufficient tools to be competent and accountable when serving any client group in any setting. Workers thus equipped can go on to teach others to apply and evaluate behavioral intervention methods. In this manner, the programmatic and professional advantages of behavioral social work will multiply as our illuminati spread their practice wisdom.

The first three chapters speak to the development of clinical competence and credibility needed for behavioral practice. Jeff Edleson and Sheldon Rose outline an instructional format for acquiring interviewing expertise—a prerequisite to the clinical implementation of any therapy. Among other techniques, the educators show the relevance of modeling, behavior rehearsal, and feedback when helping social workers learn to interview. Stan Witkin moves his teaching into the social agency and demonstrates how caseworkers can learn marital counseling procedures. Such in-service training creates a bridge between formal classroom instruction and continuing education. The contribution from Bill Butterfield and Judi Werking depicts a forefront of behavior modification and a forum for social work. Behavioral medicine and social work in primary health care present new opportunities for innovative practice with problems and allied professionals not usually part of our bailiwick.

The pair of chapters on evaluation procedures complement each other and close the section. My paper on individual case evaluation recognizes means to document practice efficacy when resources needed for control-group research are not available. Since most chapters have drawn upon individual case evaluation, the operations of small sample research are by now familiar. Richard Gorsuch's coverage of program evaluation likewise reflects data from earlier chapters. His steps of program evaluation will guide workers around obstacles to large-scale research. Coupled with behavioral methods and methods for gaining professional competence, these accountability procedures complete a viable model of social work practice. Social workers who energize the model will symbiotically benefit their clients, colleagues, and profession.

14

Developing Skills for the Interview

Jeffrey L. Edleson
and
Sheldon D. Rose

Social workers rely on clinical interviews for diagnostic information and as a format for intervention. Social workers use interviews to develop relationshiops with clients, elicit relevant information, and assist clients in choosing strategies for change. For direct-service workers, interviewing is the single most frequently employed social work method (Kadushin 1972). Social work interviewing incorporates at least two skill areas: interpersonal skill, the ability to facilitate relationships with clients, and interviewing skill, the ability to obtain relevant information from clients. Assessment and intervention strategies can be most effectively employed after students learn both sets of skills (Combs, Avila and Purkey 1971; Truax and Carkuff 1967). And, suggested relationships between counseling skills and client success or failure have increased attention as to how social workers are taught interpersonal and interviewing skills (Fischer 1973, 1976, 1978; Geismar 1972).

Various approaches have been proposed for improving different social work skills. Balgopal (1974) and Papell (1972) suggest sensitivity training for improving practitioners' interpersonal skills. But little empirical evidence supports the effectiveness of this training paradigm. Others have reported successful use of skills-training focusing on direct practice. Larsen and Hepworth (1978) increased interpersonal skills using a program of instructor modeling, formulating student responses to simulated clients, practicing responses in roleplay inteviews, and feedback from instructors and videotapes. Wells (1975) also reported success in teaching interpersonal skills using direct practice.

Similar programs for teaching interviewing skills have been reported by Ivey (1971) and Schinke, Smith, Gilchrist, and Wong 91978). Ivey's micro-counseling program emphasizes direct practice and self-evaluation. Students first engage in diagnostic roleplays with simulated clients. Next, students read manuals describing skills to be learned and view videotapes of experts utilizing specific skills. Students then view videotapes of their interviews and, with an instructor's help, identify performance strengths and weaknesses. With self-evaluation in mind, students engage in repeat roleplays with simulated clients and are given feedback by an instructor. Schinke and his colleagues (Schinke, Smith, Gilchrist, and Wong, 1978) have also outlined a practice-oriented training program. In their program, instructors introduce and model specific interviewing skills. In groups of four, students practice each skill and receive feedback on their performance from the instructors and from other students.

These and other investigators have increased both the interpersonal and interviewing skills of human service practitioners (Carkuff 1969; Ivey 1971; Wells 1975; Larsen and Hepworth 1978; and Schinke, Smith, Gilchrist, and Wong 1978). Common to these approaches have been instructor modeling, skills practice, and performance feedback. In addition to being effective, evidence shows training participants prefer these procedures (Canfield, Eley, Rollman and Schur 1975). Based on this growing body of literature, the program described here employs modeling, practice and feedback to teach competence in interpersonal and interviewing skills.

Our training program is divided into three phases: 1) interpersonal skills; 2) interviewing individuals; and 3) interviewing families and small groups. Outlining each phase in detail, we offer solutions to problems encountered during training and suggest methods of transferring learned behavior to practice environments, concluding with a description of measures used to assess worker improvement and a presentation of our findings.

TRAINING PROGRAM

Training involving weekly, two hour, small-group sessions, has been offered a total of four times in the past two years. Most recently, thirty-five senior and graduate social work students completed the training as a professional degree requirement. Another eleven students who were not trained served as a comparison group.

The instructors were trained in two stages over six months, at first following the same program given to participants before focusing on problems likely to be encountered in training sessions: encouraging participation, increasing group cohesion, confronting disruptive participants. In the second stage, instructors co-led training session made up of social work and psychiatric nursing students.

Interpersonal Skills Phase

During the first phase students receive intensive training in both verbal and nonverbal interpersonal skills, including identification and expression of feelings, giving and seeking clarification, expression of opinion, response timing, eye contact, appropriate affect, voice volume, and fluency. Following a common format, each session begins with a review of homework assignments. Weekly homework includes keeping a diary to note profession-related problem situations, student responses, subjective discomfort ratings, personal satisfaction ratings for responses, situation goals, and alternative responses. Instructors encourage discussion of past situations and those anticipated in coming weeks. An excerpt from one homework review process follows:

> *Instructor:* Jay, will you start, and tell us about the situations you recorded in your diary this week?
>
> *Jay:* Okay. Well, the first situation I have deals with a client of mine. He has been making what I think is a slow progress on his problems. This week he came in and told me that he had not even attempted what we discussed the week before.
>
> *Instructor:* What was your response when he told you that?
>
> *Jay:* I'm afraid I wasn't too effective. I was really mad and I guess the only way I expressed it was with a disapproving facial gesture. I just went on and asked him what he wanted to talk about this week.
>
> *Instructor:* Can you tell the group what your goals were for the situation and how you think you could have responded more effectively?
>
> *Jay:* I wanted to get across the idea that it is important to follow through on what we discuss. Sometimes I'm afraid to confront him because I think he is making some progress and he might react strongly if I criticize him...he could just give up. He's at a good place and I want to be careful.

The session continues with Jay and other students going over their diaries. Review of the diary assignment reinforces self-observation to facilitate problem solving. It helps specify the situation's "critical moment," formulate goals, and suggest alternative, more effective responses.

After each student has reviewed at least one diary situation, the remaining time is spent practicing new responses, as illustrated in the typical interaction below. Practice covers seven basic steps: 1) covert exercises, 2) goal setting, 3) modeling, 4) roleplaying, 5) feedback on roleplay effectiveness and possible improvements, 6) re-rehearsal, and 7) additional feedback.

> *Instructor:* Nancy, do you want to try roleplaying one of the situations you wrote in your diary?

Nancy: Sure. I'd like to work on the one with my supervisor because I think I'll be in the same situation again this week.

Instructor: Okay. Could you read the description to us again?

Nancy: I know how I want to work with a certain client but my supervisor thinks I'm wrong and tells me to do it her way.

Instructor: Before we set goals and begin roleplaying, let's all briefly practice our own responses to this situation. I'll give you thirty seconds to think of how you would respond to Nancy's supervisor. Raise a finger when you're finished so I know when everyone has had time enough to think.

Instructor: Now that everyone has indicated that they've finished covert practice, let's set a goal for this interaction. Nancy?

Nancy: Well, I want to tell my supervisor that I've seen the client and feel confident proceeding the way I've decided.

Rick: Since you have to carry on a long-term relationship with your supervisor, don't you think you should take her opinions into account?

Nancy: Yeah, I couldn't just shut her off because she is really helpful; I do use her feedback. Maybe I should add to my goal that I should somehow recognize feedback she gives at other times.

Instructor: Okay, Nancy. Summarize all that.

Nancy: I want to tell my supervisor that I feel I'm correct, but at the same time let her know I appreciate her feedback and find it useful.

In this first step, Nancy read her problem situation aloud to the group. Following the reading, all students were instructed to imagine their own response to this situation. Such covert practice increased group involvement and generated a variety of alternative responses to the situation. Aided by other group members, Nancy then developed an outcome goal for achieving a more effective interaction.

Often, one or more alternative responses are modeled in roleplayed demonstrations. After the student roleplays and rehearses the situation, group members give feedback on verbal and nonverbal behavior. Following the same example, the process continues.

Instructor: (to Nancy) Now that you've seen Rick model an alternative response, do you think you're ready to try it out?

Nancy: Sure. I liked the way he did it. I'll try it.

(Roleplay proceeds with another member as supervisor. Feedback starts following completion of the roleplay.).

Instructor: Good. Let's begin feedback by commenting on parts of the roleplay Nancy did well.

Rick: First of all, nonverbally, I think you came across very confident. You were calm; your eye contact was great; most of all, your voice was really firm!

Instructor: I can't agree more. Does anyone else have positive feedback for Nancy?

Karen: I thought the way you let your supervisor know that you appreciated her feedback was very good; this way she saw it as a disagreement rather than a put-down. You stated your right to work with this client the way you want; at the same time, you didn't hurt the relationship with your supervisor.

(Positive feedback from other group members continues.)

Instructor: Now, how about feedback for Nancy on how she might have been even more effective?

Susan: You could have been more concise. At times I thought you were rambling, not getting to the point. Although your content was good, you could have said it in a lot fewer words.

Jay: I agree. Sometimes you sounded almost apologetic for not changing your strategy with this client.

Instructor: (After additional feedback) Nancy, could you summarize the feedback you've received?

Nancy: Well, on the positive side, I was calm; my voice was strong, eye contact good. The way I took my supervisor's feedback into account but still stood up for my intervention strategy was pretty effective. I could have been more concise and let my supervisor know that I found her feedback useful in the past.

Instructor: Very good. Let's go on to someone else's situation.

Here, feedback first focused on positive aspects of Nancy's roleplayed performance, made specific recommendations regarding both verbal and nonverbal behavior, and focused on alternative means of achieving the goal. Feedback indicated that individual preferences dictate different responses, and that a variety of responses are equally competent.

Students frequently wanted to rehearse situations a second time to incorporate feedback suggestons. Following rehearsal, others commented on improvements made and remaining weaknesses. Homework assignments to prepare for meetings and facilitate transfer of learning ended each training session. In addition to keeping a diary of problem situations, members also agreed to try out newly learned behaviors when feasible.

Interviewing with Individuals

Our second phase focuses on teaching verbal and nonverbal interviewing skills. Verbal skills include starting an interview, putting the client at ease, developing questions that require more than one response, seeking concrete examples, summarizing, paraphrasing, reflecting client statements, making transitions from one topic to another, prompting briefly to encourage client speech, and finding constructive confrontations. Nonverbal skills are silence to elicit client statements and attending behavior to show interest. Although interviewing skills are of primary focus, the interpersonal skills earlier outlined are also considered during feedback.

In addition to modeling, roleplay and feedback, training in interviewing uses videotaped modeling films at the start of each group session. Tapes present skilled interviewers with a roleplayed client, are replayed, and discussed. To help students acquire new interviewing behavior, we develop such client situations as the following.

> INSTRUCTIONS TO INTERVIEWER: You are a mental health counselor seeing a client, Gloria Bittner, for the first time. Ms. Bittner has been referred by a physician who views her constant fatigue as of psychological origin since all tests showed no organic cause.
>
> DEMOGRAPHIC BACKGROUND: Gloria Bittner, Age: 41. Children: Thomas Jr., 22; Sandra, 18. Husband: Thomas, Sr., 45, is a printer in a small company. Education: High school.
>
> INSTRUCTIONS TO THE CLIENT (READ ONLY BY THE "CLIENT"): You are concerned because your doctor has been unable to find a physical reason for your fatigue. You do not want to see a "therapist" because you are afraid you may be told that you are causing your own problems. You are very defensive about any questions that seem to point to your experiencing stress or feeling depressed. Your daughter has just moved out of the house to go to college. You find yourself at loose ends and have nothing to do a lot of the time. Your husband has work chums with whom he bowls two nights a week. During these evenings you watch TV and go to bed early. On nights he spends with you, you seldom have any energy to do things. This irritates him and he often nags you for being no fun. You don't hear much from Tom Jr. and feel lonely.

To apply diverse interviewing skills with such practice situations require an extension of roleplay periods up to thirty minutes. Although only two or three situations are practiced each session, the benefits of longer, more complex roleplays and more comprehensive group and video feedback seem to warrant extra time.

The following transcript is a portion of a roleplayed interview using the client simulation. Group member Carole played the social worker and another student played Ms. Bittner. Other members watched for specific strengths and weaknesses in student performance.

> *Worker:* Hi, Ms. Bittner. My name is Carole Stern. Let's go into my office and sit down... Well, the way I like to start an interview is by giving some information about me, what I do here at the mental health center, and some general information about our services. (Worker gives brief information.) I've been talking a lot; now I'd like to hear about you. But first what Dr. West told me: She said you've been quite tired lately and that she can't find anything causing the fatigue. Does that sound about right?
>
> *Client:* Yeah. So far she hasn't found the cause.
>
> *Worker:* To help me understand, can you give me some examples of when you've felt tired?
>
> *Client:* Well, there aren't particular times. I just feel a lot more tired than I used to.
>
> *Worker:* Than you used to?
>
> *Client:* Well...I used to be more active. But lately I just haven't felt up to my old self.
>
> *Worker:* You say you used to be much more active...What did you do

when you were more active?

Client: Well, I had a lot of stuff to do for the kids, you know, being the taxi driver, cook, look after them and their friends, and so on. I did a lot with the school and was involved with our neighborhood association.

Worker: (Silence and nodding.)

Client: Now the kids have moved out; and because of being tired all the time, I just haven't been as active.

Worker: It sounds like you have a lot of free time now.

Client: Yes, but I just sit around.

Worker: I'd like to get a better idea of how you spend your time these days; can you just tell me what you did yesterday, starting with when you woke up? (The inteview continues.)

As in the first phase, others offer feedback to the student on positive and negative aspects and of the interview. To facilitate specific feedback, a list of interviewing procedures and their definitions is distributed. Role-plays are often videotaped, with highlights shown during feedback. Due to length, students seldom have an opportunity to rehearse the interview a second time. Three examples of feedback follow.

Karen: I really like the way you put the client at ease in the beginning by introducing yourself, giving information about the agency and telling her what the doctor told you. If your client was anxious about the appointment, your introduction might have relaxed her.

Rick: I liked the way you used questions. They were general enough at first to give latitude in answering. When you wanted more specific information, you got it by asking Ms. Bittner to describe her day in detail. The only improvement I think could have made would be to ask fewer questions and just wait her out...What I mean is that when you did use silences, she kept on talking; the same when you used prompts like nods and "uh huh." You probably should try to use more of those and fewer questions, at least in the beginning when you want her to talk about herself.

Nancy: One thing I liked was your selective reflecting...like when you picked up on her saying she used to be more active: you said something like "Than you used to?" Also, you helped her be specific by asking her to detail what she used to do. My only critical remark is that you could vary the phrasing of your questions. You often use, "Well could you..." or "it sounds like..." I'll try to point these out on videotape.

Portions of the videotapes were then shown to further illustrate skill strengths and areas needing attention.

Interviewing with Families and Small Groups

Designed to facilitate practice of family and group interviewing, skills stressed in this phase differ from those taught earlier in several ways. Clearly, the increase from one to several clients alters the interviewing environment. Differences between group and family interviewing are also considered. Families have established modes of communication; groups, at least in early meetings, do not. Many families have "hidden agendas" known to everyone except the worker. Individual clients in groups may withhold relevant information they do not feel comfortable about disclosing to strangers. Because social work with groups and families often involves co-therapists, additional skills are demanded: co-therapists must mutually set goals in advance, divide tasks during meetings, and maintain consistency between themselves.

The training format is identifical to that of the second phase. As before, extended practice of simulated client situations is used. The situation is read, general and specific outcome goals are set, roleplay proceeds, and group member and videotaped feedback are given. A typical situation follows.

> INTERVIEWER INSTRUCTIONS: An initial interview with the Brook family was initiated by David Brook who wanted to "discuss a problem." The family consists of David Brook, 40, engineer, Michelle Brook, 38, homemaker, Andrew Brook, 16, 10th grade, Mary Brook, 12, 7th grade. Your goal is to identify the family's problems.
>
> INSTRUCTIONS TO MR. BROOK: You arranged this meeting because of concerns about your children. Andrew has started staying out late at night and won't tell you what he's been doing. You're afraid he's going to get into trouble and are pretty sure he and his friends are drinking or taking drugs. Andrew doesn't care much about school; good school achievement is important to you. Mary is quiet and shy and doesn't seem to have many friends. Lately she has been really moody and won't talk to you. You think both your children should "act more like adults" and help out more around the house. Your wife is too easy on the kids and doesn't demand enough of them. She lets them have their own way too often. Lately you have been depressed about your family problems and have started drinking more than usual; but you do not want the counselor to know this. You talk freely and interrupt others to get your ideas across.
>
> INSTRUCTIONS TO MS. BROOK: You don't agree with your husband about the kids' problems. Andy is just going through a stage and will grow out of it; the same is true for Mary. You think the kids do pretty well both at school and at home. You would rather not see problems and feel that things will work out okay. You are really worried about your husband's drinking. He has been late to work recently, and you are afaid he will lose his job. David doesn't discuss this issue with you at all, telling you it is none of your business. You are reluctant to talk about the drinking; but if asked you will share your concerns. You respond to close-ended questions with one-word answers, only divulging information if made to feel at ease.
>
> INSTRUCTIONS TO ANDREW BROOK: You are not happy about being here. You are angry and worried. You have really "had it" with your dad always on your back about everything; he seems to think you should be perfect. Mom's okay. You like your friends because you belong to an "in

group." Your grades in school have been going down because you have been cutting classes. You are worried that this interview (or future ones) will reveal that you may be in trouble at school. You do not talk freely with the counselor. You look at the floor and are not very responsive. When Dad gets on you during the interview, however, you will argue with him—especially about his drinking.

INSTRUCTIONS TO MARY BROOK: You sit by your mother and contribute very little. When asked a question, you either agree with your mother, say that you don't know, or shrug your shoulders. You laugh at your brother when Dad starts putting him down.

To illustrate use of this case material, a portion of a transcript follows. Students divided their task by giving Sandy a major responsibility for asking questions; Ken was responsible for summarizing what was said by family members and setting norms. The transcript illustrates the first disagreement between Mr. Brook, Ms. Brook, and Andrew, and how Ken handled the situation.

Mr. Brook: You know Andrew just runs around with these wierdos. I don't know what they do...He's going to get in a lot of damn trouble if he sticks around with them.

Ms. Brook: I guess I just disagree. I don't think Andy is any different than you were when you were young...(Andrew interupts).

Andrew: Yeah, you drank all the time when you were a kid...and you still drink all the time.

Ken: I'd like to just stop for a second. Each of you has things to say and it appears that what you're talking about is getting everyone pretty upset. Let's try to have one person talk at a time. Ms. Brook let's start with you.

Here, the student responsible for setting norms broke in when he saw family members interrupting each other. Feedback on his action went as follows:

Marilynne: Ken, it was very useful when you stopped the bickering before it got out of hand. I also liked how you identified feelings of concern and how you indirectly set a norm of letting one person talk at a time. I think you could have been more explicit about the norm by saying something direct like "During our meetings it is very important that everyone gets time to talk and finish what he or she is saying..."

Feedback continues, and each interviewer summarizes the feedback. Videotapes reviewed during feedback help document specific points.

The three phases cover use of interpersonal and interviewing skills in a variety of professional contexts. Although interpersonal and interviewing skills are separate areas of ability, throughout the three phases practice and feedback are not limited to skills particular to each phase. Many rehearsed situations call for a combination of both interpersonal and interviewing skills.

GROUP PROBLEMS

Roleplay Repetitiveness

Roleplaying can become repetitive over time, resulting in students' loss of interest. To prevent this, a number of training variations are introduced. For example, videotape provides feedback on nonverbal and verbal responses, and focuses group feedback on observable behavior. Another variation involves the roleplayed client leaving the room during group feedback, returning for the second rehearsal, giving impressions on changes in student performance. In other sessions, outsiders are used as antagonists to make situations more realistic. To increase roleplay difficulty, members coach the client. Finally, once students are familiar with one another, each develops a situation relevant to another. Situations are assigned and roleplayed on short notice. This procedure adds an element of surprise, so students can employ new skills without preparation.

Dividing Instructor Supervision

Another problem is how to structure group time. With up to twelve students in one group, it is impractical to use the entire group when rehearsing. To facilitate adequate supervision, smaller practice groups, and transfer of leadership, two alternative modes of group structuring are utilized. One method divides the group into three subgroups. Advantageous because it gives students opportunity to rehearse at least two situations each group session, this method necessitates splitting instuctor time over three small groups. When instructors become adjusted to a subgroup, there is often just enough time to supervise one or two roleplays. Moreover, instructor and student evaluations have indicated that although supervision of the small groups is helpful, it is too brief. A second mode of group structure appears to more adequately increase group supervision and still provide a small group experience. Here, the larger group of twelve is divided into two subgroups of six. This allows the instructor to spend one hour with each subgroup while the other group is self-led.

Transfer of Learning

Transfer of interpersonal and interviewing skills to practice environments is expressly designed into our program. Through homework assignments, students perform rehearsed situations in the natural environment. In the first training session, students are supplied with a package of twenty-four situations from which to choose relevant vignettes. As previously noted, diaries are brought in to group and used for practice. To optimize the use of extra-group time a "buddy" system lets students call each other and set up between-meeting practice situations.

Leadership functions are deliberately transferred to students. This has proved important since students will ultimately be independent of the instructor or group and because transfer of leadership produces a model to facilitate similar transfer in client groups. Such transfer of leadership and group functions takes place gradually as instructors delegate responsibility. Initially, instructors design roleplays, conduct discussions, model responses and give homework assignments. By the end of training, these functions are performed solely by group members.

MEASURING PROFESSIONAL SKILLS

Many professional skills programs similar to ours do not include an evaluation component. Other than subjective judgement, evidence of learning rarely appears. Thus, evaluation of our training program has consistently occurred via all students completing a roleplay test prior to and following the first phase. Developed by Rose, Cayner and Edleson (1977), the test consists of situations common to social work practice. Each situation requires students to interact in roleplays and record their levels of performance, discomfort, and satisfaction. Using criteria devloped by expert judges, student's responses are rated on overall effectiveness, identification and expression of seeking and giving, clarification, expressing opinions, timing of responses, persistence, appropriate affect, voice volume, and speech fluency.

The roleplay test is preferred for two reasons: First, students are evaluated on explicit performance criteria. Second, students interact with role played clients in situations seen earlier as difficult or stressful. Though not exactly like observations in the natural environment, roleplay tests can closely simulate diverse social work settings.

Our roleplay test to evaluate students' interviewing skills involves six vignettes, each representing a typical client problem and situation. Students are given vignette descriptions with which to prepare. When tested, one situation is randomly selected for a ten minute roleplay. Another person plays the client and supplies additional background information. Instructors judge students' interviewing skills on scales that cover introducing the interview, putting client at ease, using questions, seeking concreteness, summarizing, paraphrasing, and using transitions, constructive confrontation, verbal prompts, attention, and silence.

Findings

One just completed evaluation of our interview training approach examined the aforementioned groups of thirty-five trained students and eleven untrained students who served as a contrast sample. Compared on their previous experience, age and pretraining roleplay test scores, between-group differences were found only for age. The mean age of the training group (M = 25.46) was significantly higher (t = 2.03, df = 44, $p < .05$) than that of the comparison group (M = 22.27). Linear regression of age against improvement in test scores showed small correlation (r = 0.07). With the relative equivalence of the two groups established a substantive question can be asked about the efficiency of training.

Does practice interviewing increase skills? Based on changes of roleplay test scores from pretraining to posttraining, yes. As can be seen in Table One, statistically significant differences between trained and untrained groups were found (t = 2.47, $p < .01$).

Change scores indicated that performance discomfort ratings for those who were trained also lessened (t = 1.78, $p < .05$). Ratings of personal satisfaction with performance during roleplay situations did not differ between the two groups.

Table 1

Change-Score Means and t-Ratios on Outcome Measures Comparing Trained and Untrained Students

	Trained (n=35)	**Untrained (n=11)**	**t-ratio**
Roleplay Test	+8.11	-0.50	2.47**
Discomfort Rating	-0.56	-0.12	1.78*
Satisfaction Rating	+0.40	+0.21	0.68

*$p < .05$ **$p < .01$

SUMMARY

Initial results show our interviewing phase effective to teach social workers skills of critical importance for professional behavior. Despite the lack of empirical data on each technique used, observations show the total training program increasing professional skills over a brief period, indicating that short-term, intensive skills training can supplement allied components of social work education (cf. Schinke, Gilchrist, Smith, Wong, in press). Our data indicated that social work students given specific instructions, modeling, and practice will improve their skills and will concurrently reduce their discomfort in clinical situations. Lack of change in students' satisfaction with their own performance may mean that over time they raised their expectations about their own behavior.

An addition to this training program could engage students to complete one or more client interviews outside the training environment. Transcripts from these interviews might be analyzed for skills shown in students' responses, their reasons for using certain techniques, the strengths of each skill component used, and alternative responses. In vivo exercises would then help students' new learning transfer to nontraining milieus, and would provide another source of feedback for instructors and students. By following the guidelines and suggestions outlined in this chapter, social workers who employ behavioral and nonbehavioral procedures will equally profit. In these ways, our profession can become more effective, responsive, and accountable.

15

Preparing for Marital Counseling in Nontraditional Settings

Stanley Witkin

Public agency social workers are the front-line caregivers in the human services professions. Often burdened by heavy caseloads, public agency workers are asked to provide services to a population excluded, punished, or ignored by society. Despite the seriousness and complexity of the problems they face, these workers are often the most poorly trained in our profession. It is not uncommon, for example, to find workers in department of social services (DSS) agencies with literally no behavioral or social science training.

One response to this lack of expertise among DSS workers has been a proliferation of in-service training programs. Such programs usually attempt to upgrade knowledge and skills to improve job performance; however, the attainment or evaluation of this objective is difficult. In public social services, for instance, training programs developed by "outside experts" may have only limited applicability to the workers' needs.

Program developers may have had little contact with target audiences before training and thereby fail to incorporate workers' needs and problems into the in-service curricula. Even when prior contact is made, trainers may be unwilling to cover suggested topics not directly addresssed by their particular approach. Finally, some training programs come in package form and consist of set curricula presented to all audiences regardless of background or need.

These training approaches risk being viewed as irrelevant or only marginally useful. Although workers might achieve cognitive mastery of training material, they may perceive its content as too difficult to use. In short, in-service programs reflecting the latest ideas and best intentions often have little impact on posttraining activities, a failing reinforced by a paucity of training program evaluations, perhaps reflecting a disinterest or lack of evaluation skills on the part of program planners and instructors, and further hampered by the organizational context of many public social services. The evaluation climate tends to be less than optimal.

The present chapter describes a training program aimed at helping social service workers acquire skills for marital interventions. In planning, implementation, and evaluation, the program addresses the issues above. Process and outcome data show the program to be an innovative approach to training and evaluation with public agency social workers.

SETTING AND POPULATION

A ten session course in assessing marital conflict and effecting intervention was taught to fourteen caseworkers employed in a county department of social services. The department is located in a city of 175,000 and serves the needs of a large rural area. Demographic information on the caseworkers revealed thirteen females and one male, with a median age of 28.9 years and median years of education of 16.0. Nine held B.A. degrees in either social work, sociology, or psychology; four held degrees in other nonsocial science fields. Median DSS employment was 5.3 years. Seven workers worked in child welfare services, five in family and adult services, and two in medical services. Earlier training in marriage and family intervention was limited: approximately half of the workers had never taken a course in the area. Based on this information, training was designed at an elementary conceptual level with strong focus on practical application.

TRAINING NEEDS

Prior to the first training session, two meetings were held—one with supervisory personnel and one with the prospective traineers—in which specific problem areas and training needs were solicited. The author's own past experience as a DSS worker proved helpful in establishing rapport with staff, eliciting discussion of problem areas, and developing curricula. Discussions disclosed that most client marital problems were in areas of communications and sexuality, a finding documented by the literature on marriage (Greene, 1970). Incidence of violence and alcoholism were also noted. Supervisors and caseworkers felt that training should also address child-management problems since these were prevalent in cases of marital conflict and in many one-parent families.

In general, agency clients represented lower socioeconomic and educational levels. Many families receiving agency services were nonvoluntary clients, so low levels of motivation were often evident. Moreover, most couples did not possess the introspective orientation or skills found in middle-class, well educated couples—the population that much intervention is aimed toward.

Organizational factors further hindered workers from carrying out effective intervention. For example, staffing patterns led to heavy caseloads for each worker, resulting in a "crisis orientation" where workers responded mainly to cases with acute and highly visible problems. Thus, workers needed relatively short-term interventions to ameliorate present difficulties and equip clients to deal with future problems.

Besides heavy caseloads, the agency lacked the resources to assist workers with difficult cases; the minimal supervision was geared toward administrative matters. Marital and family intervention expertise was absent; few workers had training in such areas, so most cases identified as "marital problems" were referred to other agencies, which may seem a constructive approach to handling cases of marital conflict. However, the middle-class orientation of many receiving agencies left them unprepared to help lower-class clients.

Workers verbalized their uncertainty in dealing with marital problems. They had exaggerated perceptions of the effectiveness of marital counseling, assuming other professionals had highly developed procedures to alleviate marital distress. Part of this discomfort was due to their lack of assessment and evaluation tools. Most workers had no systematic method for assessing couples' strengths and weaknesses, nor for evaluating results of these interventions. Attempts were thus made to integrate such skills into training.

DESCRIPTION OF PROGRAM

Training was partitioned into three major units: 1. Introduction to conceptualizations of marital conflict and an overview of outcome studies. 2. Assessment and evaluation. 3. Substantive issues such as: a. communications and problem solving b. sexuality c. marital violence.

Using an informal seminar format, training sessions consisted of didactic presentations, modeling, roleplaying, and discussion. In addition, homework encouraged trainees to try out skills. The major course assignment was applying skills to an actual case. Ongoing throughout training, this assignment provided workers with first-hand experience in assessment and intervention techniques. The homework generated case material for class discussion and exposed workers to a variety of problem situations. Following is a description of the content and instructional techniques in each of the three units.

Unit 1: Introduction and Overview

Objectives were: 1. to provide workers with current information on the efficacy of marital intervention; 2. to introduce the behavioral approach to marital conflict and address similarities and differences with other approaches; and 3. to teach procedures appropriate for nonvoluntary clients.

Reviews of the marital intervention literature (Gurman, 1973; Beck, 1975) gave workers a current state-of-the-art overview. It was emphasized that research on marital intervention was relatively recent and limited in scope, that the relative efficacy of various forms of intervention—concurrent, conjoint, individual, group—was uncertain, and that the couples studied were generally not representative of DSS clients. This dubious picture of marital intervention encouraged workers to explore a variety of intervention strategies and to adapt procedures to clients' needs. Further, the paucity of data highlighted the importance of individual case assessment and evaluation.

Although social learning analysis was the major conceptual focus, workers were introduced to the advantages and disadvantages of alternate perspectives. The psychoanalytic approach, for example, seems to have limited applicability in the DSS setting due to its lengthy intervention phase and its emphasis on introspection and insight (Martin, 1976). In contrast, the communication/systems approach (Haley, 1963; Sluzki, 1978), emphasizing marital interaction and rules regulating interactions, leads to useful assessment and intervention. For example, since current interactions are seen as most important, the communication/systems practitioner has a "here-and-now" orientation. This results in an active change strategy and does not require recollection and analysis of past events. Another focus of the approach is on the marital relationship rather than on each spouse's deficiencies. Defining the relationship as the problem makes both spouses responsible for desired changes, helping replace destructive blaming with constructive problem-solving.

The discussion of social learning built a foundation for later instruction in behavioral intervention. While remaining focused on marital and family units, assessment and evaluation were more specific than in previous approaches and emphasized observable behavior. The teaching of social-learning concepts was supplemented by the self instructional text *Families* (Patterson, 1975).

After becoming familiar with basic concepts of social learning theory, workers were introduced to the behavioral conception of marital discord. From this perspective, marital problems result from inadequate attempts to resolve conflicts and frustrations inevitable in long-term, intimate relationshiops (Weiss, Hops & Patterson, 1973). Underlying these difficulties is excessive reliance on aversive change strategies. For example, a husband responds to his wife's unwillingness to attend a party with nagging and threats. The wife, unable to withstand his unpleasantness, reluctantly agrees to comply with his demands. The husband then learns that nagging and threats produce desired consequences, and the wife learns that compliance will terminate her spouse's nagging. According to learning principles, this mutual reinforcement increases future likelihood of such tactics when the couple is confronted with similar situations. Over time, such transactions generalize to predictable patterns.

INCREASING INTERPERSONAL INFLUENCE Following suggestions by Goldstein, Heller and Sechrest (1966), workers were taught to enhance effectiveness with clients by increasing interpersonal attraction. Emphasis was on observable learning through modeling. Modeling was particularly germane for present clients since it does not depend on verbal or introspective skills. Another advantage is that clients can learn modeled behavior such as appropriate compliments when sufficient incentives for immediate performance may be lacking. Moreover, workers are not limited to themselves as models, but may use other community persons clients perceive as having high status.

Unit 2: Assessment and Evaluation

In this unit, workers were introduced to methods of assessing marital and family functioning and evaluating an intervention's effectiveness. Assessment procedures were subdivided into self-report and observational methods.

SELF-REPORT METHODS Three types of self-report methods were discussed. The first was the global, marital adjustment or satisfaction questionnaire (e.g. Locke and Wallace, 1959). Typically, spouses complete these questionnaires separately, with scores averaged for an overall satisfaction score. Many questionnaires have available mean scores of distressed and nondistressed groups of couples that can be used as norms. Convenient to administer, these measures often suffer from response biases such as portraying one's relationship as consistent with socially approved responses (Edmonds, Withers, and Dibatista, 1972).

Further, since most use normative data of middle-class couples, scores may not reflect true measures of global satisfaction when used with lower-class persons. Finally, global results do not point to specific areas for intervention.

This latter shortcoming is addressed by a second type of self-report measure asking couples to specify problem behaviors (e.g. Stuart and Stuart, 1972). With pragmatic advantages over global measures, these measures are relatively new and have unknown reliability and validity.

A third type of self-report method is obtained by spouses recording each others' behavior. Weiss, Hops and Patterson (1973) for example, had couples record frequencies of pleasing and displeasing behavior. This method has advantages of pinpointing specific problems and providing data on occurrence rates. But, the observational and recording skills necessary to implement such methods are not easily learned.

OBSERVATIONAL METHODS Characterized by direct observation and recording of client behavior by persons other than themselves, use of these methods vary across setting and situational context. Four possible combinations of settings and situations are illustrated in Figure One.

Example of Settings and Situations
Used in Observational Assessment

Situation	Setting: **Agency**	Setting: **Client's Home**
Role play	Workers ask couple to pretend they desire to participate in different weekend activities and to resolve differences	Husband and wife show how they get children ready for bed using worker as role-played child
Husband-Wife interaction	Husband and wife discuss marital relationship problems	Worker observes family interactions during dinner

FIGURE 1

ASSESSMENT METHODOLOGY Workers were taught to implement an observational assessment. Prerequisite skills for using this method are an understanding of the elementary principles of behavior (e.g. Patterson, 1975), ability to specify behavioral referents of problem areas, and knowledge of recording methods. These skills were taught by modeling and practice. A homework assignment to conduct an observational assessment in the home of a friend or colleague provided further practice and indicated workers' ability to apply learning. Using a simple observational form (Figure Two, workers were encouraged to formualte functional hypotheses by circling rows containing target behavior and looking for trends in antecedents, responses, and consequences.

Observational Assessment Chart*

Time	Antecedent	Response	Consequence
7:00		Husband (H) requests wife (W) to bring him a beer	W replies "Get it yourself"
	H remains seated picks up magazine	W says "I thought you wanted a beer"	H says "Quiet I'm trying to read"
7:02	W walks into kitchen	W brings beer	H says "Thanks"

Recording Rules:

1. Describe only actual observation, not interpretation.
2. Record nonverbal and verbal behavior.
3. Note time of new interaction
4. Use abbreviations or shorthand notation.

* (From Hartmann and Gelfand, 1975)

FIGURE 2

After demonstrating competence with standardized measures, workers were encouraged to adapt assessment procedures to individual case situations. Often this meant modifying measurement instruments and recording methods to fit the problem. Decisions concerning the context of observation, appropriate response characteristics, level of measurement, and recording technique must all be balanced against factors of cost, inconvenience and problem frequency and severity.

EVALUATION Assessment was presented as ongoing, providing data to worker and client on the intervention's progress. Evaluation extended this process by measuring the intervention's efficacy. Unfortunately, time limitations and the workers' lack of prior preparation did not permit a thorough examination of all the design and analysis options available. Evaluation methods were limited to graphical representations of data in the context of single-case designs (see Chapter 17). Single-case designs required workers to define client problems in measurable terms and to collect related data. Teaching clients self monitoring skills was encouraged because it gives increased responsibility and control over change procedures.

Unit 3: Substantive Issues

COMMUNICATION Workers were taught a skill-training approach to communication. Three problem categories were discussed, each with corresponding communication skills. These categories are briefly described below.

1. Accuracy: Communication problems in this area result from discrepant message interpretation—the intent of the spouse expressing the message is interpreted differently by the partner. One reason for this problem is a tendency to talk in vague, global terms, with multiple meanings—"I expect you to do your share around here." Thus, an important communication skill is the ability to express messages—especially requests for change—specifically "I expect you to wash the dishes after dinner." A second cause of accuracy problems is mind-reading: or the attribution of a message to another person based on presumed thoughts, feelings, or behavior (Gottsman, Notarius, Gonso and Markman, 1976), as in the following illustrative dialogue:

> Husband: I think I'll take it easy today and let you watch the kids.
> Wife: You're angry at me for buying those new clothes.
> Husband: No, I'm not. You're just feeling guilty about spending money.

Here, wife and husband both were mind-reading, each assuming feelings and motives. To the extent that these assumptions are incorrect, couples process and act on false information. Mind-reading problems are avoided by requesting specific information. "Does 'take it easy' mean you're not going to take the kids to the movies as planned?" By indicating the behavioral referents of interpretations, "Your clenched fist tells me you're angry about something." Or by reporting one's own feelings, "I'm upset over you not wanting to watch the kids."

2. Openness: The richness of language and uniqueness of personal experience makes perfectly accurate communication highly unlikely. Sharing message interpretations is thus important for spouses' understanding of their partner's perceptions and reactions. Communication openness refers to this aspect of communication, explicitly sharing message interpretations and their consequences. Openness is exemplified by feedback, informing a person of the interpretation and impact of his/her message, thereby providing opportunity for message clarification or confirmation. Feedback is also related to accuracy since it clarifies misinterpretations.

3. Quality: Accurate and open communication gives valuable information about self and others. In addition, the positive and negative consequences of communication provide incentives to approach or avoid future interaction. This positive/negative dimension determines quality. Problems arise when communication is perceived as aversive and contributes to relationship distress. Aversive communication also affects accuracy and openness since it is usually characterized by unclear messages and poor feedback. Because quality does not correspond to one specific skill, improvement is difficult. Quality appears to result from learning what one's partner or family members find aversive and pleasant, and using such information in positive, systematic ways. For example, when a wife asks her husband to wash the dishes, a satisfactory outcome is more likely if the request is expressed in a way to not elicit negative feelings, and the husband perceives a payoff for engaging in requested behavior.

PROBLEM-SOLVING Conflicts are inevitable in any close, enduring relationship. Communication skills alone are not sufficient to help couples deal with problems and conflicts. For this reason, workers were taught a problem-solving strategy to use with clients. Helping clients become problem-solvers, or "personal scientists" (Mahoney, 1974), involved six steps: orientation to the problem, problem definition, problem analysis, solution generation, evaluation, and graduation. These steps give clients a systematic methodology for solving current and future problems and are thus likely to be superior to procedures clients with marital difficulties have employed in the past. Workers were also introduced to problem-solving aides including the "Tune-up Checklist," a form helping couples identify and deal with problems before they become distressing and "Consequence Cards" (Witkin and Caynor, 1980), helping determine costs and benefits of problem solutions. Communication and problem-solving training provided fundamental intervention strategies applicable to most couples and families and reflected a preventive orientation so clients could deal with problems independent of agency assistance.

SEXUAL PROBLEMS Training workers to intervene with sex-related difficulties was a particularly sensitive area. Apparently such sensitivity resulted from worker anxiety about sexual topics and limited knowledge of sexual behavior and intervention procedures. Because many clients did not share the predominately middle-class sexual values and beliefs held by workers, differences in perceived values represented an additional source of worker concern.

Accordingly, training began with a discussion of relativity: diverse forms of prevailing sexual values and conduct. Examining the impact of factors such as social class, race and religion on sexual attitudes and behavior helped workers understand the societal and cultural context of sexuality. The importance of learning to sexual behavior was also emphasized. To overcome anxiety associated with discussing sex-related topics, several in-class exercises were introduced. Exercises allowed workers to verbalize sexually explicit terms in an atmosphere of acceptance, to share with others their own beliefs, misunderstandings, and attitudes about sexuality, to examine sources of sexual beliefs and effect on behavior, and to increase understanding of how clients feel when asked to discuss sexual matters. An illustrative exercise on sexual myths follows.

After a short discussion of sexual myths and misunderstandings most people learn (McCrary, 1971), workers related their own sexual myths, their source, and impact on behavior. Initially eliciting considerable anxiety, this exercise was a learning experience for most workers. In addition to exposing a range of sexual beliefs, anecdotes demonstrated how beliefs affect behavior. For example, one woman told of a belief that too much sex was unhealthy. This conviction led to serious problems in her marriage, eventuating in its dissolution. Not until some years later, at a church-sponsored seminar on sexuality, had the woman courage to voice her belief. Much to her surprise the seminar leader blithely replied, "On the contrary, have sex as much as you possibly can."

The remainder of the sexuality unit was devoted to basic information concerning sexual organs and physiology. Again, diversity of sexual responses was emphasized. Presentation of common sexual dysfunctions was followed by a description of interventions including relaxation training, desensitization, anxiety extinction, the roleplaying of exaggerated orgasms, the use of discriminative stimuli, masturbation, sexual aids, sexual assertion rehearsal, generalization training, information, and influencing fantasy and cognitions (Sayner and Durrell, 1975). Discussion of these techniques provided workers with a comprehensive, but brief overview of intervention procedures.

MARITAL VIOLENCE The final topic introduced was marital violence. Unfortunately, time limitations allowed only an introduction to this serious problem. This unit's objectives were to familiarize workers with current thinking on marital violence and possible intervention strategies to use when confronted with appropriate cases. Workers were encouraged to view marital violence as resulting from multiple, interrelated variables. Thus, factors of external stress, alcoholism, and a patriarchical social system (Martin, 1976) appear to contribute to abuse, with no single factor sufficient to precipitate violence.

A second focal area was the difficulty in working with marital violence cases. Workers examined societal proscriptions deterring outside intervention, norms concerning rights of family members, sexism, and privacy. The reasons for which abused wives remain with their husbands were especially relevant since there appears to be a relationship between the lack of resources (e.g. unemployment) and an unwillingness to seek help (Gelles, 1976). Finally, the relationship of marital violence and family violence was explored. Gelles (1976), for example, has shown that women who observed conjugal violence or were victims of parental violence as children were likely to be victims of marital violence as adults.

A multi-level approach to intervention in cases of marital violence was proposed. In addition to pragmatic procedures (removal of weapons) and long-term objectives (legislative and social change), workers were taught to direct intervention toward the antecedents and consequences of violence. Previously learned course material on increasing interpersonal influence and improving communication and problem-solving proved useful. Cognitive procedures for coping with stress (Meichenbaum, 1977) were discussed as a way of helping abusers recognize and control violence. Finally, the use of interpersonal contracts to manipulate consequences was discussed (e.g. Saunders, 1977). Contracts can provide a woman with specific guidelines to follow when threatened with abuse and can prescribe negative consequences for her spouse. Further, contracts can also help couples attain positive outcomes for engaging in constructive interactions. The unit concluded with a discussion of community services for battered women and appropriate referral procedures.

PROGRAM EVALUATION

Training effectiveness was assessed in two ways: by workers completing four questionnaires prior to and following training, and by having each worker formulate, implement, and evaluate a client intervention program.

Staff Training Questionnaire

This twenty-six item questionnaire, based on material from Patterson (1975) and Witkin and Caynor (1980), covered fundamental principles and techniques of behavior management, communication, and problem solving.

Attitude Measure of Sexual Behavior

A twelve item semantic-differential instrument developed by Fretz (1975) requested workers to express attitudes toward sexual behavior. Each item is followed by seven bipolar adjectives representing three factors: evaluation, dynamism, and understanding.

Sex Knowledge Inventory

The Sex Knowledge Inventory is an eighty item questionnaire dealing with psychological aspects of sexual relationships (McHugh, 1968). From five possible responses to each question, workers were instructed to choose the best. Topics of sexual techniques, physiology, causes of poor sexual adjustment, and birth control are covered.

Job Satisfaction Questionnaire (JSQ)

To assess job-attitude change as a result of training, workers were asked to complete an eighteen item job satisfaction questionnaire (Brayfield and Rothe, 1951). Each item was rated on a five-point Likert scale ranging from strongly agree to strongly disagree.

Client-Intervention Program

Each worker or worker pair applied training content to an actual case. Cases were described in writing and submitted to the instructor at the last training session. Although reports did not yield outcome data in a traditional sense, they proved useful as an evaluation of worker performance and ability to generalize learning. Class discussion of the cases plus class and instructor feedback during the course yielded ongoing evaluative data and stimulated discussion.

RESULTS

Improvements following training were assessed by analyzing pretest to posttest changes on evaluative measures. *T*-tests for correlated samples detected statistically significant gains. Resulting data are summarized in Table One. Examination of these results reveals that workers made significant improvements on the Staff Training Questionnaire and the Sex Knowledge Inventory. Scores on the Attitude Measure of Sexual

Table 1

Means (*M*) Standard Deviations (*SD*), and *t*-Test Results (*t*) on Evaluation Measures at Pretest and Posttest

Measure	**Pretest**		**Posttest**		
	M	*SD*	*M*	*SD*	*t*
Staff Training					
Questionnaire	11.89	3.39	20.13	1.92	8.79**
Sex Knowledge					
Inventory	59.08	5.72	63.92	3.01	4.03*
Attitude Measure of Sexual Behavior					
Evaluation	158.57	31.06	154.00	33.64	1.40
Dynamism	108.39	13.85	103.00	11.74	2.02
Understanding	110.73	24.27	113.14	20.98	0.25
Job Satisfaction					
Questionnaire	63.57	11.59	64.36	10.25	0.40

* $p < .01$

** $P < .001$

Behavior failed to reveal significant posttest increases on any of the three factors; in fact, mean scores decreased from pretraining on two factors. Job Satisfaction scores showed upward but non-signficant changes.

Worker Intervention Programs

All workers were able to carry out assessment and intervention with a marital or family case. Although success rates are difficult to ascertain because of time constraints and differences in severity and complexity of client problems, most workers documented improvement in at least one behavior. Following are brief descriptions of three representative case examples.

Case one was a multiproblem family consisting of a husband (Mr. A), wife (Ms. A), and two children, Tom aged seven, and Cheryl aged four. Most pressing difficulties centered around Tom's behavior (hitting parents and breaking things) and arguments between husband and wife. Both problems were successfully treated; however, only marital problems are discussed here.

Following home observation, the worker was able to determine salient behavior precipitating marital spats. Arguments usually stemmed from Mr. A's complaints about his wife's neglect of child care and household tasks, and from Ms. A's complaints about her husband's infrequent family interactions. After sharing these perceptions, the worker held a joint session to help the couple negotiate a behavior change agreement. Mr. A worked on increasing the frequency of conversations with his wife and the initiation of play with the children. Ms. A agreed to more frequently help the children dress and have dinner ready at a specified time. This agreement was formalized by a contingency contract in which performing the target behavior earned privileges for each spouse (e.g. a back rub and a "night off"). As illustrated in Figures Three and Four, intervention appeared highly successful.

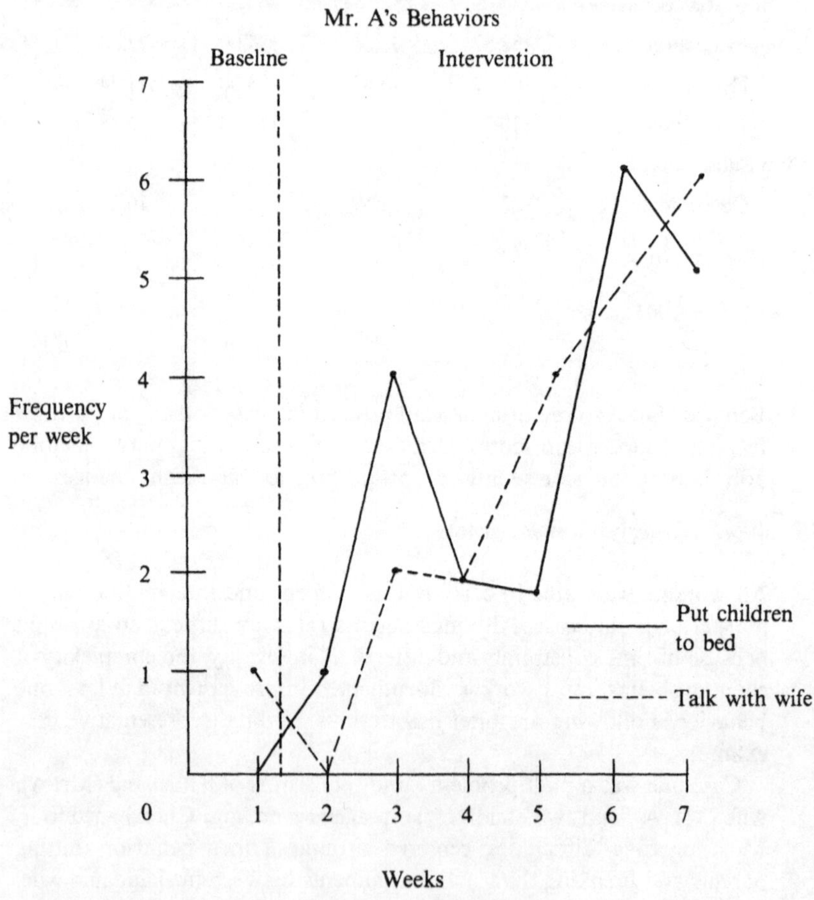

FIGURE 3

Case two involved the T family, a couple with two girls, aged three and one. Home observation and information from the Marital Pre-Counseling Inventory (Stuart and Stuart, 1972) indicated problems with communication—an inability to discuss differences without yelling—and performance of household tasks. The latter behavior was further specified, and chosen for initial monitoring and intervention. Ms. T was to increase washing breakfast dishes, cleaning the kitchen, and making lunch. Mr. T agreed to take out the garbage, put his dirty clothes in the hamper, and close dresser drawers. Spouses were taught to monitor each other's performance of these tasks and arrange for rewards and sanctions for their fulfillment or nonfulfillment. Results of this intervention are shown in Figure Five.

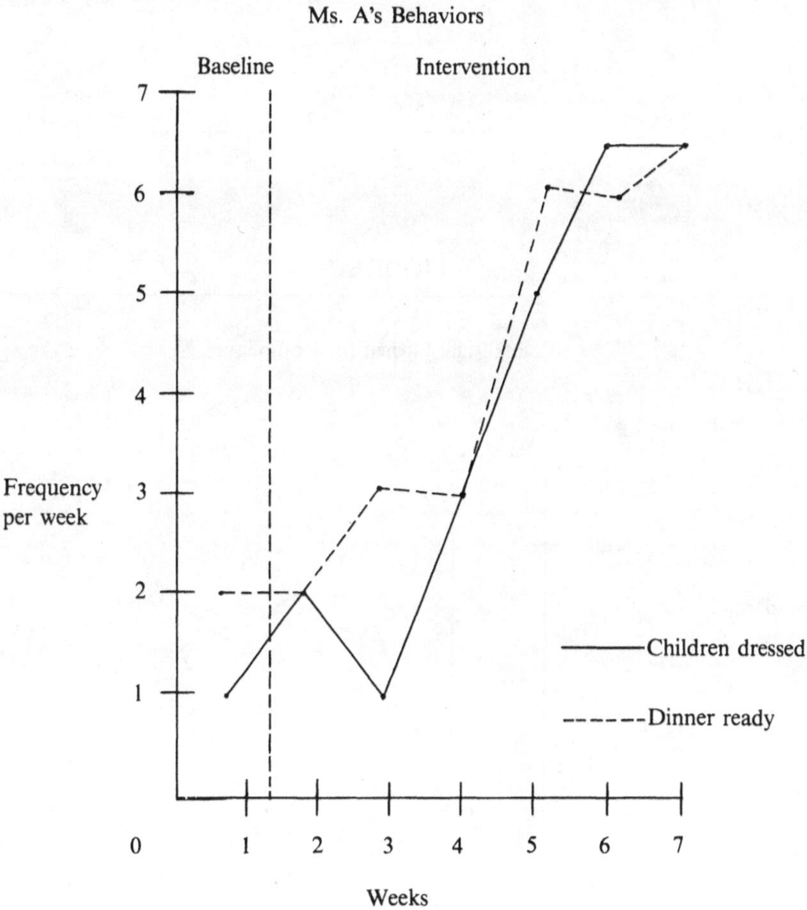

FIGURE 4

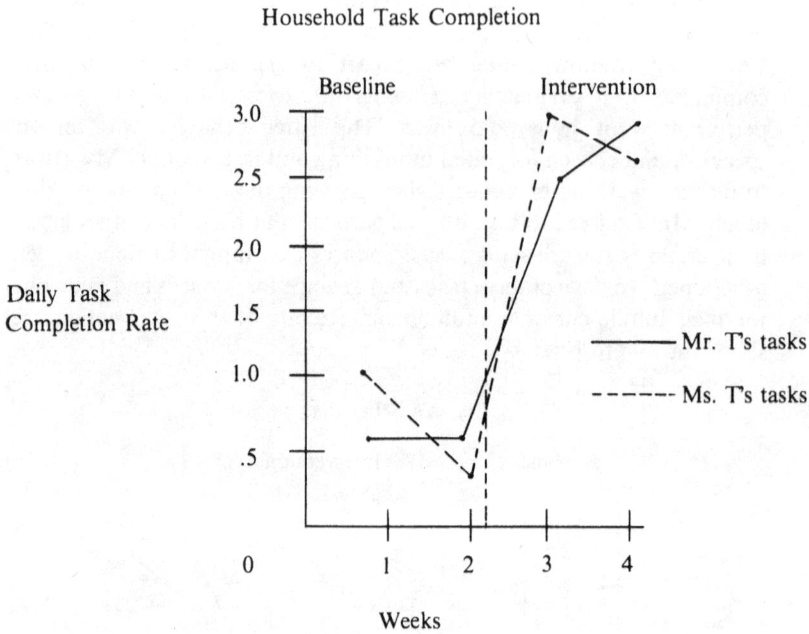

FIGURE 5

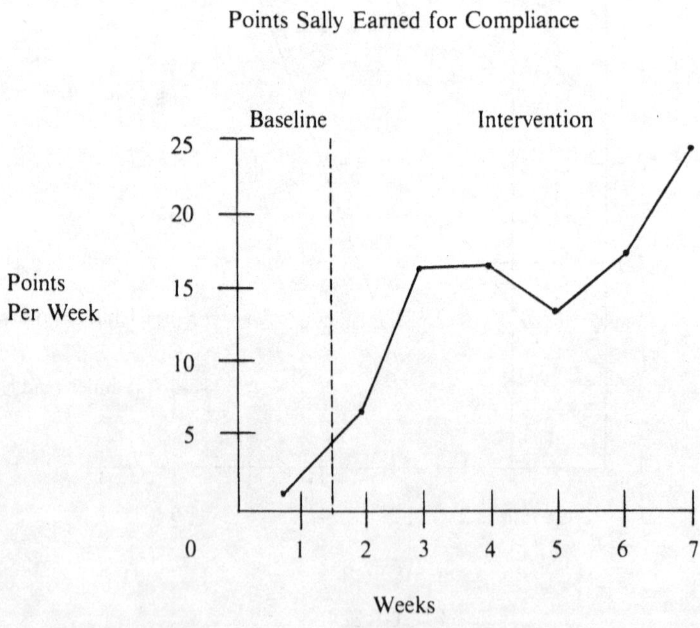

FIGURE 6

Case three was another multiproblem family in which both marital and child management difficulties were causing distress. The present discussion focuses on child-related problems. Ten year old Sally Y was referred for noncompliance—refusing to pick up toys, not keeping her room clean, refusing to go to bed when told. Aversive measures including spanking were not successful in altering the child's behavior. In fact, discipline had contributed to the deterioration of the parent-child relationship and was the topic of frequent husband and wife arguments. Guided by the worker, Mr. and Ms. Y specified positive behavior they wanted their daughter to increase. A contract to this end enabled Sally to earn points for such privileges as staying up an hour later. Social reinforcement from the parents for desirable behavior was also used. Depicted in Figure Six, improvement in Sally's behavior following intervention was rapid. Moreover, the worker noted a more positive relationship between mother and daughter and a decrease in reported arguments between Mr. and Ms. Y. Thus, modifying the family interaction system may have yielded other benefits.

DISCUSSION

This chapter describes a marital and family intervention training program for public social service workers. Grounded in social-learning theory, the program taught workers to assess, intervene, and evaluate services with marriage and family conflict, interpersonal communication, sexuality, and marital violence. Program evaluation showed workers better able to serve marital and family discord after training than before. Significant pretest to posttest improvement on Staff Training Questionnaire and Sex Knowledge Inventory scores indicated workers acquired factual knowledge of intervention methods and determinants of marital and family discord

In the area of human sexuality, evaluation data revealed inconsistencies between knowledge and attitudes: increases in Sex Knowledge Inventory scores were not paralleled by increases on the Attitude Measures of Sexual Behavior. Closer examination of attitudinal responses suggest changes may be partially explained as workers' presenting a stance of evaluative neutrality, a greater willingness to admit lack of understanding, and differences in connotative meaning of terms used on the measure.

Pretest to posttest decreases in job satisfaction was not totally unexpected. In a training program for group home workers, Schinke, and Wong (1977b) found a decrease in job satisfaction although increases in knowledge and skills were attained. The consistency of such decreases across training programs suggests workers increasing their repetoire of practice skills may find organizational constraints to implementing skills frustrating, a notion supported by a negative correlation of -.75 ($p < .001$) between pretest and posttest changes on Stafff Training and Job Satisfaction Questionnaires. This suggestion underscores need for program planners to become familiar with the organizational contexts of service provision. For instance, Witkin, Shapiro, and McCall (in press) note, "Agencies are often expected to serve both humanistic and social control functions while conserving public funds. As a result, workers find themselves accountable for meeting the organizational goal of effectiveness in providing human services while fulfilling the onerous requirements of a government bureaucracy" (p.4).

In addition to pretest and posttest measures, workers' intervention efforts provided information on training process as well as outcome. Implementation of training material to an actual case increased the likelihood that learned skills would be transferred to nontraining environments. The high number of successful intervention programs demonstrated worker learning. Further, workers not completely successful in intervention attempts gained practice experience under close supervision.

Trainee Evaluations

Further information on the training program came from anonymous posttraining questionnaires requesting information on course content, instructor, and subsequent worker performance. Responses were based on a five-point scale, with one indicating the most favorable response. Workers viewed course and instructor positively, with mean scores of 1.88 and 1.75. Mean ratings of self-performance were also high (2.31) although many saw job pressures interfering with their ability to devote time to the course.

This chapter recounts how in a marital intervention training program for social workers in a public agency, the use of a behavioral approach to marital assessment, intervention and evaluation was highly compatible with the exigencies and needs of the workers and couples served. Assessment was clear and provided clients and workers with ongoing feedback. Intervention was directive and action-oriented; evaluation was straightforward and relevant.

Program evaluation suggests this model offers a promising approach to social work training in public agencies. Workers increased their knowledge of common areas of relationship problems and were able to implement this knowledge in actual cases. Measurement of intervention efficacy provided accountability data.

16

Behavioral Methods In Primary Health Care

William H. Butterfield
and
Judith Werking

In most health-care settings social work intervention has generally focused on social and emotional problems. Recent experience indicates that social workers can also significantly enhance the effectiveness of medical interventions (Brockway, Werking, Fitzgibbons, & Butterfield, 1976). The purposes of this chapter are to introduce selected examples of behaviorally oriented intervention in health care settings relevant for social work practice, discuss theoretical concepts of particular importance in such settings, and provide practical information about medical social work.

BEHAVIORAL MEDICINE

Broadly defined, behavioral medicine is the application of experimentally derived principles of behavior change to medically related problems. (For a further discussion of the origin and definition of behavioral medicine see Pomerleau, 1979.) This section examines three facets of behavioral medicine: the improvement of patients' compliance with medical regimens, and the prevention, and treatment of disease and disability.

Prevention

Until recently few attempts have been made to apply behavioral principles to preventing disease and disability. Published reports focus on altering the behavior of at-medical-risk populations and can roughly be divided into primary and secondary prevention models. Programs attempting to avoid problems from occurring are considered primary prevention. Secondary prevention programs attempt to treat conditions in the initial stages so that they do not develop into serious problems (cf. Poser, 1979).

One program of primary prevention, developed by Reiss, Piotorski and Bailey (1976), was designed to encourage low-income families to seek dental care for their children. Families, with children attending a rural elementary school were divided into three groups: parents in the first group received a note listing dental screening data on their children, families in the second group received similar notes and were contacted by phone and in person by a dental hygienist who urged them to take their children for a dental examination, the third group received the note and a $5.00 coupon redeemable after their children received dental examinations. Outcome measures included: number of initial dental visits, number of follow-up visits, number of families completing treatment, intervention costs. The results shown in Table One, clearly document the relative superiority and cost effectiveness of the money-coupon incentive.

Table 1

Dental Visits, Completed Treatments, and Intervention Costs for Each Experimental Group

Note Only **Outcome**	**Note and Contact** **(n =)**	**Note and Coupon** **(n =)**	**(n =)**
Number of Initial Visits	3	6	8
Number of Follow-up Visits	6	1	18
Families Completing Treatment	1	1	5
Costs ($)			
Families contacted	.20	11.85	4.14
Families seeking treatment	.88	19.75	6.21

Weiss and Engel (1971), developed a secondary prevention program which focused on hospitalized patients with premature ventricular contractions (PVC)—a heart condition associated with increased probability of sudden death, diminished coronary artery and cerebral blood flow. During daily experimental sessions patients lay in their beds in view of a meter and a vertical display of three lights. The lights provided heartrate feedback cues when the rate was too high or too low and signaled reinforcement when patients produced correct heart rates. Total time at the correct rate was registered on the meter.

The use of this technique allowed patients to develop control over the occurrence of PVCs in the laboratory and on the ward; most treated patients were also able to control PVCs at home.

Treatment

Interventions which prevent problems from occurring or from developing into more serious problems are relatively rare in behavioral medicine. Most treatment has focused on the alleviation of disease and disability. Representative examples from the literature include the treatment of asthma, epileptic seizures, hysterical paralysis, and vomiting.

Asthma affects between four and five million individuals in the US (Purcell & Weiss, 1970; Reckless, 1971; Rowe & Rowe, 1963). Typical symptoms are episodes of labored breathing, shortness of breath, and coughing and wheezing. Asthma can be fatal, with four to seven thousand deaths reported each year (Gottlieb, 1964). Initiated by allergies, environmental irritants, or emotional responses to such stimuli, treatment can entail one or more levels of intervention, reducing the effectiveness of the stimuli initiating the attacks; reducing anxiety stemming from and exacerbating attacks; training in bronchodilation; helping family members minimize potential secondary gains from asthmatic symptoms; and inducing positive expectancies for treatment and realistic symptom evaluation. Thus, antecedents, and consequences of asthma may be the therapy focus.

Case material on behavioral intervention of asthma is provided by Neisworth and Moore (1972) who employed an operant strategy to treat a seven year old boy whose attacks appeared to be controlled by attention and concern. Intervention consisted of withdrawing parental attention and medication during bedtime attacks and reinforcing incompatable behavior (not coughing). The results provide compelling evidence for the environmental control of the child's disorder. Follow-up data showed a near zero rate of asthmatic attacks ten months after the intervention.

A respondent procedure was used by Sirota and Mahoney (1974) to treat a forty-one year old woman with a thirty-four year history of asthma. Trained to use muscle relaxation to combat stress and anxiety, the patient also learned to delay the use of bronchodilator. When she experienced breathing difficulties, the patient set a kitchen timer for three or four minutes, practiced relaxation, and after the timer went off inhaled bronchodilators only if necessary. Prior to treatment the patient used the medication about eight times a day. After intervention use rapidly decreased. A two month follow-up revealed discontinuance of cortisone therapy, and an eighty percent reduction in the use of bronchodialators. Reports showing similar results for behavioral intervention with asthma have been published by Katz and Zlutnick (1975), Moore (1965), Alexander (1972), Alexander, Miklich, and Hershkoff (1972), Sargent and Yorkston (1969), and Knapp and Wells (1978).

Behavioral control of epileptic seizures has been viewed as unlikely. In a recent series of case studies, however, a number of investigators have demonstrated operant control over the frequency of epileptic episodes. Zlutnick, Mayville and Moffat (1975), for example, treated four patients with a punishment procedure consisting of shouting "No" and grasping and shaking the patient's shoulders. A fifth patient was treated with a differential reinforcement of other behavior (DRO) procedure. Because this patient apparently triggered epileptic seizures by raising her arms, treatment consisted of moving her arms back to her sides and praising her and giving her an M&M candy when she lowered her own arms. Single-case research designs showed four of the five patients realizing immediate and lasting reductions in seizure frequency. Other programs supporting behavioral control of epileptic seizures are reported by Johnson and Meyer (1974), Lubar and Bahler (1976), Mostofsky and Balaschak (1977), and Stanulis and Glaros (1976).

Although relatively uncommon in outpatient populations, hysterical illness presents special challenges. An early study by Hilgard and Marquis (1940) illustrated how control can be developed over hysterical behavior that on first analysis did not seem responsive to environmental manipulation. The investigator treated a thirty-two year old woman whose left arm had been paralyzed without feeling since an automobile accident six years earlier. Prior to intervention, the patient reported no sensation when her left hand was shocked. By preceding an electric shock to the right hand with a shock to the paralyzed left hand, however, authors reasoned that sensitivity might return to the left hand since the patient could prevent shock to her right hand by withdrawing it from the electrode when the left hand was shocked. Gradually, sensitivity did develop in the left hand and the patient was able to avoid shocks to her right hand. Since functional use of her left hand was important, the authors then reversed the procedure: a shock to the right hand signaled that a shock to the left hand was about to occur. The second shock could be avoided by moving the left hand. The patient gradually regained control over the left hand's movement and with additional physiotherapy regained full use of the left arm.

Behavioral intervention has also been used by Malmo, Davis, and Barza (1952), to treat hysterical deafness and by Brady and Lind (1961),

Zimmerman and Grosz (1966), and Parry-Jones, Santer-Westgate, and Crawley (1970) to treat hysterical blindness.

Chronic vomiting, a serious problem leading to dehydration, malnutrition, lowered resistance to disease, and ultimately death (Walen, Hauserman, & Lavin, 1977) can often be controlled by removing attention given the vomiting response. Wolf, Birnbrauer, Williams, and Lawler (1965), for example removed attention for vomiting and eliminated the problem with a nine year old retarded child. Vomiting was seen as an operant, reinforced by classroom attention and by the child being returned to the dormitory when she vomited. The teacher, therefore, was asked to continue the class as usual when the child vomited and to not send her back to the dormitory until after class. Within thirty class days, vomiting ceased. But, the following year when the child vomited once she was sent back to the dormitory. Her vomiting then increased to where it was occurring in about a third of her classes. Extinction again helped reduce the vomiting behavior. The last two months of school the child vomited only once. Also using extinction, Alford, Blanchard and Buckley (1972) obtained similar results with a seventeen year old girl with a ten year history of vomiting.

A more intrusive technique for controlling vomiting is reported by Sajwaj, Libet, and Agras (1974). They treated a six month old child, in danger of dying because of persistent vomiting, by squirting between five and ten *ccs* of lemon juice into the child's mouth when vigorous tongue movements were detected. Data were collected for thirty-three days, including two days of baseline, six days of lemon juice therapy, one day's suspension of therapy (reversal), and twenty-four days of reinstatement of therapy. Vomiting had not reoccured at a one year follow-up. Results are reported in Table Two which is taken from Sajwaj, Libet, and Agras (1974).

Table 2

Mean Number and Duration of Rumination Episodes Across Experimental Conditions

Condition	Number	Duration (Seconds)
Baseline	9.6	60.6
Lemon Juice Therapy	4.5	33.4
Reversal	6.0	106.0
Reinstatement of Lemon Juice Therapy		
First Half	2.8	26.4
Second Half	0.9	9.8

Lang and Melamed (1969), used a still more intrusive technique with a nine months old infant in critical condition, who routinely regurgitated food within ten minutes of feeding. During treatment, when vomiting occurred, it was followed by a one second shock continued at one second intervals until vomiting ceased. The problem behavior was eliminated in five sessions.

Compliance

Behavioral intervention to improve compliance with medical regimes represents a recent and promising area of behavioral medicine. This use of behavioral techniques focuses on helping patients comply with intervention strategies developed by health care teams. Studies by Barnes (1976) and by Werking are illustrative of the interventions in these areas.

Barnes (1976) treated a forty two year old male having extreme difficulty in complying with dietary restrictions made necessary because of renal failure. During the fifth month of medical treatment the patient had to be hospitalized because of pulmonary edema, congestive heart failure and high blood pressure. The patient agreed to participate in a token economy program where points could be earned for proper dietary behavior, and for keeping his daily weight gain to less than two pounds. Points could be used to purchase up to 800 *ccs* of water each day. After initation of the program, weight gain between dialysis periods and blood pressure readings began to decrease, permitting the removal of a kidney, further reducing the patient's blood pressure. The patient continued to use the token program and to successfully control his diet after discharge.

A case drawn from the second author's work further illustrates behavioral assessment and intervention procedure with a medical compliance problem: Amy B. was a three year old suffering from marked femoral anteversion. This disorder is marked by internal rotation of the thigh and knee, and can result in "knocked-knees" and a "pigeon-toed" gait, often disabling and certainly unattractive. Many afflicted children cannot run well or keep up with friends at play; some children are so hampered they trip over their own feet. Although the etiology of the condition—an internal rotation of the thighbone—is unknown, in Amy's case, her pediatrician felt the condition might be reversed if the child's habitual sitting position were changed.

Characteristically, children with femoral anteversion adopt the reverse tailor, or "W" position when sitting on a flat surface. (See Figure One). With the knee bent and the lower leg resting flat on the floor to either side of the trunk this position rotates the thigh and knee inward. Physicians disagree about whether the sitting position is causal or the result of a congenital malformation. Conventional treatment usually includes an admonition to parents not to let the child sit in the "W" position and to encourage their child to adopt the tailor position (See Figure One).

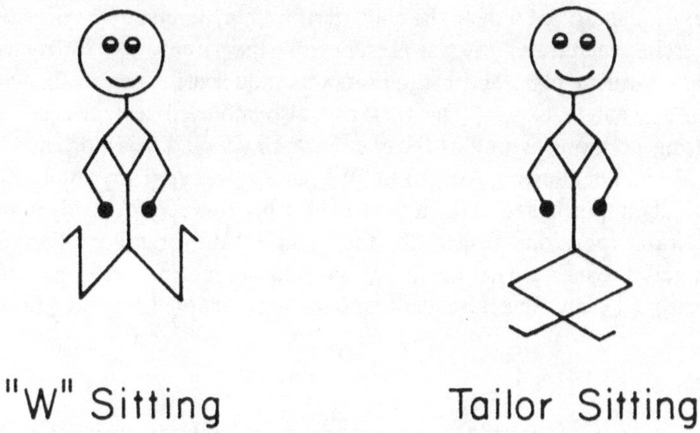

FIGURE 1. Illustration of Tailor and "W" Sitting Position

If rotation is severe, the physician may place the child in leg casts for several weeks to relieve torsion on the hip joints and to change the habitual sitting position. Amy's program, a behavioral one, follows.

Assessment

At initial contact the social worker asked Amy's parents to observe her for one week, noting how many times she sat in the "W" position, and what she was doing at the time. On the next visit the parents reported that they had ceased counting the frequency of the "W" sitting since "Amy never adopted any *other* position." They had noticed that Amy was usually playing on the floor or watching TV when she sat in the "W" position. A physical examination showed that Amy's knees and feet were markedly turned in; her gait was clumsy and she had difficulty climbing stairs. Asked to sit tailor fashion, she was unable to lower her knees a third of the way to the floor.

Intervention

Since Amy always adopted the "W" position while engaging in a favored activity, a time-out procedure was developed. Whenever she was observed in the "W" the parents were instructed to remove her from the favored activity location and to place her on an adult-sized chair in another room for one minute. The parents were also instructed to praise Amy lavishly whenever she adopted any other sitting position. Further,

her mother agreed to help the child perform ten minutes of the prescribed exercises each day. Amy was present while the parents were instructed in the treatment plan, and a time out was modeled for her so she would know what to expect. The therapist also modeled several acceptable sitting positions as well as the exercises Amy would be doing each day.

While not allowing Amy to sit "W" fashion was very important, it was equally important to make it possible for her to sit comfortably in more desirable positions—especially the reverse "W" or tailor. Therefore, exercises to increase her flexibility and range of motion were a part of the treatment plan. Several ballet exercises were adapted for this purpose.

Outcome

The parents continued the program for eight weeks, by which time Amy was averaging between one and three time outs per week, but was spontaneously adopting alternate sitting positions most of the time. The physician reported a normal gait with feet and legs straight. With no assistance or difficulty, Amy was now able to lower her knees halfway to the floor when asked to sit in the tailor position. At a two month follow-up, time outs were occurring at the rate of about one every other week. The parents, the pediatrician and Amy were extremely pleased with her program. Amy also reported she felt more comfortable with friends and schoolmates. Figure Two shows the results of treatment.

A third illustration of an attempt to ensure compliance is a study by Sackett, Haynes, Gibson, Taylor, Roberts, and Johnson (1977). In this study the authors report some preliminary results of attempts to avoid the long-term effects of hypertension (high blood pressure). Two-hundred-forty-five men who had hypertension and who failed to take assigned medication were randomly assigned to an experimental group receiving instruction about hypertension and its effects on health and life expectancy or to a control group receiving no instruction. Evaluation showed patients in the experimental group had learned information contained in the instructional material. At follow-up, however, they were no more likely to take their medication than patients receiving no instruction. Making their medical treatment more available by providing care at their work site also failed to change their medication-taking behavior.

Thirty-eight men from the above trial, who had not achieved compliance, were used in a second experiment. Here, control group patients received no treatment. Experimental group members were taught how to measure their own blood pressure, record it and medication usage, and how to build medication taking into their daily routines. A para-professional was also used to "reward" these patients for improvements in their compliance to blood-pressure control regimens.

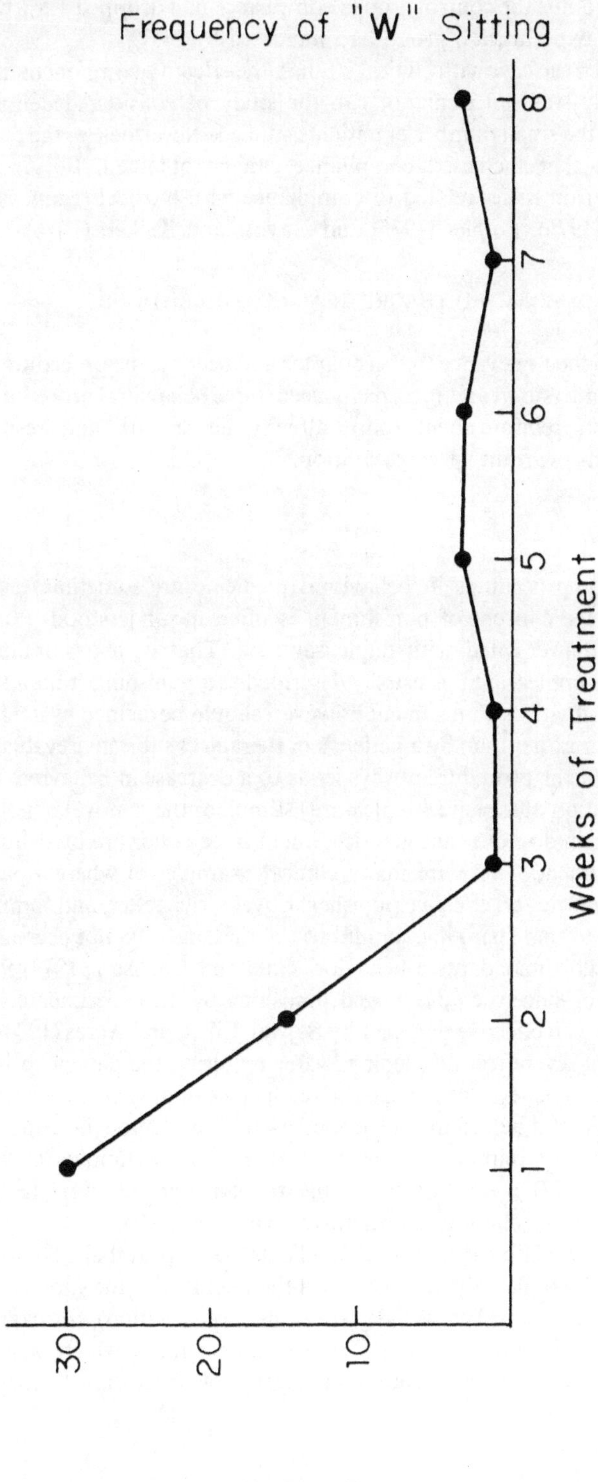

FIGURE 2. Effect of time out on the frequency of Amy sitting in the "W" Position

After six months the control groups compliance had dropped 1.5% while that of the experimental group had increased by 21.3%.

As is often the case with clinical studies, the effective component in the above study was not clear nor can the study be considered definitive because of the small number of patients studied. Nevertheless, the results do suggest that increased compliance can be obtained. For further information on issues related to compliance with medical regimens see Blackwell (1976), Pothier (1975) and Haynes and Sackett (1976).

SELECTED THEORETICAL CONSIDERATIONS

Because of their relevance to this chapter and because the procedures are often misunderstood and incorrectly used, three behavioral procedures—punishment, reinforcement (both already illustrated), and response deprivation—warrant special attention.

Punishment

Punishment procedures in behavioral medicine are sometimes useful. However, the concept of punishment is often misunderstood. Punishment is often equated with unpleasantness. That is, if a stimulus or situation is unpleasant it is usually described as a punishing stimulus or a punishing situation. Punishment however, should be defined by its effects on behavior rather than by a patient's or therapist's subjective evaluation: the punishment procedure always leads to a decrease in behavior. Thus the application of aversive (unpleasant) stimuli or the removal of positive stimuli which do not result in a decrement in behavior are by definition not punishment. There are many clinical examples of where a painful stimulus was not an effective punisher. Lovaas, Schaeffer, and Simmons (1965) found that spanking, painful to the therapist, did not decrease an autistic child's maladaptive behavior. Gale and Carlsson (1977) found that a lemon-juice therapy, judged punishing by the experimenters and shown to be an effective punisher by Sajwaj, Libet, and Agras (1974), did not control severe teeth clenching. After requiring the patient to ingest lemon juice whenever he engaged in teeth clenching, teeth clenching did not decrease and indeed may have increased. Thus, lemon juice appeared to be acting as a reinforcer rather than as an aversive stimulus. Gale and Carlsson (1977) were, however, able to gain control over the teeth clenching by switching to another aversive stimulus.

An opposite effect can also occur: clients may report that a stimulus is neutral or even pleasant yet when used therapeutically, the stimulus may be an effective punisher. Whaley (personal conversation), for example, reported, with some retardates that electric shocks which were not perceptible to the experimenter and clearly not unpleasant to the child reduced self-mutilating behavior. Thus by definition the shock was a punisher even though it was not unpleasant to worker or client.

Reinforcement

Reinforcement is commonly equated with pleasure or satisfaction. As with punishment, however, the correlation between reinforcement effects and the clients subjective evaluation is far from perfect. The authors have worked with many clients who reported certain activities as pleasant and enjoyable and yet, when the activities were employed as reinforcing events, clients did not show increases in behavior.

For example, the senior author once worked with a client who reported reading as a very pleasurable activity. But attempts to use reading as a reinforcer for increased social activity resulted in less reading and no increase in the social activity.

Another important variable in the use of punishment and reinforcement is the fact that their effects are situationally determined. For example a study by the senior author illustrating the situational specificity of reinforcement showed that schizophrenic patients able to earn a variety of extrinsic rewards for engaging in simple manual tasks generated high stable rates of the manual behavior. But when the task was changed to making a verbal response to a word or picture projected on a screen, the patients did not respond. Lack of response was not a result of the patient's lack of ability: many ultimately did speak; the controlling variable was the nature of the task not of the extrinsic reward.

The examples illustrate two important points: first, a stimulus must be defined as a reinforcer or a punisher on the basis of its behavioral effects, not on the basis of pleasantness or unpleasantness; second, the behavioral effects of a stimulus are situation specific and must be redetermined when the situation changes. These facts are of great importance in medical settings.

Patients often have problems that they find unpleasant and want to eliminate or alleviate, yet in many cases these very problems are major sources of reinforcement to the patients. Table Three, taken from Reese and Woolfenden (1973), provides a helpful summary of various punishment and reinforcement operations.

The literature on the medical application of behavioral principles is replete with attempts to get clients to comply with medical regimens that were unsuccessful until a behavioral analysis of the controlling conditions led to altered interventions. It is not uncommon for medical staff, for example, to attempt to control patient misbehavior with verbal threats or other methods of coercion, often unsuccessfully. In fact, careful analysis frequently shows that these subjectively unpleasant attempts at control in fact reinforce the problematic behavior. Most commonly, what is

Table 3

Procedures for Changing Respiration Rate

Procedures	Open	Consequences	Affect Upon Respiration Rate
Positive	Reinforcement	Presentation	Increase
Negative	Reinforcement	Removal	Decrease
Positive	Punishment	Presentation	Decrease
Negative	Punishment	Removal	Decrease

occurring is that the patient is receiving much attention (albeit unpleasant) for inappropriate behavior and little attention for appropriate behavior. A simple modification of the contingencies (that is attention for appropriate behavior and no attention for inappropriate behavior) often produces dramatic changes in patient behavior.

In summary, the clinician working in a medical setting will often discover that unpleasant stimuli may be reinforcing and on occasion that pleasant stimuli are not reinforcing. Thus it is crucial that the subjective evaluations by clinicians, patients, or staff not be used as the basis for intervention.

Response Deprivation

Response deprivation is a concept that fostered many important clinical techniques, including the Premack Principle already detailed in Chapter Three. First proposed by Timberlake and Allison, (1974), the response deprivation procedure can be summarized as follows: for any pair of behaviors, A and B, the probability of A can be increased or decreased if the performance of B is not allowed to occur at baseline rates and if A must occur for B to occur. The opposite relationship also holds. In a given situation, the rate of B can be increased (or decreased) if the performance of A is limited and if B must occur for A to occur. Specific steps needed to establish these contingencies are:

1. Establish base-rates of Behavior A and B.
2. Decide which behavior is to be increased (or decreased) and designate that response the instrumental response.
3. Prevent the base-rate performance of the noninstrumental response and designate it the dependent response.
4. Establish conditions under which the instrumental response must be performed for the dependent response to be performed.

The response deprivation hypothesis is very important to clinicians since it has wide utility and reduces the need for extrinsic reinforcers or punishers.

To date, the primary clinical use of the response deprivation hypothesis has been to increase the likelihood of new behavioral responses. A typical use is in the treatment of depression.

Depressed patients have a high probability of manifesting behavior that prolongs their depression—talking about how badly they feel. Depressed people have a low probability of behaving in ways that counter depression. Social interaction is one such countervailing behavior. The response deprivation procedure has been used to increase low probability behavior in the following manner. A high probability response—talking to the therapist about feeling depressed—is made contingent on a social activity—attending a swimming class, choir rehearsal, or a party. The probability of the client successfully completing the social activity is enhanced by requiring partial performance of the instrumental behavior in the beginning, and then gradually increasing the response requirement. Success is further facilitated by helping the client anticipate and prepare for agreed-upon activities (Anton, Dunbar, & Friedman, 1976). A future application of the response deprivation procedure might be helping a client reduce a problem behavior. (A special issue of the *Journal of Experimental Psychology* [Vol. 108, 1979] discusses the theroretical underpinnings of the hypothesis. The article by Staddon [1979] in that issue is particularly informative.)

Medical Social Work

Regardless of how sophisticated the intervention techniques, social work effectiveness also depends on how well professionals are able to work within the health care system. As with all learned responses, those comprising social work practice are shaped by environmental contingencies. The usual setting for medical social work are hospitals and private clinics. The latter are distinctly different from nonprofit, education-oriented medical centers: such differences affect use of time, record-keeping, and collegial relationships. Our experience in private and public medical settings may help others understand the values predominating in each.

In the private clinic, workers are often struck by the extremely limited amount of free time. When the physician, nurse, and social worker are on the job, maximum efficiency demands that each quarter-hour segment of the day be scheduled with a patient or patient-related activity. Everyone is busy; there is little time for lengthy discussion or consultation. Although time can usually be scheduled for significant discussions regarding a patient or a problem, rarely do staff have time for leisurely perambulations. Chatty individuals may find themselves placed on extinction schedules. When workers request a colleague's time, therefore, they should come prepared with a concise statement of purpose and well-defined questions. Unless the practice setting maintains a collection of reference works, it is a good idea to purchase a standard text in general medicine or a subspecialty such as pediatrics. Reference works on behavioral intervention should also be available.

In public and medical school affiliated health-care centers, with educational and research foci, there is often time to teach colleagues and to learn from them. Problems encountered are frequently less routine; and workers are encouraged to explore new and experimental methods. Consultation is also readily available. Patients are more likely to be seen by a team, with professionals sharing intervention responsibility, and maintaining a high level of communication. Because most medical social workers are trained in these environments, the terseness and solitude of private practice can be disconcerting.

Another set of factors contributing to isolation in private settings involves philosophical differences and attitudes. Many physicians enter medicine because they desire a service profession; others enter the field for its high status. For both groups the remuneration—social and financial—can be substantial. Contrariwise, people are often attracted to social work by the public service opportunities rather than by prospects of high pay. Consequently, physicians may look at private practice as a business, with social workers less familiar and less comfortable with thinking about practice in such terms.

The number of patients seen in any medical setting depends largely on referral rates. Especially in private settings, workers will receive substantial referrals only after the referring physician finds the worker competent and trustworthy. This process should not be viewed as insulting; social workers often feel the same way about referring their clients to other professionals. Since trust is established with feedback, it is well worth the time to discover the feedback mechanisms valued by each referring physician. Some physicians wish to know only outcome results; others prefer a more detailed analysis. A courtesy not to be confined to social workers, this should not be seen as demeaning.

Lest the world of academic practice sound utopian compared to the grim realities of the marketplace, emerging professionals should consider some positive points of private medical settings:

1) Salaries are usually better and the administrative process easier to deal with. Raises and benefit packages are individually negotiated with the business manager and based on performance. Workers in private clinics are not usually dependent upon grant support, state budget appropriations, or tax revenues.

2) If the need for additional help can be documented, hiring new staff is relatively simple.

3) Duties and the expectations of the private clinic are clearly defined. In an academic setting with multiple expectations—teaching, direct service, research, publication, and frequently administration, one ends up with several jobs and discovers that the multiplicity of expectations are difficult to define and meet.

4) Private settings present multiple opportunities to sharpen skills. A good volume of clients means more problems of a specific kind will be seen in a shorter period of time. The repetition of basic problems leads rapidly to finely honed expertise.

Regardless of setting, the patient record is of enormous importance. Records are subject to subpoena by courts of law and are open to scrutiny by several groups, including insurance companies and the patient. When handling records, workers must be constantly aware of two rules: Enter all information necessary to document variables evaluated in any intervention including contracts established with patients, patients' response to intervention, plans for termination, and consultations obtained. Second, information recorded should be actually necessary for an adequate data base. Comments should be descriptive, not judgmental. Gratuitous information that might potentially embarrass the patient or worker should not be recorded.

Finally, the workers should guard against accepting problems requiring skills they do not have. The mark of a professional is knowledge of personal limits. When workers have no experience dealing with a particular problem, or have not dealt with the problem for some time, they should ask a colleague to provide supervision or refer the case to someone else. Developing informal consultation contacts is vital to isolated social workers practicing in clinics. Sometimes it is necessary merely to check out one's direction; often it is wiser to have a colleage review the planned intervention, the results, and perhaps to see the client. When faced with having no peers available for consultation, workers can explore several options. A nearby university may have behaviorally oriented training programs. Catalogues generally list what courses are taught, and by whom. The Association for Advancement of Behavior Therapy maintains a consultation service open to all members. The Social Work Group for The Study of Behavioral Methods also can identify available consultants.

CONCLUSION

In this chapter we have illustrated how the concepts and techniques of behavioral medicine are applicable to social work problems in health-care settings. With Gordon and Schutz (1977) we concur that social workers uniquely deal with the interface between individuals and their environments.

The patient's social environment has traditionally been the turf of the social worker, a pattern that started in settlement work and public health and now extends to most medical intervention. Indeed, the holistic approach to caring for people within the social system seems the only way to adequately treat health problems.

Since behavioral methods stress the person/environment interaction, they offer social work tools for analyzing an interaction and for developing intervention plans. The social worker's skill in identifying and assessing environmental resources and the behaviorist's skill in controlling variables is an ideal admixture. We hope more of our colleagues will adapt the techniques of behavioral medicine to better serve clients in health-care settings.

17

Individual Case Evaluation

Steven Paul Schinke

The scientific emphasis cutting across these eighteen chapters provides a delightful status report on the place of research in behavioral social work. Such commitment to research has not always marked social work practice nor that of allied professions, regardless of intervention modality and setting. In no small way, stepped-up evaluation efforts in the human services are due to recent methodological advances. New and reworked methods of research design, measurement, information management, and data analysis alike have preceded rigorous and responsive evaluations.

This chapter is devoted to a promising methodology for evaluating social work with individual cases. For present purposes, individual cases are defined as single clients, couples, families, groups, intact classrooms, entire agencies, and whole communities. A background section distinguishes individual-case evaluation from traditional case study and group research. Limitations of the latter two are then highlighted. Next detailed are fundamentals of individual-case evaluation. Examples from this worker's practice illustrate two common individual evaluation designs. Benefits of the approach for social work are outlined as are practice implementation problems and guidelines for their resolution.

BACKGROUND

Evaluation through individual-case research transcends multiple academic and applied fields. From social work, psychology, sociology, education, psychiatry, biology, economics, history, and political science come field applications of individual-case evaluation. Current individual-evaluation techniques originate from examinations of Congressional voting patterns, traffic fatalities before and after relevant legislation, and changes in monetary indices (Campbell, 1969). Theorists and empiricists recognizing the potential of such research for evalution in human services have increased the methodology's armamentarium.

Individual-case evaluation is best understood when set apart from two other concepts sometimes confused with the approach: case studies and group research. Case studies on the observation and analysis of a clinical event have unquestionably enriched our knowledge base. Representative are detailed notes on a single client, clinical problem, etiology, therapeutic regimen, therapy, progress, and outcome. Landmark works by Breuer and Freud (1957), Pavlov (1928), and Piaget (1963), are illustrative. The production of future data on numerous overt and covert events will carry on the case study's long and proud history.

Still, inherent features of the case study constrain its application and restrict use of its findings. Every case study is unique to one client, presenting problem, practice milieu, worker, social situation, and environmental setting. Accordingly, it is not possible to characterize the role assumed by each of these factors when accounting for positive or negative client change. Which factor was responsible for the outcome? Was the therapy modality critical? Were worker sex, race, age, and cultural background key factors? Did change occur because of the hour of the day, day of the week, and physical environment in which therapy took place? Or, are the client's new attitudes, thoughts, and actions attributable to a combination of many factors? Even intense post hoc analysis of the case study cannot answer these and other key questions. Without prior controls, case studies remain descriptive, and do not approximate clinical research.

Group research has dominated behavioral and social science evaluations. The approach relies on random assignment to place clients within various experimental conditions or groups (Campbell & Stanley, 1963; Kazdin, 1980; Kerlinger, 1979). Comparing pretest to posttest change or a clinical outcome judges the effects of being in these conditions. Since group-research designs generally relegate at least one subset of clients to a control condition, the paradigm is also called control-group research. Results of group research are averaged for clients in the separate conditions. These data are tested by inferential statistics to find the probability that between-condition differences happened because of intervention and not by chance. The next chapter details the strengths of group research and its use in community-based behavioral social work. Germane to the purposes of this chapter are limitations posed by group research.

Group-research methods require investigations to fit within certain constraints. The initial restriction is that the clinical phenomenon of interest be experienced by enough clients to comprise intervention and control groups. The difficulties applied researchers experience in finding several clients suffering the same problem, wishing help, and willing to participate in a research project may be prohibitive. Anyone who has tried to draw together a group of clients for any purpose has felt the encumbrances of logistics, limited time and transportation, and competing personal, social, and job demands. Group research necessitates that identical intervention be appropriate for all clients assigned to the same experimental condition. Further, the clinical viability of group research is questioned by the ethics of randomly putting clients in nonintervention control conditions.

Additional confinements of group research are felt when analyzing and interpreting data. Regarding the first issue, clients in one condition who change for the better and others who change for the worse will average to an overall difference that accurately reflects neither subgroup. Comparisons through inferential and parametric statistics can be misleading if clients do not represent the at-risk population, if clients in the same group are more different than similar, if too few clients end up in one group, or if the total cohort numbers less than forty people (Hays, 1973). Interpretations are further limited by statistical averages or means. Differences are registered in terms of a mean client, difficult to portray as to her/his mean sex, race, marital status, social class, and other descriptors. Given these practical and methodological limitations, the dearth of applied group research in natural settings is understandable.

FUNDAMENTALS OF INDIVIDUAL-CASE EVALUATION

The rationale that underlies individual-case evaluation is the same as the one that guides group research. Both approaches permit controlled examination of the manner in which intervention affects outcome. Both can examine the same intervention. For example, task-centered casework with child-abusing families could be studied by either approach. Both research paradigms will probably look at the same outcome—e.g. parental attitudes toward corporal punishment, incidence of child abuse, and parent/child interactions. Pre- to postinterventive changes are conjointly of interest in research conducted under these two approaches.

Group research and individual-case evaluation differ in the way each attempts to control alternative explanations of outcome. Rather than randomly assigning clients to intervention and control groups, individual-case evalution pits clients against themselves as their own research controls. From this concept the paradigm derives its several labels: single-subject, ideographic, time series, single group, N = 1, and individual case. Seeing the origins of these labels sheds light on how the notion of individual corresponds to a person, group, family couple, agency, city, state, or collective body like the U.S. Congress. Individual-case evaluation is a framework to quantify the effects of intervention on any single unit without separate comparison and control groups.

The approach establishes research control through relatively standard phases. To begin, preintervention baseline data are gathered. The discovery of adscititious assessment information at this point can be beneficial. Stable baseline data can then launch intervention. Intervention may involve routine agency services, a new treatment technique, or different data-gatering methods. Before a procedure is studied through individual-case evaluation, group methods, or any research paradigm, however, it must first be deemed ethical, grounded in the scholarly literature, and familiar to worker and supervisor (Schinke, in press-a).

Evaluation of intervention efficacy can commence as soon as intervention begins, or evaluation can wait until intervention has proceeded through additional phases of a research design. Though data collected during baseline and intervention will juxtapose the two phases, to conclude that the intervention caused a specific outcome is tenuous and cannot rule out other explanations. Would the outcome have resulted simply from the passage of time and no intervention per se? Was intervention the contributing cause or was it the placebo effect of increased attention given to the client and to the presenting problem?

Viable and competitve explanation for change are controlled by systematically delivering intervention within a research design. The scores of individual-case designs that contrast data gathered before, during, and after intervention fall into two categories: 1) Designs requiring continual data collection on the same individual, problem, and clinical context. 2) Designs wanting data on different individuals who have similar problems, data on one individual's problem as manifested in different contexts, or data on several problems of a single individual. Applications of these designs are illustrated later.

Analyzing results from individual-case research resembles the procedures that follow group research. After data have been collected within either paradigm, results are compared across phases, contexts, and clients. Data from one or more clients in individual-case evaluation generally preclude the inferential statistical tests done with results from group research. This feature has led to graphic displays of individual-case data and to analyses by visual inspection or by descriptive statistics.

This departure from traditional analytic methods has not been without controversy. Critics and defenders alike have articulated their arguments over the last dozen years (Edgington, 1967, 1975, 1980; Elashoff & Thorensen, 1978; Jayaratne, 1978a; Kazdin, 1976, 1978b; Levin, Marascuilo & Hubert, 1978). And, treatises voiced at professional conferences and written in the literature evidence little hope for resolving issues about the correctness of statistical tests versus visual analyses of individual-case evaluation data (Baer, 1977; DeProspero, Cohen,

Kennen, & Edelstein, 1975; Gentile, Roden, & Klein, 1972; Parsonson & Baer, 1978). Such heated debate notwithstanding, practitioners will avoid nonproductive data-analytic issues by critically examining individual-case results, recognizing alternative explanations for change, and conservatively reporting their findings.

APPLICATIONS TO PRACTICE

The application of individual-case evaluation is best described by the relationship between social casework practice and methods of scientific inquiry. This association was early put forth by such pioneer social workers as Mary Richmond (1922) and attendees of the 1923-1928 Milford Conference (American Association of Social Workers, 1929). A decade ago Briar and Miller (1971) show parallel perspicacity.

> Stemming from the tradition of science is the paradigm of observation-hypothesis-experiment. This model is analogous to the traditional social casework formula of study, diagnosis, and treatment. A social study is merely a special instance of careful observation on the basis of which certain hypotheses (diagnoses) are formulated. The diagnostic assessment is put to test during the course of treatment. To the extent that the therapeutic laboratory casts doubt on the diagnostic formulation or hypothesis, the latter is revised and put to the test again. Thus, in outline, the model of study, diagnosis, and treatment becomes, for every caseworker, similar to the operations undertaken by any scientist who attempts the solution of a problem. (p. 81)

The fundamental bases of individual-case evaluation are therefore operationalized in every social work practice situation. Instances of individual-case evaluations are plentiful and come from the many settings of contemporary social work. For purposes of this chapter, examples from my practice will amplify components of the most common individual-case research designs: the reversal design, and the multiple-baseline design.

Reversal Designs

Margaret C. and her fifteen year old son, Michael, were well acquainted with the University of Washington Child Development and Mental Retardation Center. As a child, Michael was diagnosed as the victim of mild mental retardation. Despite great strides in special education and habilitative programs, Michael's adolescence was proving tumultuous. The youth's independence, his attempts to be equal rather than subordinate to Ms. C., and his faltering trials at new adult roles had caught Ms. C. unprepared. Recent separation from Mr. C. even more detracted from the woman's willingness to cope with her son's ever changing, sometimes obstreperous, behavior.

I responded to Margaret C.'s plea for services by offering to help the family dyad reduce the level of their unpleasant interactions. Arguments between mother and son became our initial focus. The first step of behavioral practice and individual-case evaluation was to collect assessment data. This involved Ms. C.'s use of the form in Figure One. Here she noted the occurence of arguments—defined as unpleasant verbal exchanges between her and her son. Keeping records of the frequency of arguments and times she and Michael were together allowed computation of occurrence rate. In fact, whenever data are collected during periods that vary, a per-minute or per-hour rate of behavior is more accurate than is a simple frequency count. Ms. C.'s records for one week seemed sufficient to establish a preintervention baseline, the second step of practice evaluation.

WEEKLY RECORD: Recording Sheet and Ms. C.'s Baseline Data

Name: *Margaret C* Date: *Sept 9th to Sept 15th*
Event Recorded: *Arguments with Michael*
Time: *Anytime they happen; Write down when we're together.*

	SUN	MON	TUES	WED	THUR	FRI	SAT
A.M.	9-noon 111	7-8 11	7-8 11	7-8 11	6:30-8 11	7-8 11	9-1 111
P.M.	2-9pm 1111 111					3-3:15 1	
EVE.		6-9:30 11	5-10pm 1111	6-10 111	6-10 1111	6:30-11 111	9-10pm 11
TOTAL	11	4	6	5	6	6	5

FIGURE 1

Arguments within the client dyad appeared to center on Michael's chores and privileges. Intervention, the third step of a reversal design, was a daily contracting routine that required Ms. C. and her son to spell out their expectations of each other. "Michael will bring in the garbage cans, feed the cat, and can stay up until Johnny Carson comes on TV," and, "Michael doesn't have to be home from school until 6:00 PM, and Mom feeds Snuggles (the cat)," are two contracts evidencing this process.

The fourth step of individual-case evaluation is need for reasonably stable data following intervention. The criterion of data stability kept intervention in effect with Ms. C. and Michael until consistent change occurred during ten of eleven days of contracting. So far, clinical practice with the C. family was identical to any behavioral social work program.

The use of clinical-research procedures not differing from those of routine social work practice provides an impetus to individual-case evaluation though this correspondence neither masks nor otherwise distorts the nature of the approach. Quite the opposite. Each phase of the research design is laid out and negotiated with clients and mediators prior to implementation. From the onset and throughout our work together Ms. C. and Michael were advised that efforts for change would be evaluated in terms of a predetermined plan. The stepwise progression of data collection and intervention were presented as integral to our ability to determine the reasons for a positive or negative outcome. In such a mannner, equal importance was placed on the next step of a reversal design: the halting of intervention.

Failure at the start of the program to apprise clients of this and every other evaluative step runs the risk of some procedures being viewed as extraneous or as departures from common practice. Seen as optional, evaluation may be cut short. Immediate, positive changes soon after intervention begins can falsely give license to not interrupting the program of intervention. Paradoxically, belief that initial changes are permanent can lead to prematurely stopping intervention. These assumptions are scientifically refuted or confirmed only after the reversal design goes through replication phases of a second baseline and redelivery of intervention. As I arranged with Ms. C. and Michael, explicit agreement to complete all phases of the research plan signifies a commitment to systematic and objective evaluation.

Ms. C.'s and Michael's return to baseline meant the elimination of daily contracting. Family arguments climbed back to a frequency near that recorded at preintervention. Comparable and consistent data throughout the one week reversal suggested a causal relationship between daily contracts and reduced arguments. Redelivery of intervention

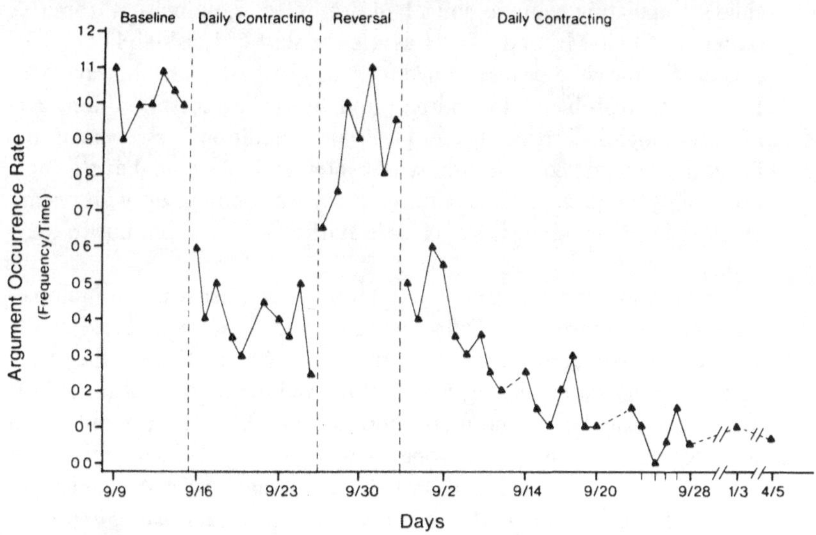

FIGURE 2. Reversal in Individual Case Evaluation: Program to Reduce Arguments Between Ms. C. and Her Son

confirmed the relationship. Few arguments were reported for twenty-two of the next twenty-five days and at three-and six-month follow-ups. Margaret C.'s records for the individual case evaluation are graphed in Figure Two.

Multiple Baseline Designs

Practice situations may contraindicate disrupting intervention. Presenting problems of adults that go against individual-case evaluation through reversal designs include alcoholism and drug abuse. Adolescent problems of delinquency and truancy may not lend themselves to evaluation, permitting a return to baseline. Social work with children who hurt themselves by self-mutilation or who physically aggress calls for quick and uninterrupted intervention. Continuous treatment might also be warranted with any client group or problem dependent on intervention delivered by outside mediators. Noted in my earlier contribution, the assistance of third-party mediators such as teachers, employers, and paraprofessionals is often critical to efficient and efficacious social work. Mediators, compared with clients' families, friends, and close associates, should be expected to show less tolerance if intervention is intentionally ceased—especially if the program is working positively.

Clinical circumstances counter evaluation by a reversal design obtained with a family who came to our agency. Five year old Lois H. was brought in by her parents because of the child's diurnal enuresis. The family was referred to the Child Development and Mental Retardation Center by the daycare center Lois attended for halfday sessions. The child's nonabating enuretic bouts had prompted an ultimatum from the center staff that Mr. and Ms. H assure the staff of Lois's ability to stay dry, or that the child be disenrolled from daycare. At intake, Mr. and Ms. H. related the problem's long history and, by medical corroboration, lack of physiological origin. These facts, plus additional assessment information, suggested that behavioral intervention would have a high probability of success. Of central concern was coming up with results quickly, in order to convince daycare staff to let Lois continue in their care.

Intervention and evaluation were brought together within a multiple-baseline research design. Data on Lois' enuresis were collected at the daycare center and at the child's home. When Mr. H. came to the center to pick up his daughter, daycare staff relayed the number of times Lois was wet during the four-hour afternoon session. Ms. H. kept similar data at home each morning. After one week's baseline, an intervention that rewarded Lois for urinating in the toilet and a matter-of-fact changing of her wet pants was started at home. Five days' data manifesting improved bladder control indicated that the same procedures could be effective if implemented at daycare. Given baseline and postintervention records of

Lois' enuresis in both settings, daycare staff agreed and began intervention. Supplemental findings on this multiple-baseline evaluation include a two-month follow-up. Portrayed in Figure Three, outcome results compellingly support our intervention.

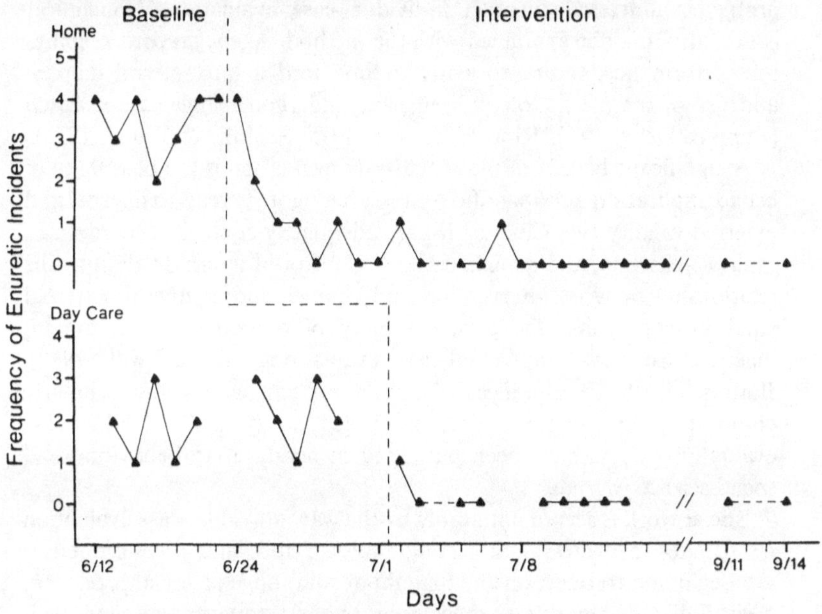

FIGURE 3. Multiple-Baseline Example: Evaluating Intervention with Childhood Enuresis

BENEFITS

These examples evidence the clinical viability and research integrity of individual-case evaluation. Social workers who use reversal, multiple-baseline, and variants of the two designs will discover many direct and indirect benefits. When clinical applications are preceded by in-depth study of other source materials, such benefits expand in number and scope (Gottman & Markman, 1978; Hersen, in press; Hersen & Barlow, 1976; Jayaratne & Levy, 1979; Kratochwill, 1978; Thoresen, in press). The next paragraphs detail the major benefits of individual-case evaluation for social work practice, research, administration, and education.

A foremost advantage to professional practice is the wide applicability of the evaluation methodology. Few social work situations are closed to individual-case evaluation. Barring unusual constraints, small sample research is rigorous at micro-, mezzo-, and macropractice levels. Social work roles of direct service, consultation, administration, and policy analysis are equally suited to individual-case evaluation. A congeries of presenting problems is no barrier to practice applications of the approach. Child abuse, depression, sexual dysfunction, marital distress, underachievmeent at school, incorrigibility, underemployment, addictions, and many foci from the present volume highlight the disparate problems addressed through individual-case evaluation. Nonclinical issues, also, may be examined with the method. Agency record keeping, job performance, getting to work on time, feedback to referral sources, and use of the methodology itself have undergone single-case research (Repp & Deitz, 1979; Rinn & Vernon, 1975; Schinke & Wong, 1978).

A significant benefit of individual-case evaluation is the possibility of broad application at no sacrifice to research rigor. Threats to internal and external validity (see Chapter 18) are adequately controlled by reversal, multiple-baseline, and similar designs. Control of internal validity—the relationship between intervention and change, and control of external validity—concerning the generalizability of outcome results, are indigenous to most individual-case evaluations (Kratochwill, 1978). Buttressing the acceptance of the approach within the scholarly community are copious findings based solely on individual-case evaluation. These have been published in nearly every behavioral and social science journal.

Social work is served admirably by the way individual-case evaluation contributes to professional accountability. Public and private interests are beginning to question the magnitude and range of social programs, their dollar expenditures, their poor budget management, and their marginal gains (Schinke, 1979a, 1979b). The burden now falls on social service professionals to justify their work or to face allocation cuts. As federal agencies and other funding bodies are better able to distinguish good research from bad, the value of individual-case evaluation grows. Methods of individual-case evaluation, still in their infancy, have yet to examine a sizable social program. Doubtless, investigators charged with documenting the impact of future projects will employ these methods when studying program process, outcome, and cost-effectiveness (Yates, 1979). Concurrent with this auspicious trend, we should witness less reliance on group research and on qualitative evaluations (Bernstein & Freeman, 1975).

The educational benefits of the evaluation methodology have special meaning for the practice orientation of social work. Conceptual underpinnings and procedural components are logical, not difficult to learn, and readily applied in the field. At all three professional levels—B.S.W., M.S.W., D.S.W.—students and enfranchised workers can grasp the methodology and try it out in social agencies and in constituent communities. Minimal prerequisities for learning its research components favor the approach. A background knowledge of research design, descriptive and inferential statistics, and data handling, though preferable, are not crucial. Formats for acquiring individual-case-evaluation skills can break out of traditional classroom environments in which group research methods are taught. Optimally, individual-case-research skills are learned in the applied settings of field-practice placements, in-service seminars, or continuing education workshops (Schinke, Smith, Gilchrist, & Wong, in press). Informal peer supervision and collegial consultation are ideal settings for professionals to learn from one another about individual-case evaluations.

PROBLEMS IN FIELD IMPLEMENTATION

The evolution of this evaluative approach is akin to the growth of any practice or research concept. Real-world implementation uncovers difficulties not considered in the methodology's theoretical formulations. Expatiated here are problems of practical applications and means for solving them. Stressed are troubles that take place in the design, conduct, and analysis of research on social work practice.

Investment in planning individual-case evaluations determines success. The aforementioned necessity of apprising clients of all phases of reversal design is important. Correct use of multiple-baseline designs also rests on client knowledge of why and how data collection and intervention are going to happen. Unclear plans will produce fuzzy lines separating data collection and intervention, and will jeopardize later analysis. Consequently, workers must assume that clients and mediators are ignorant of reasons and mechanisms for practice evaluation, data collection, and intervention delivery. Simply previewing these steps is insufficient. All referents deserve verbal and diagrammed outlines of the treatment program, chances to question and discuss the plans, and veto power over every part of the proposed program.

Noxious and longstanding problems need extra care during program design. Clients struggling with their own or someone else's aggravation are eager to move from baseline collection to intervention. Short-circuiting baseline in favor of intervention should be anticipated if mediators and clients are not fully briefed. Time and efforts devoted to program design can be lessened by joint-planning sessions with clients, families, mediators, and colleagues.

Conducting individual-case evaluations brings problems with data collection to the surface. Worker admonitions aside, few clients are ready for the demands of this activity. Consistent data collection is neglected as clients handle competing tasks. Conscientiously gathering daily information on the same problem is tedious, boring, and easily supplanted by more attractive things. Anticipation of such trouble will alleviate some of the onus of data collection. It is thus critical for workers to have firsthand and ongoing involvement with data collection and each intervention phase. Lacking support and empathy, clients will revert to familiar ways of coping with target problems. Needless to say, these methods rarely involve objective data collection. No matter how it happens—by telephone or face-to-face contact, initiated by client or worker—client and mediator support should be systematic and predictable. Routinely with all key actors, the worker must review program progress to date, collected data, future steps, objectives to be reached by next contact, and arrangements for that contact. Moreover, feedback, guidance, and reinforcement should be given to anyone who has simply pursued the intervention and evaluation program; reinforcement should not be reserved for success per se since such success is impossible to ensure.

Through generally rewarding, the analysis of results from individual evaluations can be disappointing. Data that depict slow and small postinterventive changes are not atypical. By recording and graphing their data, clients are susceptible to giving up programs that have unremarkable outcomes. Workers must provide a perspective on gradual changes by forewarning clients of gradual results. After data collection, clients should be alerted to the possibility of having higher standards or different expectations for the target problem. Successful completion of one individual-case evaluation should be marked with a celebration—regardless of results. At this juncture clients are reminded that any experience with the process can guide future and more dramatic programs.

Concerned professionals are hardly immune to the frustration of individual-case results. Even positive findings may not bring enthusiastic responses from workers. Workers who share their impact on a client, social problem, or organizational system with colleagues will receive mixed reactions. Past association with behavioral methods can implicate individual-case evaluation as limited to behavior modification. Critics having research acumen may impugn the generalizability of findings derived from evaluation with a single client unit. Others may ask why differences between baseline and intervention are not tested statistically. Such criticisms can usually be met by relating individual-case evaluation to earlier discussed strengths of research control and validity (Jayaratne & Levy, 1979; Kratochwill, 1978; Kratochwill & Brody, 1978). Convincing counterarguments are further built by replications of successful intervention and evaluation, by combining results with those of colleagues, and by using the published literature (cf. Hersen & Barlow, 1976).

In sum, professionals committed to conscientious and accountable practice prepare themselves and their clients for the setbacks, criticisms, and minor triumphs that attend individual-case evaluation. Weighing the benefits of practice-level research against its problems should eventuate in myriad other social workers taking on this commitment.

18

Evaluation At The Community-Program Level

Richard L. Gorsuch

Program evaluation is concerned with large-scale outcome assessment of an entire intervention effort instead of intervention and outcome assessment with individual clients or groups of clients. Although extending the behavioral model to large-scale evaluation presents somewhat different possibilities and problems than evaluation with individual clients, the basic process of behavioral analysis remains similar. Behaviors to be changed need to be identified, and then the intervention given while the process is appropriately monitored over time to determine if goals are met. Using illustrative case material drawn from a YMCA project designed to prevent alcohol abuse in early adolescence, this chapter reviews a behavioral approach to large-scale program evaluation.

For present purposes, the evaluative process is divided into six steps. Step one is Initial Task Definition, during which perceptions of program goals are explored. Seldom are goals from task definition sufficiently clear to be considered measurable outcomes. Instead, goals are translated into behavioral indicators at step two, Specification of Outcome Criteria. Once program goals are operationalized into outcome criteria, an

The author would like to thank Richard Batchelder, David Arno, and the editors for their helpful comments.

intervention is developed in step three, Intervention Development. In step four, Intervention Delivery, services are given according to a plan developed to provide the clearest determination of program effects. Collected information is compiled and compared in step five, Data Analysis. But even with data analysis complete, evaluation is incomplete until the results are translated into statements about program impact. Step six, Interpretation of Results, therefore, is the final step of the evaluation process. Table One summarizes these six steps for outcome assessment.

Table 1

Steps in the Evaluation Process

Step 1—Initial Task Definition

How are goals perceived by different groups involved?
How can several goals be merged?

Step 2—Specification of Outcome Criteria

What behavioral criteria indicate goal achievement?
Are appropriate measures available?

Step 3—Intervention Development

What intervention does prior research suggest?
Should another intervention also be tried?

Step 4—Intervention Delivery

How and by whom will intervention be delivered so outcome effects can be isolated?
Can alternative explanations for change be controlled?
Was intervention consistently delivered?

Step 5—Data Analysis

How can collected information be summarized?
What statistical comparisons will give meaningful results?

Step 6—Interpretation of Results

What conclusions can be drawn about program impact?
How will findings be presented?

The basic evaluative steps of Table One form an outline for this chapter's next six sections. The author's experiences in a YMCA program evaluation are used to illustrate each step and as an entree into more general issues of evaluating community-based behavioral programs. The last section discusses how external and internal evaluation both enhance social work program effectiveness.

STEP ONE: INITIAL TASK DEFINITION

In most community-based intervention programs, a number of interested groups have initial definitions of program tasks. Interested groups include funding sources, the agencies or organizations sponsoring the program, those carrying out the program, and program recipients. Naturally, initial task definitions vary from one group to another and are likely to be incompatible. One role of the evaluator is to negotiate a consensus on the task.

To begin negotiations, the tasks identified by each group are brought into the open and discussed with the interested parties. Because people frequently disagree on fundamental program tasks, this must be done tactfully. Considerable perceptiveness is also needed since people often "talk past" each other. Vague language—for example, "to prevent alcohol abuse"—obscures implicit disagreements needing explications. In our work with the YMCA program, "alcohol abuse" varied in meaning from any alcohol use through being drunk or antisocial behavior under the influence of alcohol all the way to having a health-related problem after twenty years of drinking. Until all involved discuss actual behaviors underlying vague language, few realize that disparate desired outcomes were implied by the same phrase.

Negotiation of the task definition is further complicated since many participants will be deeply concerned about the topic under study. Indeed, people deeply concerned about the project are those most likely to provide input and to be involved. Unfortunately, deeply concerned people may have little tolerance for positions different from their own (cf. Sherif & Sherif, 1969). As these people move from generalities to specifics, negotiating program tasks becomes more difficult.

Being responsive to the multiple initial task definitions generally requires defining the task as affecting multiple behaviors. The multiple behaviors selected for outcome assessment need to include the particular concerns of each group among them.

In our evaluation, two major constituencies took part in the initial task definition. The first was the National Institute of Alcohol Abuse and Addiction (NIAAA), funders of the grant for a program preventing alcohol abuse. The second constituency was the grant recipient, the National YMCA. In addition to being concerned with alcohol abuse prevention, YMCA administrators saw the project fitting a more general goal of developing "valuing" people. Batchelder summarized the concept of a valuing person for the National YMCA as "one who recognizes the value dimension of a problem, accepts responsibilitiy for his/her own value decision-making, identifies viable alternative solutions, weighs the consequences of each solution, examines the most promising solution in light of his/her already established system of values, makes suitable use of other resources, decides consciously to choose and implement one of the alternatives, acts upon the decision, keeps him/herself open to future growth in value development, and relates constructively to other people" (Glashagel, 1974, p. 2). The YMCA position was that valuing people are less likely to misuse alcohol, and so developing such people prevents alcohol abuse.

Discrepancies between what granting agencies think they are funding and what organizations hope to accomplish can be major. With the YMCA, however, we were fortunate to have in-house expertise on research and evaluation—Richard Batchelder and his associates—who helped integrate the goals. Integration centered on preventing alcohol abuse among teenagers through helping children become valuing people as preteenagers. For both agencies, then, developing appropriate valuing people was seen as a mutually acceptable program goal in part because it would affect adolescent alcohol abuse.

STEP TWO: SPECIFICATION OF OUTCOME CRITERIA

After initial tasks are established, they are translated into observable behavior serving as outcome criteria. These criteria become the actual record-keeping instructions for collection of information to evaluate the program. This specification of collectable criteria is a crucial step because even if initial task definition is clear, the program will be improperly evaluated unless outcomes are properly recorded.

In addition to the relationship to record-keeping, the specified outcomes step also differs from the initial task definition step in precision and in its behavioral nature. Outcome criteria are only sufficient if they allow several people observing the same individual and the same situation to agree whether or not the criterion behavior occurred. Technically, this requirement is referred to as *interrater reliability*. Raters are individuals observing the situation; to be reliable means the raters reach the same conclusion. Reliability is usually measured by percentage of agreement between two people observing the same event simultaneously and is considered acceptable if the percentage of agreement is above 80%.

Outcome criteria need to explicitly define even the obvious. After working through the initial task definition, some outcomes will be clearly appropriate. For example, part of the YMCA program was to train leaders in strategies for increasing valuing; therefore, one immediately specified outcome was the number of children reached by the program. Such obvious measures are surprisingly easy to overlook.

To accurately reflect an entire project, evaluation requires adding more complex measures to the simple counting of who was where when. For example, simple counting seldom provides a basis for examining positive and negative effects of a program. "How much impact did the YMCA program have on children's value orientations?" and, "Was the program likely to prevent alcohol abuse several years later?" were such questions in the YMCA project.

Criteria for children's valuing were developed in the YMCA project by examining the research literature. Fortunately, most areas of interest to social work are covered in professional literature. Many instruments and techniques are available in the literature but the studies do vary in quality and relevance, and expert consultation may be needed to effectively evaluate the literature. Nevertheless, techniques to measure almost any behavior can be found if the literature is thoroughly searched. Some references useful in such a literature search are in Table Two. The instruments and techniques which are best for task definition are those having documented evidence of change in similar past programs and showing high reliability.

Table 2

Scores of Measurement Instruments

Banks, J., & Rardin, R.L. Measurement practice in intensive and special adult probation. *Evaluation Quarterly,* 1978, *2,* 127-140.

Beere, C.A. *Women and women's issues: A handbook of tests and measures.* San Francisco: Jossey-Bass, 1979.

Buros, O.K. (Ed.). *The mental measurements yearbook.* Highland Park, New Jersey: Gryphon Press, 1965.

Buros, O.K. (Ed.). *Tests in print.* Highland Park, New Jersey: Gryphon Press, 1961.

Buros, O.K. (Ed.). *Reading tests and reviews.* Highland Park, New Jersey: Gryphon Press, 1968.

Buros, O.K. (Ed.). *The eighth annual mental measurements yearsbook,* Vol. I & II. Highland Park, New Jersey: Gryphon Press, 1978.

Cattell, R.B., & Warburton, F.W. *Objective personality and motivation tests.* Urbana, Illinois: Institute for Personality and Ability Testing, 1967.

Chun, K., Cobb, S., & French, J., Jr. *Measures for psychological assessment: A guide to 3,000 original sources and their applications.* Ann Arbor, Michigan: Institute for Social Research, 1975.

Comrey, A., Barker, T., & Glaser, E. *A sourcebook for mental health measures.* Los Angeles, California: Human Interaction Research Institute, 1973.

Cone, J.D., & Hawkins, R.P. *Behavioral assessment.* New York: Brunner/Mazel, 1977.

Educational Testing Service. *Tests in microfiche: Annotated index.* Princeton, New Jersey: Educational Testing Service, 1975.

Flagherty, E.W., Barry E., & Swift M. Use of an unobstructive measure for the evaluation of interagency coordination. *Evaluation Quarterly,* 1978, *2,* 261-273.

Goldman, B.A., & Saunders, J.L. *Directory of unpublished experimental mental measures: Volume I.* New York: Human Sciences Press, 1974.

Horst, P. *Psychological measurement and prediction.* Belmont, California: Wadsworth, 1966, 261-294.

Hudson, J. Problems of measurement in criminal justice. In L. Rutman (Ed.), *Evaluation research methods: A basic guide.* Beverly Hills, California: 1977.

Hult, S.J., & Hult, C. *Direct observation and measurement of behavior.* Springfield, Illinois: Charles C. Thomas, 1970.

Johnson, O.G. *Tests and measurements in child development: Volume I.* San Francisco, California: Jossey-Bass, 1971.

Johnson, O.G. *Tests and measurements in child development: Volume II.* San Francisco, California: Jossey-Bass, 1976.

Jones, R.J., Reid, J.B., & Patterson, G.R. Naturalistic observation in clinical assessment. In P. McReynolds (Ed.), *Advances in clinical assessment (Vol. 3).* San Francisco, California: Jossey-Bass, 1975.

Kazdin, A.E. Artifact, bias, and complexity of assessment: The ABC's of reliability. *Journal of Applied Behavior Analysis,* 1977, *10,* 141-150.

Kratochwill, T. R., & Wetzel, R. J. Observer agreement, credibility, and judgment: Some considerations in presenting observer agreement data. *Journal of Applied Behavior Analysis,* 1977, *10,* 133-139.

Lake, D.G. (Ed.). *Measuring human behavior: Tools for the assessment of social functioning.* New York: Teachers College Press, 1973.

Linehan, M.M. Issues in behavioral interviewing. In J.D. Cone & R.P. Hawkins (Ed.), *Behavioral assessment.* New York: Brunner/Mazel, 1977.

Lord, F.M. & Novick, N.R. *Statistical theories of mental test scores.* Reading, Massachusetts: Addison-Wesley, 1968.

Miller, D.C. *Handbook of research design and social measurement* (3rd edition). New York: Longman Press, 1977.

Nunnally, J.C. *Psychometric theory.* New York: McGraw-Hill, 1967.

Nunnally, J.C. Psychometric properties in evaluation measures. In M. Guttentag & E. L. Struening (Eds.). *Handbook of evaluation research* (Vol. I.) New York: Russell Sage Foundation, 1975.

Oakland, T. (Ed.). *Psychological and educational assessment of minority children.* New York: Brunner/Mazel, 1977.

Palmer, J. M., & McGuire, F.L. The use of unobtrusive measures in mental health research. In H.C. Schulberg & F. Baker (Eds.), *Program evaluation in the health fields* (Vol. II). New York: Human Sciences Press, 1979.

Reid, J.B., (Ed.). *Observation in home settings.* Eugene, Oregon: Castalia,
1978.

Robinson, J.P., & Shaver, P.R. *Measures of social psychological attitudes* (revised). Ann Arbor, Michigan: Insititue for Social Research, 1973.

Robinson, J.P., Athanasion, R., & Head, K. *Measures of occupational attitudes and occupational characteristics* (revised). Ann Arbor: Michigan: Institute for Social Reserch, 1973.

Sattler, J. *Assessment of children's intelligence.* New York: Saunders, 1974.

Shaw, M.E., & Wright, J.M. *Scales for the measurement of attitudes.* New York: McGraw-Hill Book Co., 1967.

Stanley, J.C. Reliability. In R.L. Thorndike (Ed.), *Educational measurement.* Washington D.C.: American Council on Education, 1971.

Survey Research Center. *Interviewer's manual* (1976 revision). Ann Arbor, Michigan: Institute for Social Research, 1976.

Thorndike, R.L. Reliability. In D. N. Jackson and S. Messick (Eds.), *Problems in human assessment.* New York: McGraw-Hill, 1967.

Tyler, L.E. *Tests and measurements.* Englewood Cliffs, New Jersey: Prentice-Hall, 1963.

Walls, R.T., Werner, T.J., Bacon, A., & Zane, T. Behavior checklists. In J.D. Cone & R.P. Hawkins (Eds.), *Behavioral assessment.* New York: Brunner/Mazel, 1977.

Webb, E.J., Campbell, D.T., Schwartz, R.D., & Sechrest, L. *Unobtrusive measures: Nonreactive research in the social sciences.* Chicagoo: Rand McNally, 1966.

Webster, H., & Bereiter, C. The reliability of changes measured by mental health scores. In C.W. Harris (Ed.), *Problems in measuring change.* Madison: University of Wisconsin Press, 1967.

It is best to use established instruments. Instrument construction is generally a complex task and appears easy only to the uninitiated or to those willing to accept superficial measures of outcome. Useful and reliable instruments usually take years to develop and require a significant commitment to that task alone. Of course, it is sometimes possible to develop appropriate instrumentation when initial task definitions include clear and readily observable behaviors. For example, the number of completed arithmetic problems, whether a child has wet the bed, and other overt behavior lends itself to straight-forward measurement. But subtleties in observation and recording can complicate a seemingly unambiguous outcome indicator. Asking the child, mother, and father if the child has wet the bed, for instance, may lead to different answers. In short, program evaluators should make every effort to avoid complications by using established measurement instruments: only if that is not feasible should expert consultation be sought on developing new measures.

Fortunately for the YMCA project, the area of value development had a number of available and proven instruments. These included measures used by Jessor, Graves, Hansen, and Jessor (1976), Schwartz (1968), and Hoffman and Saltzstein (1967), who quantified value development along the following dimensions: the extent to which children hold values most children generally see as desirable and which adults generally hold more strongly than children at this age; whether children have positive or negative attitudes toward such values; the degree to which culturally defined deviant acts are seen by children as deviant; whether children feel their friends would see such acts as deviant; children's use of internalized values in their thinking as contrasted to using values based on external circumstances; whether children accept personal responsibility in making value-related decisions; and the degree to which children anticipate their actions' consequences for others.

Comparing these value measures with YMCA goals for value development—summarized earlier by Batchelder—reveals little direct correspondence. YMCA program goals had originated without specific references to previous research and, therefore, to existing measures. But evaluating the alcohol abuse prevention project demanded well defined and immediately usable measures. Most evaluation studies are caught in this dilemma between the initial task and available criteria. Resulting discrepancies can be minimized by careful task definition with initiating groups. For example, had the YMCA staff drawing up the grant proposal been more knowledgeable of past research in the target area, the project could have been better tailored to readily specified outcomes.

Although the specification of the YMCA's intial task definitions was relatively simple because of the existing literature, the granting agency's goals were not easily put into operation. NIAAA's concern for *preventing* alcohol abuse during teenage years was admirable, but measuring behavior that has not yet occurred is a difficult mandate! Delaying outcome evaluation three or four years to measure subsequent alcohol abuse was possible neither fiscally nor in the program's terms. Hence the granting agency's goal could not be directly evaluated.

In the YMCA study as well as in many other evaluations of preventive programs, it is necessary to use indirect outcome assessment. This requires a literature search for variables preceding the behavior to be prevented. The literature on predictors of alcohol abuse from childhood to adolescence is sparse, but attitudes are related to behavior under special circumstances (Schwartz, 1968), and a correspondence between values and alcohol abuse has been shown (Bowers, 1968; Arno & Gorsuch, 1974; Gorsuch & Butler, 1976). Proceeding under the assumption that this literature could be generalized to our population allowed use of value measures for the program. Measures of alcohol abuse were more difficult to derive since none were found in the literature and scale development for children is particularly hazardous (Gorsuch, Henighan, & Barnard, 1972). It was necessary to revise our new scales toward alcohol use and toward alcohol abuse several times during the longitudinal evaluation. The considerable effort, time, and resources invested in developing these scales, however, warrants reiterating the preference for using extant measures whenever possible.

Often overlooked in the Specification of Outcome Criteria step is the need for identifying possible negative consequences of a program. A recent example of this need is supplied by McCord (1978) who traced 500 men for thirty years after an extensive delinquency prevention program. Involving many advanced techniques still being recommended as part of social prevention, the program had negative effects. As compared to a randomly selected control group, persons in the prevention program more often committed more than one crime, had more indicators of alcoholism, died at a younger age, and were less likely to hold white collar jobs. McCord also noted limitations of self-report measures, for in this study the men receiving intervention felt they had benefitted and were less delinquent than men in the control condition even though behavioral data showed the opposite.

Specifying outcome criteria for possible negative effects of the YMCA program was easily completed. Other than the unnecessary involvement of the children's and leaders' time, most potential negative effects were already being measured. If the program produced a reaction against valuing, it would show up in the value scales; if the program left attitudes toward values undeveloped, this would also be measured. Hence, additional instruments evaluating possible negative side effects did not seem necessary.

Ideally, initial task definition should be sufficiently clear and unambiguous so specification of outcome criteria is unnecessary. As administrators learn the value of program evaluation techniques, specifiable outcomes may become part of task definition. Although preferable, such a process is not likely to occur in most contemporary program evaluations. Thus, evaluators will still have a crucial role in both initial task definition and specification of outcome criteria.

STEP THREE: INTERVENTION DEVELOPMENT

Intervention development can be related to the outcome criteria specification in several ways. When criteria are first associated with appropriate measures, intervention staff can become thoroughly acquainted with the measures and select intervention procedures directly affecting the criteria. Intervention is then based on the same body of research as the outcome criteria. Or an intervention may be developed first, with evaluation staff then seeking outcome criteria likely to be affected by it. Another approach is to develop both intervention and outcome criteria from the initial task definition. This last arrangement is only possible if initial task definitions are very clear, if evaluation and intervention staff agree on how to accomplish goals, and if considerable resources are available.

Unless initial task definitions, outcome criteria, and intervention are exceptionally clear, advantages seem to lie with specifying criteria first and then developing an intervention. At a minimum this—unlike the other two approaches—assures measureable criteria. Choosing outcome criteria first also focuses the project on initial task definitions with the intervention becoming those procedures most likely to affect criteria operationalizing the task. The second approach—developing intervention first and then specifying criteria—is desirable only if there exist well developed and established intervention techniques that need not be implemented immediately. In this case, resources can be devoted to developing specialized instruments having a high possibility of being affected by the intervention. As noted above, however, instrument development demands skills and time not available to many program evaluators.

For the YMCA evaluation, intervention and outcome criteria were simultaneously developed. Despite shared theoretical paradigms, however, interfacing intervention and outcome was often difficult because of varying interpretations of program goals. Moreover, distance between intervention and evaluation teams inhibited routine interactions. One untoward consequence was that intervention and measurement procedures were not integrated early enough to pilot-test program components. Had earlier integration been possible, program segments could have been evaluated by preliminary forms of measurement instruments, with intervention and criteria being revised for maximum congruity (see last section).

The YMCA program of preventive intervention was based upon value literature similar to that used in instrument development. Drawing from value clarification literature (Raths, Harmin, & Simon, 1966) and research on moral development and behavior (Licona, 1976), intervention procedures helped children identify values, make value decisions, and incorporate these decisions into behavior. Small group sessions, twenty to forty minutes long, were used for group discussion, modeling, roleplay, behavior rehearsal, coaching, reinforcement, and feedback.

STEP FOUR: INTERVENTION DELIVERY

Empirical documentation that the persons delivering an intervention are adequately trained and will consistently implement intervention procedures is necessary, for evaluations of social programs can fail because the intervention as planned did not occur. A complete evaluation needs to separate program failure per se from failure caused by vagaries of the intervention staff's knowledge and abilities to implement procedures consistent with underlying theoretical orientation and preestablished protocol. A possible weakness in the YMCA program evaluation was that group-leader training and intervention delivery were not rigorously measured because of budgetary constraints and a belief that leaders were relatively homogeneous and committed to value development regarding alcohol abuse.

After assuring that the intervention can be and is delivered, the single most important step in any evaluative endeavor is determining who receives what and when it is received—in short, developing the *research design.* The goal of a research design is to eliminate any other possible explanations of the outcome so that the program's most severe critic will be forced to acknowledge its effectiveness. If the research design is poor, it will be possible to "explain away" the results as due to some factor other than the intervention itself.

Developing a research design begins with asking what possible explanations might be offered for a favorable outcome beside the intervention. A classic volume by Donald Campbell and Julian Stanley,

Experimental and Quasi-Experimental Designs for Research (1963), separates potential alternative explanations into several categories. One category, *selection,* identifies problems occuring when persons sharing a high probability for success are screened into a program while persons sharing a chance for failure are screened out, a process which makes even a poor program seem good and would be a reasonable alternative explanation if not eliminated by a design including all possible types of people. Effects of *history,* another alternative explanation, occur when program participants experience an extraneous event concurrent with intervention—change of seasons, for example—that could account for observed changes. *Maturation* effects, certainly germane to the young participants in the present case, are suspected when people undergo life-development changes simultaneously with the implementation of the social program.

Research designs providing experimental control over various potential problems can eliminate, or at least reduce, the likelihood of these and other alternative explanations for change. The control group design, with participants randomly assigned to an intervention group or to a control group which receives no intervention, is appropriate because it controls for most alternative explanations of change. For example, if the intervention group improves more than the control group—which is the result generally hypothesized—selection cannot be producing differences because participants are assigned randomly. Maturation could not produce differences between the two groups because it would affect them equally. Effects of history are also controlled since outside events would affect both groups equally. Thus, greater improvement in the intervention group than in the control group means that no other explanation except the effectiveness of the program applies.

If it is difficult to randomly assign participants to groups, quasi-experimental designs—in which nonrandomly assigned groups are compared—become viable options. Comparison groups help control for alternative explanations of change. The alternative explanation of maturation in the YMCA project was checked by comparison groups composed of children not given intervention. The wisdom of this approach was proved when one attitude scale showed comparison group children becoming increasingly tolerant of deviant acts as they grew older. Because children in the YMCA program did not show the maturational trend, intervention was successful in preventing development of tolerance of deviance. If no comparison group had been included, a conclusion that the intervention did not affect the children could have been erroneously drawn.

Since prevention training was delivered within more general YMCA programs, results may have been a function of other YMCA efforts rather than the intervention. To check this alternative explanation (of the history type), one study used children from other YMCA programs as the comparison group. Data showed greater improvement for the intervention group than for comparison groups, indicating that the positive effects were not attributable to the more general programs.

Unfortunately, using other YMCA groups for comparison meant going outside the neighborhood where intervention was being conducted, thereby introducing a variant of the selection alternative explanation: differences in neighborhoods from which groups were selected might have made intervention appear effective when it was not. To control for this, a comparison was made with other children in the same classrooms as children receiving intervention. The data showed effects to be independent of neighborhood and school, with children given intervention changing more positively than their school peers.

Without random assignment, comparison groups cannot control for systematic differences among participants before the program begins. Of the many reasons for children being in a YMCA group, some are probably related to values. YMCA participants do differ from other children, who would be in the comparison gruops. If outcome is only measured once after intervention, a critic could argue that observed postintervention differences were carried over from differences existing before intervention. This alternative explanation was controlled for by measuring children's values before and after the program. Finding differences only after the intervention—and not before—eliminates this alternative explanation.

Although pretest measurement reduces some alternative explanations, pretests themselves can produce special problems. A pretest could have alerted children that the YMCA was interested in values. The pretested children might then have paid more attention to intervention, producing an interaction between pretest and intervention. To reduce this possible alternative explanation, testing was conducted in school classrooms so that children would not view the measures as part of the YMCA program.

Controlling for these alternative explanations helped determine whether intervention had an effect on the participating children, thus establishing the study's *internal validity.* Also of interest is *external validity* of study's findings, that is, whether the intervention could be generalized to other YMCA settings and other groups of children. External validity was examined by involving children from several grade levels and children enrolled in summer camps. The results showed intervention effectiveness with different age groups, although not when implemented for only brief periods of time. Similar to many other social intervention efforts, the YMCA program was therefore validated internally and proved to be externally valid in circumstances for which it was designed but not necessarily in other circumstances.

Note that the evaluations of the YMCA project could only be accomplished by careful selection of who received what intervention and determining when it was delivered, a crucial step that must be thoughtfully planned. The research design therefore is an integral part of the design for the delivery of the intervention, and can never be "tacked on" afterwards. Proper delivery of intervention to satisfy the requirements of a reasonable research design is readily accomplished if planned in advance. Close cooperation of evaluation and delivery teams before decisions are made by either is crucial.

STEP FIVE: DATA ANALYSIS

Data analysis generally serves two functions. First, analysis is used to summarize data in *descriptive statistics.* Descriptive analysis yields basic information about how many people participated in the program, what their demographic characteristics were, what scores they obtained on various measures, and other variables related to program process. Usually, descriptive analytic techniques involve frequency counts, means, standard deviations, and simple measures of association.

Second, analysis is used to determine the likelihood that differences among program participants are due to random chance. Termed *inferential statistics,* such procedures indicate the probability that observed change from pretest to posttest, observed differences between intervention and control groups, and observed correlations among outcome measures could have happened by accidents of sampling or other chance events. If the odds are low that the observed statistics occurred by chance, interpretation begins.

Analysis of YMCA data was accomplished by the general linear model, within which appear better-known statistical procedures such as analysis of variance and regression analysis as special cases (see Ward & Jennings, 1973; Cohen & Cohen, 1975). This quite flexible statistical procedure permitted tailoring statistical procedures to the several quasi-experimental evaluation designs.

The inferential analysis showed that:

1. Intervention produced a shift toward values children and adults view as desirable.

2. Although children become increasingly tolerant of deviant acts as they grow older, intervention participants stayed relatively intolerant of

deviant acts.

3. Boys receiving more intervention showed greater changes than did those receiving only occasional training.

4. Group leaders with a higher degree of value internalization had more impact than did leaders with less value internalization.

5. Results varied considerably among groups, suggesting that the nature of the small groups in which value education occurred was an important component of the intervention.

6. Of all groups, the highest rejection of alcohol abuse was for those boys involved in the intervention program for the longest time.

In total, the findings indicated a generally successful intervention. The fifth and sixth findings, however, point to a lack of standardization throughout the program and further emphasize the need for evaluating leader training and for monitoring delivery.

STEP SIX: INTERPRETATION OF RESULTS

An evaluation is conducted to obtain an interpretation based upon objective procedures rather than subjective opinion. An objective interpretation begins with clearly stated results. Clearly stated results leave little room for speculation, centering interpretation on actual program outcomes instead.

Interpretation asks two questions of the results. First, why did the observed results occur? Answering this question involves, in part, analysis of delivery design to determine if all major alternative explanations were indeed controlled. Occasionally a new alternative explanation is found which was not controlled for in the delivery and research design. All uncontrolled alternative explanations are discussed in the results to help readers evaluate the usefulness of the intervention for their own purposes.

The second question is that of the importance of the statistically signficant results. Some results may be unimportant because effects were very small. (Note that statistical significance is not the same as importance; both are needed.) In that case, the effects are noted but are not stressed in the interpretation. Results seldom found in similar situations are also noted as are results commonly found elsewhere but which did not occur here. In this manner interpretation places the results of the study in perspective so that they can be appropriately utilized.

Objectively interpreting results can be a difficult step for the evaluation team. By this point they are intimately involved in details of the research process, its problems, and the data it yields. As essential as such involvement is to assure a good evaluation, involvement does present a danger: loss of perspective on the program's major goals and trends. Loss of perspective can be a major reason why results are presented in a manner confusing to readers. Involvement of others in the final interpretation is a useful corrective.

Following these caveats, the interpreting and presenting of results at the conclusion of the YMCA prevention program developed from a conference format including the evaluative team, the intervention staff, and others with a broad view of the project not directly involved with either intervention or evaluation. Focused discussion helped all interpret and understand potentially conflicting findings, such as overall intervention effectiveness as compared to differential leadership effects. Mixed findings—the rule rather than the exception in most programs—demonstrate that a carefully planned program for interpreting results is a crucial step for accurate evaluation. Indeed, developing improved subsequent programs can best occur when evaluators, administrators, and planners together critically examine evaluations of current programs.

EXTERNAL AND INTERNAL EVALUATION OF SOCIAL PROGRAMS

Examination of the YMCA alcohol abuse prevention program, conducted by researchers outside the organization seeking to document program impact, was an example of *external evaluation.* Ensuring objectivity, external evaluation provides critical feedback to funding agencies, service providers, and clients. Methodologies and resulting findings of such evaluation are usually viewed as credible simply because of the research staff's assumed lack of bias. In short, given adequate funds, time, and resources, external evaluation is an effective means of determining social program impact.

External evaluations have the continuing problem of being seen as a threat to those conducting the intervention, a legitimate concern when the goals of the program personnel are not central to evaluation criteria. Often, however, much concern occurs simply from being evaluated. In part the anxiety arises because most program administrators give verbal reports of their own impressions. Verbal reports are inexact and vague, which allows everyone to interpret them as they see fit. It is only human to prefer that kind of evaluation to objective criteria that might show the program to be wanting, and only natural for outside groups to prefer the external evaluation. In our project the National YMCA served the function of outside evaluator in part, as well as the granting agency. Fortunately, because the National YMCA was involved, the evaluation was also partially "in house" and that eased some evaluation anxieties.

Agencies themselves have needs for *internal evaluations* (also referred to as developmental research, Thomas, 1978). They provide early feedback on program strengths and weaknesses, thereby guiding modifications prior to large-scale program implementation. The internal evaluative staff may be drawn from existing agency ranks or may come from the outside, depending on resources. Typically, an internal evaluation is manifested as a series of pilot studies, each examining various phases of intervention and measurement. The results of one pilot study cause changes to be made in the intervention, and the changed intervention is then used for another pilot study. Cycles of pilot study, feedback, and revision continue until program personnel are comfortable in launching the larger social program. Ideally, the last stage of the internal evaluation should be a miniature of the expected external evaluation.

Internal evaluation requires care in its conduct and the interpretation of its findings. It is distinct from external evaluation in that final outcome criteria may not be appropriate measures for evaluating pilot efforts. Intermediate outcome criteria are specified for the internal evaluation. Rigorous research design and careful assessment of change can easily be overlooked in internal evaluation, but are just as essential as in external evaluation to prevent skewed findings because of idiosyncratic data from atypical client samples or poor intervention delivery. Without proper measures and proper design, early internal evaluation of poor quality could result in misleading predictions about future program impact.

Conducting an internal evaluation requires a program director sympathetic with and understanding of evaluation processes. Administrators also need sufficient experience with evaluation to make realistic cost estimates of internal evaluations. Personnel are needed who know both intervention and how to evaluate it. Attempting to solve internal evaluation problems by consultation from those who know little about the program can be frustrating and discouraging. Only when people involved directly with the program are somewhat familiar with evaluation techniques can the appropriate procedures be built in "from the ground up" so that they are effective.

Internal and external evaluations function much like agency budget management processes. Internal budget evaluation includes bookkeeping staff who track accounts receivable, accounts payable and available capital on a day-by-day basis. Administrators use ongoing budgetary data to revise procedures and programs. Periodically, however, external auditors with special expertise carefully review the agency's financial health, reporting their findings to the Executive Board, interested citizen groups, and certain government bureaus. Thus, both internal budget evaluation and external financial audit are essential to successful agency operations. In the same manner, internal and external evaluation both are critical for high-quality, community-based social work programs.

References & Indices

Abramson, Edward E. 1977—Behavioral Approaches to Weight Control: An Updated Review. *Behaviour Research and Therapy* 15(4):355-363.

Adams, H. E., & Hughes, H. H. 1976—Animal Analogues of Behavioral Treatment Procedures: A Critical Evaluation. In *Progress in Behavior Modification,* Vol. 3, M. Hersen, R. M. Eisler, and P. M. Miller, Eds. New York: Academic.

Akiskal, H. S., & McKinney, W. T., Jr. 1973—Depressive Disorders: Toward a Unified Hypothesis. *Science* 182(4107):20-29.

Alberti, R. E. 1977—A Statement of "Principals for Ethical Practice of Assertive Behavior Training." In *Assertiveness: Innovations, Applications, Issues,* R.E. Alberti, ed. San Luis Obispo: Impact.

Alberti, R. E., & Emmons, M. L. 1974—*Your Perfect Right.* San Luis Obispo: Impact.

Alexander, A. Systematic relaxation and flow rates in asthmatic children; relationship to emotional precipitants and anxiety. *Journal of Psychosomatic Research,* 1972, *16,* 405-410.

Alexander, A., Micklich, D., & Hershkoff, H. The immediate effects of systematic relaxation training on peak expiratory flow rates in asthmatic children. *Psychosomatic Medicine,* 1972, *34,* 388-394.

Alexander, J. F. & Parsons, B. U. 1973—Short-term Behavioral Intervention with Delinquent Families: Impact on Family Process and Recidivism. *Journal of Abnormal Psychology,* 81:219-225.

Alford, G., Blanchard, E., & Buckley T. Treatment of hysterical vomiting by modification of social contingencies; a case study. *Journal of Behavior Therapy & Experimental Psychiatry,* 1972, *3,* 209-212.

Allen, Dean A. 1971—Underachievement is many-sided. *Personnel and Guidance Journal* 49:529-532.

Allen, K. E., & Harris, F. R. 1966—Elimination of a Child's Excessive Scratching by Training the Mother in Reinforcement Procedures. *Behaviour Research and Therapy* 4(2):79-84.

Alter, H. M. 1954—A study of high school students with scores of 130 and above on the California Test of Mental Maturity. In *Bright Underachievers,* Jane B. Raph, Mirriam L. Goldberg, and Harry A. Passow. New York, N.Y.: Teachers College Press.

American Association of Social Workers. 1929—*Social case work, generic and specific: A report of the Milford Conference.* New York: Author.

Anton, J., Dunbar, J., & Friendman, L. Anticipation training in the treatment of depression. In *Counseling Methods,* J. Krumboltz & Co. Throesen, eds., New York: Holt, Rinehart & Winston, 1976.

Arno, D., & Gorsuch, R. L. *Values and value changes as they relate to the use of alcohol by children and adolescents.* Fort Worth, Texas: Institute of Behavior Research, Texas Christian University, 1974.

Ashem, B., & Donner, L, 1968—Covert Sensitization with Alcoholics: A Controlled Replication. *Behaviour Research and Therapy* 6(1):7-12.

Azrin, N. A strategy for applied research: Learning-based but outcome—oriented. *American Psychologist,* 1977, *32* 140-149.

Azrin, N., Flores, T., & Kaplan, S. J. 1975—Job-Finding Club: A Group Assisted Program for Obtaining Employment. *Behaviour Research and Therapy* 13(1):17-26.

Azrin, N., Naster, B., & Jones, R. 1973—Reciprocity Counseling: A Rapid Learning-Based Procedure for Marital Counseling. *Behaviour Research and Therapy* 11(4):365-382.

Baer, Donald M. 1962—Laboratory Control of Thumbsucking by Withdrawal and Representation of Reinforcement. *Journal of the Experimental Analysis of Behavior* 5(4):525-528.

Baer, Donald M. 1977—Perhaps It Would Be Better Not to Know Everything. *Journal of Applied Behavior Analysis* 10(1):167-1972.

Baer, D., Peterson, R. F., & Sherman, J. A. 1967—Development of Imitation by Reinforcing Behavioral Similarity to a Model. *Journal of the Experimental Analysis of Behavior* 10(5):405-416.

Baer, D. M., Wolf, M. M. & Risley, T. R. 1968—Some current dimensions of applied behavior analysis. *Journal of Applied Behavior Analysis* 1:91-97.

Baer, J. 1976—*How to Be an Assertive (Not Aggressive) Woman in Life, in Love, and on the Job.* New York: The New American Library.

Balgopal, P. R. 1974—Sensitivity training: A conceptual model for social work education. *Journal of Education for Social Work* 10:5-11.

Ballard, K. D. & Glynn, T. 1975—Behavioral and self-management in story writing with elementary school children. *Journal of Applied Behavior Analysis* 8:387-398.

Bandura, A. Psychotherapy based on modeling principles. In A. E. Bergin & S. L. Garfield (Eds.), *Handbook of psychotherapy and behavior change: An empirical analysis.* New York: Wiley, 1971. (a)

Bandura, A. Vicarious and self-reinforcement processes. In R. Glaser (Ed.,) *The nature of reinforcement.* New York: Academic Press, 1971. (b)

Bandura, Albert 1977(a) *Social Learning Theory.* Englewood Cliffs, New Jersey: Prentice Hall (a).

Bandura, A., Adams, N. E. & Beyer, J. 1977 Cognitive Processes Mediating Behavioral Change. *Journal of Personality and Social Psychology 35(3):125-139.*

Barbach, L. G. For yourself the fulfillment of female sexuality: A guide to orgasmic response. Garden City: Doubleday, 1975.

Barbee, J. R. & Ellsworth, C. K. 1973—Experimental Techniques of Job Interview Training for the Disadvantaged: Videotaped Feedback, Behavior Modification, and Microcounseling. *Journal of Applied Psychology,* 58 (October):209-213.

Barlow, David 1979—Quoted in The Sex-Change Conspiracy, R.M. Restale. *Psychology Today,* 13(2):20-25.

Barnard, J. D. Christophersen, E. R., & Wolf, M. M. 1972—Supervising

Paraprofessionals: Performance—Related Feedback. Proceedings of the 80th Annual Convention of the American Psychological Association 7:765-766.

Barnes, M. Token economy control of fluid overload in a patient receiving hemodialysis. *Journal of Behavior Therapy and Experimental Psychiatry,* 1976, *7,* 305-306.

Beck, Aaron T. 1967—*Depression: Clinical, Experimental and Theoretical Aspects.* New York: Hoeber.

Beck, Aaron T. The Development of Depression: A Cognitive Model. In Raymond J. Friendman & Katz, M. M. (Eds.), *The Psychology of Depression: Contemporary Theory and Research.* Washington: V.H. Winston.

Beck, Aaron T. *Cognitive Therapy and the Emotional Disorders.* New York: Internatonal Universities Press.

Beck, D. F. Research findings on the outcomes of marital counseling. *Social Casework,* 1975, *56,* 153-181.

Becker, Joseph 1977—*Affective Disorders.* Morristown, New Jersey: General Learning Press.

Becker, W. C. 1971—*Parents are Teachers.* Champaign, Ill.: Research Press.

Bednar, R. L. & Lawlis, J. F. 1971—Empirical Research in Group Psychotherapy. In *Handbook of Psychotherapy and Behavior Change: An Empircal Analysis,* A. E. Bergin and S. L. Garfield, (Eds.), New York: John Wiley and Sons.

Bellack, Alan S. 1976—A Comparison of Self-Reinforcement and Self-Monitoring in a Weight Reduction Program. *Behavior Therapy* 7(1):68-75.

Becllack, Alan S. 1977—Behavioral Treatment for Obesity: Appraisal and Recommendations. In *Progress in Behavior Modification,* volume four, Michel Hersen, Richard M. Eisler, and Peter M. Miller, (Eds.), New York: Academic Press.

Bellack, Alan S. 1979—A Critical Appraisal of Strategies of Assessing Social Skill. *Behavioral Assessment,* 1:157-176.

Bellin, S. S. *Relations among kindred in later years of life: Parents, their siblings and adult children.* Paper presented at the meeting of the American Sociological Association, St. Louis, September 1961.

Bem, S. L. Verbal self-control: The establishment of effective self-instruction. *Journal of Experimental Training,* Champaign, Ill.: Research, 1967.

Beneke, W. & Harris, M. 1972—Teaching Self-Control of Study Behavior. *Behaviour Research and Therapy* 10(1):35-41.

Beneke, W. M., & Paulsen, B. K. 1979—Long-Term Efficacy of a Behavior Modification Weight Loss Program: A Comparison of Two Follow-Up Maintenance Strategies. *Behavior Therapy* 10(1):8-13.

Bennett, R., & Eisdorfer, C. The institutional environment and behavior change. In S. Sherwood (Ed.), *Long-term care: A handbook for researchers, planners, and providers.* New York: Spectrum, 1975.

Berecz, John. 1976—Treatment of Smoking with Cognitive Conditioning Therapy: A Self-Administered Aversion Technique. *Behavior Therapy* 7(5):641-648.

Bergin, Allen E. 1980a—Psychotherapy and Religious Values. *Journal of Consulting and clinical Psychology* 48(1):95-105.

Bergin, Allen E. 1980b—Behavior Therapy and Ethical Relativism: Time for Clarity. *Journal of Consulting and Clinical Psychology* 48(1):11-13.

Berkowitz, B. P. & Graziano, A. M. 1972—Training Parents as Behavior Therapists: A Review. *Behavior Research and Therapy* 10:297-317.

Bernstein, D. A., & Borkovec, T. D. *Progressive relaxation training.* Champaign, Ill.: Research, 1973.

Bernstein, I. N., & Freeman, H. E. 1975—*Academic and Entrepreneurial Research.* New York: Russell Sage.

Best, J. Allan. 1975—Tailoring Smoking Withdrawal Procedures to Personality and Motivational Differences. *Journal of Consulting and Clinical Psychology* 43(1):1-8.

Best, J. A., Bass, F., & Owen, L. E. 1977—Mode of Service Delivery in a Smoking Cessation Program for Public Health. *Canadian Journal of Public Health* 68(6):469-473.

Best, J. A., Owen, L. E., & Trentadue, L. 1978—Comparison of Satiation and Rapid Smoking in Self-Managed Smoking Cessation. *Addictive Behaviors* 3(1):71-78.

Bielski, R. J., & Friedel, R. O. 1976—Prediction of Tricyclic Antidepressant Response: A Critical Review. *Archives of General Psychiatry* 33(12):1479-1489.

Bigelow, G., Cohen, M., Liebson, I., & Faillace, L. A. 1972—Abstinence or Moderation? Choice by Alcoholics. *Behaviour Research and Therapy* 10(3):209-214.

Blackman, D. K., Howe, M., & Pinkston, E. M. Increasing participation in social interaction of the institutionalized elderly. *Gerontologist,* 1976, 16(1), 69-76.

Blackwell, B. Treatment adherence. *British Journal of psychiatry,* 1976, *129,* 513-531.

Blake, B. George 1965—The Application of Behaviour Therapy to the Treatment of Alcoholism. *Behaviour Research and Therapy* 3(2):75-85.

Blake, B. George 1967—A Follow-Up of Alcoholics Treated by Behaviour Therapy. *Behaviour Research and Therapy* 5(2):89-94.

Blittner, M., Goldberg, J., & Merbaum, M., 1978—Cognitive Self-Control Factors in the Reduction of Smoking Behavior. *Behavior Therapy* 9(4):553-561.

Blythe, B. J., Gilchrist, L. D., & Schinke, S. P. Pregnancy-prevention groups for adolescents. *Social Work,* in press.

Blythe, B. J., Gilchrist, L. D., Shinke, S. P., & Burt G. A. 1979—An Interpersonal Decision-Making Approach to Preventing Smoking in Adolescents. Paper presented at the 107th meeting of the American Public Health Association, New York, November.

Bobo, N., Winget, C., & Gleser, G. C. 1970—Ego Defenses and Perceptual Styles. *Perceptual and Motor Skills* 30(2): 599-604.

Bolstad, O. D. & Johnson, S. M. 1972—Self-regulation in the modification of disruptive classroom behavior. *Journal of Applied Behavior Analysis* 5:443-454.

Bordin-Sandler, Suzanne 1976—If You Don't Stop Hitting Your Sister I'm Going to Beat Your Brains In. *Journal of Clinical Child Psychology,* 5(1):27-29.

Bornstein, P., Hamilton, S. B., Carmody, T. B., Rychtarik, R. G., & Veraldi, D. M. Reliability enhancement: Increasing the accuracy of self-report through mediation-based procedures. *Cognitive Therapy and Research,* 1977, *1,* 85-98.

Bowers, W. J. Normative constraints on deviant behavior in the college context. *Sociometry,* 1968, *31,* 370-385.

Bowie, N. E. 1979—Welfare and Freedom. *Ethics* 89(3):254-268.

Bowman, R. S., Stein, L. I., & Newton, J. R. 1975—Measurement and Interpretation of Drinking Behavior. *Journal of Studies on Alcohol* 36(9):1154-1172.

Boyd, J. Microcounseling for a counseling-like verbal response set: Differential effects of two micromodels and two methods of counseling supervision. *Journal of Counseling Psychology,* 1973, *20,* 97-98.

Brady, John Paul 1966—Brevital-Relaxation Treatment of Frigidity. *Behavior Research and Therapy* 4(2):71-77.

Brady, J., & Lind, D. Experimental analysis of hysterical blindness. *Archives of General Psychiatry,* 1961, *4,* 331-339.

Braukmann, C. J. & Fixsen, D. L. 1975—Behavior Modification with Delinquents. In *Progress In Behavior Modification,* M. Hersen, R. M. Eisler & P. M. Miller, (Eds.), New York: Academic Press.

Braukmann, C. J.,Wolf, M. M., Maloney, D. M., Fixsen, D. L., & Phillips, E. L. 1974—An Analysis of a Selection Interview Training Package for Predelinquents at Achievement Place. *Criminal Justice and Behavior,* 1(1):30-42.

Brayfield, A. H., & Rothe, H. F. An index of job satisfaction. *Journal of Applied Psychology,* 1951, *35,* 307-311.

Breuer, J. & Freud, S. 1957—*Studies on Hysteria.* New York: Basic Books.

Briar, Scott 1977—Social Work Practice: Contemporary Issues. In *Encyclopedia of Social Work,* Beatrice N. Saunders, ed. National Association of Social Workers Volume 1 (16th ed.). Washington, D.C.: National Association of Social Workers. (a)

Briar, S., & Miller, H. 1971—*Problems and issues in social casework.* New York: Columbia University Press.

Brockway, B. S. 1978—Chemical Validation of Self-Reported Smoking Rates. *Behavior Therapy* 9(4):685-686.

Brockway, B.S. Assertive training for professional women. *Social Work,* 1976, 21(6), 498-505.

Brockway, B. S., Kleinmann, G., Edleson, J., & Gruenewald, K. 1977—Non-Aversive Procedures and Their Effect on Cigarette Smoking. *Addictive Behaviors* 2(2/3):121-128.

Brockway, B., Werking, J., Fitzgibbons, K., & Butterfield, W. Social work in the doctors office. In *Social Work Practice.* B. Ross & S. Khinduka, (Eds.), Washington, D.C.: National Association of Social Workers, 1976.

Brodel, J., Ohlsen, M. M., Proff, F. & Southard, C. 1965—The effects of group counseling on gifted underachieving adolescents. In *Underachievement,* Milton Kornrich, (Ed.) Springfield, Ill.: Charles C. Thomas.

Broden, M., Hall, V. R. & Mitts, B. 1971—The effect of self-recording on the classroom behavior of two eighth-grade students. *Journal of Applied Behavior Analysis* 4:191-199.

Brolin, D., & Kokaska, C. Critical issues in job placement of the educable mentally retarded. *Rehabilitation Literature,* 1974, *35,* 1974-177.

Buckholdt, D. R., & Gubrium, J. F. 1980—The Underlife of Behavior Modification. *American Journal of Orthopsychiatry* 50(21):279-290.

Burchard, J. D. & Harig, P. T. 1976—Behavior Modification and Juvenile Delinquency. In *Handbook of Behavior Modification and Behavior Therapy,* H. Leitenberg, (Ed.), Englewood Cliffs, N.J.: Prentice-Hall.

Burgess, R. L. & Conger, R. D. 1977—Family Interaction Patterns Related to Child Abuse and Neglect: Some Preliminary Findings. *Child Abuse and Neglect* 1:269-277.

Butler, R.N. *Why survive?: Being old in America.* New York: Harper and Row, 1975.

Bybee, Rodger W. 1979—Toward Further Understanding and Reducing Violence Against Youth in Families. *Journal of Social Issues,* 35(2):161-173.

Byles, John A. 1978—Violence, Alcohol Problems and Other Problems in Disintegrating Families. *Journal of Studies on Alcohol* 39(3):551-553.

Campbell, Donald T. 1969—Reforms as Experiments. *American Psychologist* 24(5):409-429.

Campbell, D. T., & Stanley, J. C. *Experimental and quasi-experimental designs for research.* Chicago: Rand McNally College Publishing Co., 1963.

Canfield, S.F., Eley, J., Rollman, L.P. & Schur, E.L. 1975—A laboratory training model for the development of effective interpersonal communications in social work. *Journal of Education for Social Work* 11:45-50.

Carkuff, R. R. 1969—*Helping and Human Relations: Selection and Training, Vol. 1.* New York: Holt, Rinehart and Winston.

Carr, J. E., & Whittenbaugh, J. 1965—Perception of "Improvement" and Interjudge Reliability in Therapy Outcome Studies. *Proceedings of the 73rd Annual Convention of the American Psychological Association.* Washington, D.C.; 197-198.

Carr, Robert J. 1971—A comparison of the effects of three types of intervention with underachieving high school juniors. *Dissertation Abstracts Inter-*

national 32:1946A.

Carstens, Carl C. 1921—The Development of Social Work for Child Protection. *The Annals of the American Academy of Political and Social Science,* 98:135-142.

Castro, L., & Rachlin, H. 1980—Self-Reward, Self-Monitoring, and Self-Punishment as Feedback in Weight control. *Behavior Therapy* 11(1):38-48.

Cautela, Joseph R. 1966—Treatment of Compulsive Behavior by Covert Sensitization. *Psychological Record* 16(1):33-41.

Cautela, J. R. Behavior therapy and self-control: Techniques and implications. In C. M. Frank (Ed.,), *Behavior therapy: Appraisal and status.* London: McGraw, 1969.

Cautela, Joseph R. 1977—*Behavior Analysis Forms for Clinical Intervention.* Champaign: Research Press.

Cautela, J. R. & Upper, D. 1976—The Behavioral Inventory Battery: The Use of Self-Report Measures in Behavioral Analysis and Therapy. In *Behavioral Assessment: A Practical Handbook,* Michel Hersen and Alan S. Bellack, (Eds.), Oxford: Pergamon Press.

Chance, June R. 1965—Independence training and first graders' achievement. In *Underachievement,* Milton Kornrich, ed. Springfield, Ill.: Charles C. Thomas.

Cheek, D. K. 1977—Assertive Behavior and Black Lifestyles. In *Assertiveness: Innovations, Applications, Issues,* R.E. Alberti, (Ed.), San Luis Obispo: Impact.

Cheek, F. E., Tomarchio, T., Standen, J. & Albahary, R.S. 1973—Methadone Plus: A Behavior Modification Training Program in Self-Control for Addicts in Methadone Maintainence. *International Journal of the Addictions,* 8:969-996.

Child Welfare League of America 1975—*Standards for Foster Family Service.* New York.

Christophersen, E. R. 1977—*Little People: Guidelines for Common sense Childrearing.* Lawrence, Kansas: H & H Enterprises.

Churchill, S. R. 1965—Social Group Work: A Diagnostic Look in Child Guidance. *American Journal of Orthopsychiatry* 35:581-588.

Clark, R., Burgess, R., & Hendee, J. 1972—The Development of Anti-Litter Behavior in a Forest Campground. *Journal of Applied Behavior Analysis* 5(1):1-5.

Clarren, S. K. & Smith, D. W. 1978—The Fetal Alcohol Syndrome. *New England Journal of Medicine* 298(19):1063-1067.

Coates, T. J. & Thoresen, C. E. 1978—Treating Obesity in Children and Adolescents: A Review. *American Journal of Public Health* 68(2):143-151.

Cohen, J. P., & Cohen, P. *Applied multiple regression/correlation analysis for the behavioral sciences.* Hillsdale, New Jersey: Lawrence Erlbaum Associates, 1975.

Cohen, M., Liebson, I. A., Faillace, L. A., & Allen, R. P. 1971—Moderate Drinking by Chronic Alcoholics: A Schedule-Dependent Phenomenon.

Journal of Nervous and Mental Disease 153(6):434-444.

Combs, A., Avila, D. & Purkey, W. 1971—*Helping Relationships: Basic Concepts for the Helping Professions.* Boston: Allyn and Bacon, Inc.

Conger, J. J. 1977—*Adolescence and Youth: Psychological Development in a Changing World,* 2nd ed. New York: Harper and Row.

Conger, R. D., Burgess, R. L. & Barrett, C. 1979—Child Abuse Related to Life Change and Perceptions of Illness: Some Preliminary Findings. *The Family Coordinator,* 28(1):73-78.

Conway, John B. 1977—Behavioral Self-Control of Smoking Through Aversive Conditioning and Self-Management. *Journal of Consulting and Clinical Psychology* 45(3):348-357.

Conway, J. B. & Bucher, B. D. 1976—Transfer and Maintenance of Behavior Change in Children: A Review and Suggestions. In *Behavior Modification and Families,* E.J. Mash, L.A. Hamerlynck and L.C. Handy, (Eds.) New York: Brunner/Mazel.

Cooke, C. J. & Meyers, A. 1980—The Role of Predictor Variables in the Behavioral Treatment of Obesity. *Behavioral Assessment* 2(1):59-69.

Costin, Lela B. 1969—An analysis of the tasks in school social work. *Social Service Review* 43:274-285.

Costin, Lela B. 1972—Adaptations in the delivery of school social work practices. *Social Casework* 53:348-354.

Costin, Lela B. 1977—School social work. In National Association of Social Workers *Encyclopedia of Social Work,* New York 17:1237-1243.

Covi, L., Lipman, R., Derogatis, L. R., Smith, J. E. III, & Pattison, J. H. 1974—Drugs and Group Psychotherapy in Neurotic Depression. *American Journal of Psychiatry* 131(2):191-198.

Cowan, Emory L. 1978—Some Problems in Community Program Evaluation Research. *Journal of Consulting and Clinical Psychology* 46(4):792-805.

Cox, R. D., Gunn, W. B. & Cox, M. J. 1976—A Film Assessment and Comparison of the Social Skillfulness of Behavior Problem and Non-Problem Male Children. Paper presented at the Association for Advancement of Behavior Therapy, New York, December.

Cradock, C., Cotler, S., & Jason, L. A. 1978—Primary Prevention: Immunization of Children for Speech Anxiety. *Cognitive Therapy and Research,* 2(4):389-396.

Cumming, M. E. New thoughts on the theory of disengagement. In R. Kastenbaum (Ed.), *New thoughts on old age.* New York: Springer, 1964.

Cumming, M. E. & Henry, W. E. *Growing old: The process of disengagement.* New York: Basic Books, 1961.

Curran, J. P. 1979—Pandora's Box Reopened? The Assessment of Social Skills. *Journal of Behavioral Assessment,* 1(1):55-71.

Cuvo, Anthony J. 1973—Child Care Workers as Trainers of Mentally Retarded Children. *Child Care Quarterly* 2(1):25-37.

Cvetkovich, G. & Grote, B. 1976—Psychosocial Development and the Social Problem of Teenage Illegitimacy. Paper presented at the Conference on

Determinants of Adolescent Pregnancy and Childbearing. Elkridge, MD, May

Danaher, Brian G. 1977—Rapid Smoking and Self-Control in the Modification of Smoking Behavior. *Journal of Consulting and Clinical Psychology* 45(6):1068-1075.

Danford, S. *Designing arenas of influence over elderly behavior.* Paper presented at the Nova Behavioral Confernce, Port St. Lucie, Florida, May 1978.

Danish, S. J. & Hauer, A. L. 1973—*Helping Skills: A Basic Training Program.* New York: Human Science Press.

Davids, A. & Berenson, J. K. 1977—Integration of a Behavior Modification Program into a Traditionally Oriented Residential Treatment Center for Children. *Journal of Autism and Childhood Schizophrenia* 7(3):269-285.

Davidson, W. S. II, & Seidman, E. 1974—Studies of Behavior Modification and Juvenile Delinquency: A Review, Methodological Critique, and Social Perspective. *Psychological Bulletin* 81:998-1011.

Davison, Gerald 1968—Systematic Densitization as a Counterconditioning Process. *Journal of Abnormal Psychology* 73(2):91-99.

Davidson, G. C., & Rosen, R. C. 1972—Lobeline and Reduction of Cigarette Smoking. *Psychological Reports* 31(2):443-456.

Davoren, Elizabeth 1974—The Role of the Social Worker. In *The Battered Child,* Ray E. Helfer and C. Henry Kempe, (Eds.), London: University of Chicago Press.

Davoren, Elizabeth 1975—A Social Worker's View. *Children Today,* 4(3):2-43.

Dawley, Jr., H. H., & Dillenkoffer, R. L. 1975—Minimizing the Risks in Rapid Smoking Treatment. *Journal of Behavior Therapy and Experimental Psychiatry* 6(2):174.

Dean, Charles W. 1971—From a Superintendent's Perspective. Paper presented at the meeting of the American Psychological Association, Washington, D.C., September.

DeGiovanni, S., & Epstein, N. 1978—Unbinding Assertion and Aggression in Research and Clinical Practice. *Behavior Modification* 2:173-192.

Department of Health, Educaton, and Welfare, U.S. Public Health Service. 1972—*Health Consequences of Smoking.* Washington, D.C.: U.S. Government Printing Office.

Department of Health, Education, and Welfare, U.S. Public Health Service. 1973—*Health Consequences of Smoking.* Washington, D.C.: U.S. Government Printing Office.

Department of Health, Education, and Welfare, U.S. Public Health Service. 1977—*The Smoking Digest: Progress Report on a Nation Kicking The Habit.* Washington, D.C.: U.S. Government Printing Office.

Department of Health, Education, and Welfare, U.S. Public Health Service. 1979—*Smoking and Health: A Report of The Surgeon General.* Washington D.C.: U.S. Government Printing Office.

DeProspero, A. J., Cohen, S. H., Kennen, R. D., & Edelstein, B. M. 1975—Objective approach to visual inspection of intrasubject replication data.

Paper presented at the 83rd Annual Convention of the American Psychological Association, August 30, 1975, Chicago.

Derdeyn, Andre P. 1977—Child Abuse and Neglect: The Rights of Parents and the Needs of Their Children. *American Journal of Orthopsychiatry.* 47(3):377-387.

DeRicco, D. A., Brigham, T. A., & Garlington, W. K. 1977—Development and Evaluation of Treatment Paradigms for the Suppression of Smoking Behavior. *Journal of Applied Behavior Analysis* 10(2):173-181.

DiLoreto, Adolph O. 1971—*Comparative Psychotherapy: An Experimental Analysis.* Chicago: Aldine-Atherton.

Dimock, Edmund 1977—Youth Crisis Services: Short-Term Community-Based Residential Treatment. *Child Welfare* 56(3):187-195.

Disbrow, M. A., Doerr, H. A., & Caulfield, C. 1977—Measuring the Components of Parents' Potential for Child Abuse and Neglect. *Child Abuse and Neglect,* 1:279-296.

Doleys, D. M., Ciminero, A. R., Wallach, E. S., & Davidson, R. S. 1977—Responding by Alcoholics During Aversive Conditioning: Implications for Treatment. *Behavior Modificaton* 1(2):205-220.

Doster, J., & Brooks, S. Interviewer disclosure modeling, information revealed, and interviewee verbal behavior. *Journal of Consulting and Clinical Psychology,* 1974, *42,* 420-426.

Doubros, S. Behavior therapy with high level, institutionalized, retarded adolescents. *Exceptional Children,* 1966, *33,* 229-233.

Duehn, W. D., & Mayadas, N. S. Measuring spectatoring processes in sexual interaction, a cognitive behavioral approach. Paper presented at the 3rd International Congress of medical Sexology, Rome, Italy, 1978.

D'Zurilla, T. J., & Goldfried, M. R. 1971—Problem Solving and Behavior Modification. *Journal of Abnormal Psychology* 78(1):107-126.

Eagle, E. Prognosis and outcome of community placement of institutionalized retardates. *American Journal of Mental Deficiency,* 1967, *72,* 232-243.

Edinger, J. D., Nelson III, W. M., Davidson, K. M., & Wallace, J. 1978—Modification of Smoking Behaviors in a Correctional Institution. *Journal of Clinical Psychology* 34(4):991-998.

Edington, Eugene S. 1967—Statistical Inference from N=1 Experiments. *Journal of Psychology* 165(2):195-199.

1975—Randomization Tests for One-Subject Experiments. Symposium presented at the 83rd Annual Convention of the American Psychological Association, September, 1975, Chicago.

1980—Random assignment and statistical tests for one-subject experiments. *Behavioral Assessment* 2( ):19-28.

Edmonds, V., Withers, G., & Dibastista, B. Adjustment, conservatism, and marital conventionalization. *Journal of Marriage and the Family,* 1972, *34,* 96-103.

Eisler, R. Fredericksen, L. W. & Peterson, G. L. 1978—The Relationship of Cognitive Variables to the Expression of Assertiveness. *Behavior Therapy,*

9(3):419-427.

Eisler, R. M., Hersen, M. & Miller, P. M. 1973—Effects of Modeling on Components of Assertive Behavior. *Journal of Behavior Therapy and Experimental Psychiatry* 4:(3)1-6.

Eisler, R. M., Hersen, M., Miller, P. M., & Blanchard, E. B. 1975—Situational Determinants of Assertive Behaviors. *Journal of Consulting and Clinical Psychology,* 43-:330-340.

Eisler, R. M., Miller, P. M., Hersen, M., & Alford, H. 1974—Effects of Assertive Training on Marital Interaction., *Archives of General Psychiatry* 30(5):643-649.

Elashoff, J. D., & Thoresen, C. E. 1978—Choosing a Statistical Method for Analysis of an Intensive Experiment. In *Single Subject Research: Strategies for Evaluating Change,* T. Kratochwill, ed. New York: Academic Press.

Elder, S. T., Ruiz, Z. R., Deabler, H. L., & Dillen Koffer, R. L. 1973—Instrumental Conditioning of Distolic Blood Pressure in Essential Hypertensive Patients. *Journal of Applied Behavior Analysis* 6(3):377-382.

Ellis, Albert 1962—*Reason and Emotion in Psychotherapy.* New York: Lyle Stuart.

Elmer, Elizabeth 1979—Child Abuse and Family Stress. *Journal of Social Issues,* 35 (2)60-71.

Empey, L. T., & M. L. Erickson 1972—*The Provo Experiment.* Lexington Mass.: D. C. Health and Co.

Epstein, Laura 1977—A project in school social work. In *Task-Centered Practice,* William J. Reid and Laura Epstein, eds. New York: Columbia University Press.

Evans, R. I., Hansemn, W. B., & Mittelmark, M. B. 1977—Increasing the Validity of Self-Reports of Smoking Behavior in Children. *Journal of Applied Psychology* 62(4):521-523.

Everett, P. B. 1980—A Behavioral Approach to Transportation Systems Management. In *Behavioral Community Psychology: Progress and Prospects,* David Glenwick and Leonard Jason, eds. New York: Holt, Rinehart and Winston.

Fanshel, D. 1971—The exit of children from foster care: An interim research report. *Child Welfare* 50(2):65-81.

Fanshel, D., & Shinn, E. B. 1978—*Children in Foster Care: A Longitudinal Investigation.* New York: Columbia University Press.

Farquhar, John W. 1978—*The American Way of Life Need Not Be Hazardous to Your Health.* New York: W. W. Norton.

Farrar, C. H., Powell, B. J., & Martin, L. K. 1968—Punishment of Alcohol Consumption by Apneic Paralysis. *Behaviour Research and Therapy* 6(1):13-16.

Farrell, A. D., Mariotto, M. J., Conger, A. J., Curran, J. P., & Wallander, J. L. 1979—Self-and Judges' Ratings of Heterosexual-social Anxiety and Skill: A Generalizability Study. *Journal of Consulting and Clinical Psychology,* 47:164-175.

Fay, Shirl E. 1975—The Social Worker's Use of the Court. In *Child Abuse: Intervention and Treatment,* Nancy B. Ebeling and Deborah A. Hill, eds. Acton: Publishing Sciences Group.

Feldman, R. A. & Wodarski, J. S. 1974—Bureaucratic Constraints and Methodological Adaptations in Community-Based Research. *American Journal of Community Psychology* 2(2):211-224.

1975—*Contemporary Approaches to Group Treatment.* San Francisco: Jossey-Bass.

Feldman, R. A., Wodarski, J. S., Flax, N., & Goodman, M. 1972—Treating Delinquents in Traditional Agencies. *Social Work* 17:71-78.

1973—Delinquency Theories, Group Composition, Treatment Locus, and a Service-Research Model for "Traditional" Community Agencies. *Journal of Sociology and Social Welfare* 1:59-74.

Ferster, C. B., Nurnberger, J. I. & Levitt, E. B. 1962—The control of eating. Journal of Mathetics 1:87-109.

Filipczak, J., Archer, M., & Friedman, R. M. in press—In-School Social Skills Training with Disruptive Adolescents. *Behavior Modificaton.*

Filipczak, J., Archer, M. B., Neale, M. S., & Winett, R. A. 1979—Issues in Multivariate Assessment of a Large-Scale Behavioral Program. *Journal of Applied Behavior Analysis* 12(4):593-613.

Fischer, J. 1973—Is casework effective? A review. *Social Work* 18:5-20.

Fischer, J. 1976—*The Effectiveness of Social Casework.* Springfield, IL: C.C. Thomas.

Fischer, J. 1978—Does anything work? *Journal of Social Service Research* 1:215-243.

Fischer, J., & Grochros, H., (Eds.). *Handbook of behavior therapy with sexual problems* (Vol. I & II). New York: Pergamon Press, 1977.

Fixsen, D., Phillips, E. & Wolf, M. 1973—Achievement Place: Experiments in Self-Government with Pre-Delinquents. *Journal of Applied Behavior Analysis* 6:31-47.

Flaxman, Judith. 1979—Affect-Management and Habit Mechanisms in the Modification of Smoking Behavior. *Addictive Behaviors* 4(1):39-46.

Flowers, John V. 1972—Behavior modification of cheating in an elementary school student. A brief note. *Behavior Therapy* 3:311-312.

Flowers, John V. 1979—Behavioral Analysis of Group Therapy and a Model for Behavioral Group Therapy. In *Behavioral Group Therapy, 1979: An Annual Review.* Dennis Upper and Steven Ross, Eds. Champaign, IL: Research Press.

Fo, W. S., & O'Donnell, C. R. 1974—The Buddy System: Relationship and Contingency Conditions in a Community Intervention Program for Youth With Non-Professionals as Behavior Change Agents. *Journal of Consulting and Clinical Psychology,* 42:163-169.

Foy, D. W., Miller, P. M., Eisler, R. M., & O'Toole, D. H. 1976—Social-Skills Training to Teach Alcoholics to Refuse Drinks Effectively. *Journal of Studies on Alcohol* 37(9):1340-1345.

Frankel, A. J. & Glasser, P. H. 1974—Behavioral Approaches to Group Work *Social Work,* March: 163-175.

Franks, C. M., & Wilson, G. T. 1976—Assessment, Measurement and Methodology. In *Annual Review of Behavior Therapy, Theory and Practice:* 1976. C.M. Franks and G.T. Wilson, eds. New York: Brunner/Mazel.

Franks, C. M. & Wilson, G. T. 1978—Addictive Behaviors: Alcoholism, Obesity, and Cigarette Smoking. In *Annual Review of Behavior Therapy Theory and Practice 1978,* volume six, Cyril M. Franks and G. Terence Wilson, eds. New York: Brunner/Mazel.

Freedman, B., Rosenthal, L., Donahoe, Jr., C. P., Schulndt, D. E. & McFall, R. M. 1978—A Social-Behavioral Analysis of Skill Deficits in Delinquent and Nondelinquent Adolescent Boys. *Journal of Consulting and Clinical Psychology,* 46(6):1448-1462.

Fretz, B. R. Assessing attitudes toward sexual behaviors. *Counseling Psychologist,* 1975, *5,* 100-105.

Friedman, Alfred S. 1975—Interaction of Drug Therapy with Marital Therapy in Depressive Patients. *Archives of General Psychiatry* 32(5):619-637.

Friedrich, W. N. & Boriskin, J. A. 1976—The Role of the Child in Abuse: A Review of the Literature. *American Journal of Orthopsychiatry.* 46(4):581-590.

Fuchs, C. Z., & Rehm, L. P. 1977—A Self-Control Behavior Therapy Program for Depression. *Journal of Consulting and Clinical Psychology* 45(2):206-215.

Gale, E., & Carlsson, S. Lemon juice: Whose reinforcer is what? *Behavior Therapy,* 1977, *8,* 507-508.

Galinsky, M.J., Schopler, J. H., Safier, E. J., Gambrill, E. D. 1978—Assertion Training for Public Welfare Clients. *Social Work With Groups, 1* (4), 365-379.

Gambrill, E. D., & Richey, C. A. 1975—An Assertion Inventory for Use in Assessment and Research. *Behavior Therapy* 6: 550-561.

Gambrill, E., & Richey, C. 1976—*It's Up to You: Developing Assertive Social Skills.* Millbrae, CA: Les Femmes.

Gambrill, E. D., Thomas, E. J., & Carter, R. D. 1971—Procedure for Sociobehavioral Practice in Open Settings. *Social Work* 16(1):51-62.

Gannon, J. P. Second-term script: If President wins again, the nation may have a do-less government. *Wall Street Journal,* October 18, 1972, pp. 1; 20.

Garbarino, J., & Crouter, A. 1978—A Note on the Problem of Construct Validity in Assessing the Usefulness of Child Maltreatment Report Data. *Public Health Briefs,* 68 (6):598-600.

Geer, J. H., & Fuhr, R. Cognitive factors in sexual arousal: The role of distraction. *Journal of Consulting and Clinical Psychology,* 1977, *44,* 238-243.

Geismar, L. 1972—Thirteen evaluation studies. In *Evaluation of Social Intervention,* E.J. Mullen, J.R. Dumpson and Associations, (Eds.), San Francisco: Jossey-Bass.

Geller, E. Scott 1980—Waste Reduction and Resource Recovery: Strategies for Energy Conservaton. In *Advances in Environmental Psychology* (Vol. 3), A. Baum and J. Singer, eds. New York: Erlbaum, 1980.

Geller, E. Scott Applications of Behavioral Analysis for Litter Control. In *Behavioral Community Psychology: Progress and Prospects.* D. Glenwick and L. Jason, eds. New York: Praeger, in press.

Gelles, Richard J. 1973—Child Abuse as Psychopathology: A Sociological Critique and Reformation. *American Journal of Orthopsychiatry.* 43 (4):611-621.

Gelles, R. Abused wives: Why do they stay? *Journal of Marriage and the Family,* 1976, *38,* 659-668.

Gelles, Richard J. 1978—Violence Toward Children in the United States. *American Journal of Orthopsychiatry.* 48 (4):580-592.

Gentile, J. R., Roden, A. H., & Klein, R. D. 1972—An Analysis-of-Variance Model for the Intrasubject Replication Design. *Journal of Applied Behavior Analysis* 5(2):193-198.

Giebink, J. W., Stover, D. O. & Fahl, M. A. 1968—Teaching Adaptive Responses to Frustration to Emotionally Disturbed Boys. *Journal of Consulting and Clinical Psychology,* 32(3):366-368.

Gilchrist, L. D., Schinke, S. P., & Blythe, B. J. Primary prevention services for children and youth. *Children and Youth Services Review,* in press.

Gilchrist, L. D., Schinke, S. P., Blythe, B. J., & Renggli, A. J. Prevention and health promotion services for adolescents: Validation of a model. In J. R. Anderson (Ed.), *Social work in health care: Fission or fusion.* Seattle: University of Washington, in press.

Giovannoni, J. M., & Becerra, R. 1979—*Defining Child Abuse.* New York: Free Press/Macmillan Co.

Gittelman, Martin 1965—Behavior Rehearsal as a Technique in Child Treatment. *Journal of Child Psychology and Psychiatry,* 6:251-255.

Glaser, E., & Taylor, S. Factors influencing the success of applied research. *American Psychologist,* 1973, *28,* 140-146.

Glashagel, J. *Valuing youth.* Akron, Ohio: YMCA, 1974.

Glass, C. R., Gottman, J. M., & Shmurak, S. H. 1976—Response Acquisition and Cognitive Self-Statement Modification Approaches to Dating Skills Training. *Journal of Counseling Psychology* 23(6):520-526.

Glynn, Edward L. 1970—Classroom applications of self-determined reinforcement. *Journal of Applied Behavior Analysis* 3:123-132.

Goldfried, Marvin R. 1976—Cognitive Modification of Social Evaluative Anxiety. In Marvin R. Goldfried (Chair), *Recent Research in Cognitive Behavior Modification.* Symposium presented at the meeting of the Association for the Advancement of Behavior Therapy, New York.

Goldfried, M. R., & Davidson, G. C. 1976—*Clinical Behavior Therapy.* New York: Holt, Rinehart, and Winston.

Goldfried, M. R., Decentecio, E. T., & Weinberg, L. 1974—Systematic Rational Restructuring as a Self-Control Technique. *Behavior Therapy*

5(2):247-254.

Goldfried, M. R. & D'Zurilla, T. J. A behavioral-analytic model for assessing competence. In C. D. Spielberger (Ed.), *Current topics in clinical and community psychology* (Vol. 1). New York: Academic Press, 1969.

Goldfried, M. R., Linehan, M. M., & Smith, J. C. 1976—The Reduction of Test Anxiety Through Cognitive Restructuring. *Journal of Consulting and Clinical Psychology* 46(1):32-39.

Goldfried, M. R., & Sobocinski, D. 1975—Effect of Irrational Beliefs on Emotional Arousal. *Journal of Consulting and Clinical Psychology* 43(4):504-510.

Goldiamond, I. I. Self-control procedures in personal behavior problems. *Psychological Reports,* 1965, *17,* 851-868.

Goldman, N., & Ravid, R. Community Services: Sex Differences in Mental Illness, in M. Guttentag and S. Salasin (Eds.), *Families Abandoned: Mental Health in Today's Society.* New York: Academic Press, in press.

Goldsmith, J. B. Systematic development and evaluation of a behavioral program for training psychiatric inpatients in interpersonal skills (Doctoral dissertation, University of Wisconsin-Madison, 1973). *Dissertation Abstracts International,* 1973, *34,* 2305B. (University Microfilms No. 73-20, 246).

Goldstein, A. & Wolpe, J. 1972—Behavior Therapy in Groups. In *New Models for Group Therapy,* H.I. Kaplan and B. Sadock, (Eds.) New York: Jason Aronson.

Goldstein, A. P., Heller, K., & Sechrest, L. B. *Psychotherapy and the Psychology of Behavior Change.* New York: John Wiley, 1966.

Goldstein, J., Freud, A. & Solnit, A. 1973—*Beyond the Best Interests of the Child.* New York:Macmillan/London: Collier Macmillan.

Goodman, M. Role Changes Among the Aged. Paper presented at the National Conference on Social Welfare, May 1972, Chicago. n.d.

Gorden, R. *Interviewing: Strategy, techniques, and tactics,* (Rev. ed.). Homewood: Dorsey Press, 1975.

Gordon, W. E., & Schutz, M. A natural basis for social work specialization, *Social Work,* 1977, *22,* 422-426.

Gorsuch, R. L., & Butler, M. Initial drug abuse: A review of predisposing social psychological factors. *Psychological Bulletin,* 1976, *84,* 120-127.

Gorsuch, R. L., Henighan, R. P., & Barnard, C. Locus of control: An example of dangers in using children's scales with children. *Child Development,* 1972, *43,* 579-590.

Gottesman, L. Organizing rehabilitation services for the elderly. *Gerontologist,* 1970, *10,* 287-293.

Gottesman, L. & Brody, E. Psycho-social intervention programs within the institutional setting. In S. Sherwood (Ed.), *Long-term care: A handbook for researchers, planners, and providers.* New York: Spectrum, 1975.

Gottlieb, P. Changing mortality in bronchial asthma. *Journal of The American Medical Association,* 1964, *187,* 276-280.

Gottsman, J., Notarius, C., Gonso, J., & Markman, H. *A Couple's Guide to Communication.* Champaign, Ill. Research Press, 1976.

Graber-Kline, G., & Graber, B. *Woman's orgasm: A guide to sexual satisfaction.* New York: Popular, 1975.

Graziano, A. M., ed. 1975—*Behavior Therapy with Children.* Chicago: Aldine.

Green, R. K., & Cox, G. 1978—Social Work and Malpractice: A Converging Course. *Social Work.* 23 (2):399-352.

Greene, B. L. *A Clinical Approach to Marital Problems: Evaluation and Management.* Springfield, Ill. Charles C. Thomas, 1970.

Greenwood, C. R., Sloane, Jr., H. N., & Baskin, A. 1974—Training elementary aged peer behavior managers to control small group programmed mathematics. *Journal of Applied Behavior Analysis* 7:103-114.

Greenwood, Sadja Goldsmith. 1979—Warning: Cigarette Smoking is Dangerous to Reproductive Health. *Family Planning Perspectives* 11(3):168-172.

Grinnell, R., & Kyte, N. Delivering concrete environmental services in a public welfare agency *Journal of Social Welfare,* 1975, *2,* 69-82.

Grodner, B. S. 1977—Assertiveness and Anxiety: A Cross-Cultural and Socio-Economic Perspective. In *Assertiveness: Innovations, Applications, Issues,* R.E. Alberti, ed. San Luis Obispo: Impact.

Gruber, Alan R. 1978—*Children in Foster Care: Destitute, Neglected...Betrayed.* New York: Human Sciences Press.

Gubrium, J. F. *Living and dying at Murray Manor.* New York: St. Martin's Press, 1975.

Guerney, Jr., Bernard, 1977—The Great Potential of an Educational Skills Training Model in Problem Prevention. Paper presented at the annual meeting of the American Psychological Association, San Francisco.

Gurman, A. S. The effects and effectiveness of marital therapy: a review of outcome research. *Family Process,* 1973, *12,* 145-170.

Gutride, M., Goldstein, A., & Hunter, G. The use of modeling and role playing to increase social interaction among social psychiatric patients. *Journal of Consulting and Clinical Psychology,* 1973, *40,* 408-415.

Haase, R., & DiMattia, D. The application of the microcounseling paradigm to the training of support personnel in counseling. *Counselor Education and Supervision,* 1970, *10,* 16-22.

Haley, J. Marriage therapy. *Archives of General Psychiatry.* 1963, *8,* 213-234.

Hall, J. S., & Holmberg, M. C. 1974—The Effect of Teacher Behaviors and Food Serving Arrangements on Young Children's Eating in a Day Care Center. *Child Care Quarterly* 3(2):97-108.

Hall, R. G., Sachs, D. P. L., & Hall, S. M. 1979—Medical Risk and Therapeutic Effectiveness of Rapid Smoking. *Behavior Therapy* 10(2):249-259.

Hall, R. V., Christler, C., Cranston, S. S., & Tucker, B. 1970—Teachers and Parents as Researchers Using Multiple Baseline Designs. *Journal of Applied Behavior Analysis* 3:247-255.

Hart, B. M., Allen, K. E., Buell, J. S., Harris, F. R., & Wolf, M. M. 1964—Effects of Social Reinforcement on Operant Crying. *Journal of*

Experimental Child Psychology 1(2):145-153.

Hart, B., Reynolds, N., Baer, D., Brawley, E., & Harris, F. 1968—Effect of Contingent and Noncontingent Social Reinforcement on the Cooperative Play of a Preschool Child. *Journal of Applied Behavior Analysis* 1(1):73-76.

Hartman, W. E., & Fithian, M. A. *Treatment of sexual dysfunction: A bio-psycho-social approach.* New York: Jason Aronson, 1974.

Hartmann, D. P., & Gelfand, D. M. *Child Behavior Analysis and Therapy.* New York: Pergamon Press, 1975.

Hauser, Robert. 1974—Rapid Smoking as a Technique of Behavior Modification: Caution in Selection of Subjects. *Journal of Consulting and Clinical Psychology* 42(4):625-626.

Havighurst, R. J., Neugarten, B. L. & Tobin, S. S. Disengagement and patterns of aging. In B.L. Neugarten (Ed.), *Middleage age and aging.* University of Chicago Press, 1968.

Hawkins, R. P., Peterson, R. F. Schweid, E., & Bijou, S. W. 1966—Behavior Therapy in the Home: Amelioration of Problem Parent-Child Relations with the Parent in a Therapeutic Role. *Journal of Experimental Child Psychology* 4:99-107.

Hay, W. M., Hay, L. R., & Nelson, R. O. 1977—The Adaptation of Covert Modeling Procedures to the Treatment of Chronic Alcoholism and Obsessive-Compulsive Behavior: Two Case Reports. *Behavior Therapy* 8(1):70-76.

Haynes, R. B., & Sackett, D. L. An annotated bibliography. In *Compliance With Therapeutic Regimens.* D. Sackett & R. Haynes, (Eds.), Baltimore: John Hopkins University Press, 1976.

Hays, William 1973—*Statistics for the Social Sciences* (2nd ed.). New York, Holt, Rinehart and Winston.

Heaton, R. C., D. J. Safer, R. P. Allen, N. C. Spinnato, and F. M. Prumo 1976—A Motivational Environment for Behaviorally Defiant Junior High School Students. *Journal of Abnormal Child Psychology* 4:263-275.

Hedberg, A. G. & Campbell III, L. 1974—A Comparison of Four Behavioral Treatments of Alcoholism. *Journal of Behavior Therapy and Experimental Psychiatry* 5(3/4):251-256.

Hedges, Janice N. 1976—Youth unemployment in the 1974-1975 recession. *Monthly Labor Review* 99:49-56.

Heiman, J., LoPiccolo, L., & LoPiccolo, J. *Becoming orgasmic: A sexual growth program for women.* Englewood Cliffs, N.J.: Prentice-Hall, 1976.

Heitler, James B. 1975—Preparatory Techniques in Initiating Expressive Psychotherapy with Lower Class, Unsophisticated Patients. *Psychological bulletin.* 83 (2):339-352.

Hermann, J. A., deMontes A. I., Dominguez, B., Montes, F. & Hopkins, B. L. 1973—Effects of Bonuses for Punctuality on the Tardiness of Industrial Workers. *Journal of Applied Behavior Analysis* 6(4):563-570.

Hersen, Michel Single-Case Experimental Designs. In *International Handbook of Behavior Modification and Therapy: Vol. I,* A. S. Bellack, M. Hersen, and

A. E. Kazdin, (Eds.), New York: Plenum Press, in press.

Hersen, M. & Barlow, D. H. 1976—*Single-Case Experimental Designs: Strategies for Studying Behavior Change.* New York: Pergamon Press.

Hersen, M. & Bellack, A. S. 1977—Staff Training and Consultation. In *Behavior Therapy in the Psychiatric Setting,* Michel Hersen and Alan S. Bellack, (Eds.), Baltimore: Williams and Wilkins.

Hersen, M., Eisler, R. M. Alford, G. S., & Agras, W. S. 1973—Effects of Token Economy on Neurotic Depression: An Experimental Analysis. *Behavior Therapy* 4(3):392-397.

Hersen, M., Eisler, R. M., & Miller, P. M. Development of assertive responses: Clinical, measurement and research considerations. *Behaviour Research and Therapy,* 1973, *11,* 505-521.

Higginbotham, H. N., & Farkas, G. M. Basic and applied research in human sexuality: Current limitations and future directions in sex therapy. In J. Fischer & H. L. Gochros (Eds.), *Handbook of behavior therapy with sexual problems* (Vol. 1). New York: Pergamon Press, 1977.

Hilgard, E., & Marquis, D. *Conditioning and Learning.* New York: Appleton Century, 1940.

Hilts, Phillip J. 1974—*Behavior Modification.* New York: Harper's Magazine Press.

Hoffman, M. L., & Saltzstein, H. D. Parent discipline and the child's moral development, *Journal of Personality and Social Psychology,* 1967, *6,* 45-57.

Hollis, Florence 1968—...and What Shall We Teach? The Social Work Educator
and Knowledge. *Social Service Review* 42(2):184-196.

Horning, E. C., Horning, M. G., Carroll, D. I., Stillwell, R. N., & Dzidic, I. 1973—Nicotine in Smokers, Non-Smokers, and Room Air. *Life Sciences* 13(10): 1331-1346.

Howe, Michael W. 1974—Casework self-evaluation: A single-subject approach. *Social Service Review* 48:1-23.

Hoyer, W. J. Application of operant techniques to the modifications of elderly behavior. *Gerontologist,* 1973, *13*(1), 18-22.

Hoyer, W. J., Kafer, R. A., Simpson, S. C., & Hoyer, F. W. Reinstatement of verbal behavior in elderly mental patients using operant procedures. *Gerontologist,* 1974, *14* (2), 149-152.

Hoyer, W. J., Mishara, B. L., & Reibel, R. G. Problem behaviors as operants. *Gerontologist,* 1975, *15*(5), 452-456.

Huber, H., Karlin, R., & Nathan, P. E. 1976—Blood Alcohol Level Discrimination by Nonalcoholics: The Role of Internal and External Cues. *Journal of Studies on Alcohol* 37(1):27-39.

Hudson, Walter W. 1977—*A Measurement Package for Clinical Workers.* Unpublished manuscript, University of Hawaii.

Hughes, J. R., Frederiksen, L. W., & Frazier, M. 1978—A Carbon Monoxide Analyzer for Measurement of Smoking behavior. *Behavior Therapy* 9(2):293-296.

Hull, Andrew P. 1979—Increased Life Expectancy Offsets Energy Gains from Dieters. *American Journal of Public Health* 69(5):514-515.

Hummel, P. 1966—*An Evaluation of a Model for Guidance Counseling with Bright Academic Underachievers.* Cooperative research project #5-0633, U.S. Dept. of H.E.W.

Hunt, W. A., Barnett, L. W., & Branch, L. G. 1971—Relapse Rates in Addiction Programs. *Journal of Clinical Psychology* 27(4):455-456.

Hwang, P. O. 1977—Assertion Training for Asian-Americans. In *Assertiveness: Innovations Applications, Issues,* R.E. Alberti, (Ed.), San Luis Obispo: Impact.

Hynd, G. W., Stratton, T. T., & Severson, H. H. 1978— Smoking Treatment Strategies, Expectancy Outcomes, and Credibility in Attention-Placebo Control Conditions. *Journal of Clinical Psychology* 34(1):182-186.

Israel, A. C. & Saccone, A. J. 1979—Follow-Up of Effects of Choice of Mediator and Target of Reinforcement on Weight Loss. *Behavior Therapy* 10(2):260-265.

Ivey, A. E. 1971—Microcounseling: *Innovations in Interviewing Training.* Springfield, Ill.: Charles C. Thomas.

Ivey, A. Media therapy: Educational change planning for psychiatric patients. *Journal of Counseling Psychology,* 1973, *20,* 338-343.

Ivey, A. Microcounseling and media therapy: State of the art. *Counselor Education and Supervision,* 1974, *13,* 172-183.

Ivey, A. E. & Authier, J. 1978—*Microcounseling,* Springfield, Ill.: Charles C. Thomas.

Jacklin, C. N., & Mischel, H. N. 1973—As the Twig is Bent—Sex Role Stereotyping in Early Readers. *School Psychology Digest* 2:30-37.

Jacobs, L., Berscheid, E., & Walster, E. 1971—Self-esteem and Attraction. *Journal of Personality and Social Psychology* 17(1):84-91.

Jacobson, Edmund 1974—*Progressive Relaxation* (Third Edition). Chicago: University of Chicago Press.

Jacobson, Edmund. 1978—*You Must Relax* (fifth rev. edition). New York: McGraw-Hill Book Company.

Jason, Leonard A. 1977—Behavioral Community Psychology: Conceptualizations and Applications. *Journal of Community Psychology* 5(4):302-312.

Jason, Leonard A. 1978—Implementing Preventive and Environmental Community Interventions. *Evaluation and The Health Professions* 1(3):85-93.

Jason, L. A., McCoy, K., Blanco, D., & Zolik, E. S. Decreasing dog litter. *Evaluation Review* 1980, *4,* 355-369.

Jayaratne, Srinika 1977—Child Abusers as Parents and Children: A Review. *Social Work,* 22(1):5-9.

Jayaratne, Srinika 1978—Analytic Procedures for Single-subject Designs. *Social Work Research and Abstracts* 14(3):30-40.

Jayaratne, S., & Levy, R. L. 1979—*Empirical Clinical Practice.* New York: Columbia University Press.

Jeffrey, D. B. Self-control: Methodological issues and research trends. In M. J. Mahoney & C. E. Thorensen (Eds.), *Self-control: Power to the person.* Monterey, California: Brooks/Cole, 1974.

Jeffrey, D. Balfour. 1976—Behavioral Management of Obesity. In *Behavior Modification: Principles, Issues, and Applications,* W. Edward Craighead, Alan E. Kazdin, and Michael J. Mahoney, (Eds.), Boston: Houghton Mifflin.

Jeffrey, D. B., & Christensen, E. R. 1972—The Relative Efficacy of Behavior Therapy, Will Power, and No-Treatment Control Procedures on the Modification of Obesity. Paper presented at the Association for Advancement of Behavior Therapy Annual Meeting, October 1972, New York.

Jenkins, S., & Sauber, M. 1966—*Paths to Child Placement.* New York: Community Council of New York.

Jensen, Richard E. 1976—A Behavior Modification Program to Remediate Child Abuse. *Journal of Clinical Psychology,* 5 (1):30-32.

Jesness, C. F. 1969—*The Jesness Inventory Manual.* Palo Alto, California: Consulting Psychologist Press.

Jesness, Carl F. 1976—The Youth Center Project: Transactional Analysis and Behavior Modification Programs for Delinquents. *Behavioral Disorders* 1(1):27-36.

Jessor, R., Graves., T. D., Hanse, R. C., & Jessor, S. L. *Society, personality and deviant behavior: A study of a tri-ethnic community.* New York: Holt, Rinehart & Winston, 1968.

Jeter, Helen R. 1963—*Children, Problems and Services in Child Welfare Programs.* Washington: Children's Bureau Publication.

Johnson, C. A. & Katz, G. 1973—Using Parents as Change Agents for Their Children: A Review. *Journal of Child Psychology and Psychiatry* 14:181-200.

Johnson, R., & Meyer, R. Phased bio-feedback approach for epileptic seizure control *Journal of Behavior Therapy and Experimentl Psychiatry,* 1974, *5,* 185-187.

Johnson, R. P. & Geller, E. S. 1980—Community Mental Health Center Programs. In *Behavioral Community Psychology: Progress and Prospects,* David Glenwick and Leonard Jason, (Eds.), New York: Holt, Rinehart and Winston.

Johnson, S. M. & Geoffrey, W. 1971—Self-observation as an agent of behavioral change. *Behavior Therapy* 2:488-497.

Johnson, W. G. & Stalonas, P. 1977—Measuring Skinfold Thickness—A Cautionary Note. *Addictive Behaviors* 2(2/3):105-107.

Jones, Mary Cover 1924—The Elimination of Children's Fears. *Journal of Experimental Psychology* 7(5):382-390.

Jordan, H. A., Levitz, L. S. & Kimbrell, G. M. *Eating is okay!* New York: Rawson Associates Publishers, 1976.

Kadushin, A. 1972—*The Social Work Interview.* New York: Columbia University Press.

Kanfer, Frederick H. 1970—Self-Regulation: Research, Issues and Specuia-tions. In *Behavior Modification in Clinical Psychology,* C. Neuringer and J.L. Michaels, eds. New York: Appleton-Century-Crofts.

Kanfer, F. H., & Karoly, P. Self-control: A behavioristic excursion into the lion's den. In M. J. Mahoney & C. E. Thoresen (Eds.), *Self-control: Power to the person.* Monterey, California: Brooks/Cole, 1974.

Kanter, N. J., & Goldfried, M. R. 1976—*Relative Effectiveness of Rational Restructuring and Self-control Desensitization in the Reduction of Interpersonal Anxiety.* Unpublished manuscript.

Kaplan, H. S. *The new sex therapy.* New York: Brunner/Mazel, 1974.

Karnes, M. B., McCoy, G. F., Zehrbach, R. E., Wollersheim, J. P., & Clarizio, H. F. 1965—The efficiency of two organization plans for underachieving intellectually gifted children. In *Underachievement,* Milton Kornrich, ed. Springfield, Ill.: Charles C. Thomas.

Kastenbaum, R., & Candy, S. E. The four per cent fallacy: A methodological and empirical critique of extended care facility population statistics. *International Journal of Aging and Human Develoment,* 1973, *4*(1), 15-22.

Katell, A., Callahan, E. J., Fremouw, W. J., & Zitter, R. E. 1979—The Effects of Behavioral Treatment and Fasting on Eating Behaviors and Weight Loss: A Case Study. *Behavior Therapy* 10(4):579-587.

Katz, R., & Zlutnick, S. eds. *Behavior Therapy and Health Care.* Pergamon General Psychology Series. New York: Pergamon Press, 1975.

Katz, R. C., Heiman, M., & Gordon, S. 1977—Effects of Two Self-Management Approaches on Cigarette Smoking. *Addictive Behaviors* 2(2/3):113-119.

Kaufmann, L. M. & Wagner, B. R. 1972—Barb: A Systematic Treatment Technology for Temper Control Disorders. *Behavior Therapy,* 3:84-90.

Kazdin, Alan E. 1974(a)—Covert Modeling, Model Similarity, and Reduction of Avoidance Behavior. *Behavior Therapy* 5(3):325-340.

Kazdin, Alan E. 1974(b)—The Effect of Model Identity and Fear-Relevant Similarity on Covert Modeling. *Behavior Therapy* 5(5):624-635.

1974(c)—Reactive Self-monitoring: The Effects of Response Desirability, Goal Setting and Feedback. *Journal of Consulting and Clinical Psychology* 42(5):704-716.

Kazdin, A. E. Self-monitoring and behavior change. In M. J. Mahoney & C. E. Thoresen (Eds.), *Self-control: Power to the Person.* Monterey, California: Brooks/Cole, 1974. (d)

Kazdin, A. E. 1976—Statistical Analyses for Single-case Experimental Designs. In *Single Case. Experimental Design: Strategies for Studying Change,* M. Hersen and D. H. Barlow. New York: Pergamon Press.

Kazdin, A. E. 1977(a)—Assessing the Clinical or Applied Importance of Behavior Change Through Social Validation. *Behavior Modification* 1(4):427-452.

Kazdin, A. E. 1977(b)—*The Token Economy: A Review and Evaluation.* New York: Plenum Press.

Kazdin, A. E. 1978(a)—Evaluating the Generality of Findings in Analogue Therapy Research. *Journal of Consulting and Clinical Psychology* 46(4) :673-286.

Kazdin, A. E. 1978(b)—Methodological and Interpretive Problems of Single-Case Experimental Designs. *Journal of Consulting and Clinical Psychology,* 46
(4):629-642.

Kazdin, A. E. 1980—*Research design in clinical psychology.* New York Harper Row.

Kazdin, A. E. & Polster, R. A. 1973—Intermittent token reinforcement and response maintenance in extinction. *Behavior Therapy* 4:386-391.

Keil, E. C. & Barbee, J. R. 1973—Behavior Modification and Training the Disadvantaged Job Interviewee. *Vocational Guidance Quarterly,* 22 (September):50-56.

Keller, M. & P. Carlson 1974—The Use of Symbolic Modeling to Promote Social Skills in Preschool Children with Low Levels of Social Responsiveness. *Child Development,* 45:912-919.

Kempe, C. H., Silverman, F. N., Steele, B., Dregmuller, W., & Silver, H. 1962—The Battered Child Syndrome, *Journal of the American Medical Association,* 181 (1):17-24.

Kennedy, W. A., & Foreyt, J. P. 1968—Control of Eating Behavior in an Obese Patient by Avoidance Conditioning. *Psychological Reports* 22(2):571-576.

Kerlinger, F. N. 1979—*Behavioral research: A conceptual approach.* New York: Holt, Rinehart, & Winston.

Keutzer, C. S., Lichtenstein, E., & Mees, H. L. 1968—Modification of smoking behavior: A review. *Psychological Bulletin* 70: 520-533.

Kifer, R. E., Lewis, M. A., Green, D. R., & Phillips, E. L. 1974—Training Predelinquent Youths and Their Parents to Negotiate Conflict Situations. *Journal of Applied Behavior Analysis,* 7:357-364.

Kinney, Jill 1978—Homebuilders: An In-Home Crisis Intervention Program. *Children Today,* 7(1):15-35.

Kipnis, D. & Resnick, J. H. 1971—Experimental prevention of underachievement among intelligent, impulsive college students. *Journal of Consulting and Clinical Psychology* 36:53-60.

Kirchner, R. E., Schnelle, J. F. Domash, M., Larson, L., Carr, A., & McNees, M. P. 1980—The Applicability of a Helicopter Patrol Procedure to Diverse Areas: A Cost-Benefit Evaluation. *Journal of Applied Behavior Analysis* 13(1):143-148.

Klein, J. P., Quarter, J. J., & Laxer, R. M. 1969—Behavioral counseling of underachievers. *American Educational Research Journal* 6:415-424.

Klein, R. D., & Schuler, C. F. 1974—Increasing Academic Performance Through Contingent Use of Self-Evaluation. Paper presented at the annual meeting of the American Educational Research Association, Chicago, April 1974.

Klein, W. 1963—*An Investigation of the Spontaneous Speech of Children.*

Unpublished doctoral dissertation, University of Rochester.

Klerman, G. L., Dimascio, A., Weissman, M., Prusoff, B., & Paykel, E. S. 1974—Treatment of Depression by Drugs and Psychotherapy. *American Journal of Psychiatry* 131(2):186-191.

Klerman, G., & Weissman, M. Depression Among Women: Their Nature and Causes, in M. Guttentag and S. Salasin (Eds.), *Families Abandoned: Mental Health in Today's Society.* New York: Academic Press, in press.

Knapp, T., & Wells, L. Behavior therapy for asthma: A review. *Behavior Research and Therapy,* 1978, *16,* 103-115.

Knapczyk, D. R. & Livingston, G. 1973—Self-recording and student teacher supervision: Variables within a token economy structure. *Journal of Applied Behavior Analysis* 6:481-486.

Knowles, John H. ed. 1977—The responsibiity of the individual. In *Doing Better and Feeling Worse: Health in the United States.* John H. Knowles, (Ed.), New York: W. W. Norton.

Knowles, John H. ed. 1977—*Doing Better and Feeling Worse: Health in the United States.* New York: W. W. Norton.

Kratochwill, Thomas R. 1978—Foundations of Time-Series Research. In *Single Subject Research: Strategies for Evaluating Change,* T. Kratochwill, ed. New York: Academic Press.

Kratochwill, T. R., & Brody, G. H. 1978—Single Subject Designs: A Perspective on the Controversy over Employing Statistical Inference and Implications for Reserach and Training in Behavior Modification. *Behavior Modification* 2(3):291-307.

Lamontagne, Y., Gagnon, M. A., Trudel, G., & Boisvert, J. M. 1978—Thought-Stopping as a Treatment for Reducing Cigarette Smoking. *International Journal of the Addictions* 13(2):297-305.

Landau, P., & Paulson, T. 1977—Group Assertion Training for Spanish Speaking Mexican-American Mothers. In *Assertiveness: Innovations, Applications, Issues,,* R.E. Alberti, (Ed.), San Luis Obispo: Impact.

Lando, H. A. 1977—Successful Treatment of Smokers with a Broad-Spectrum Behavioral Approach. *Journal of Consulting and Clinical Psychology* 45(3):361-366.

Lang, P. J., & Melamed, B. C. Case report; avoidance conditioning therapy of an infant with chronic rumination vomiting. *Journal of Abnormal Psychology,* 1969, *74,* 1-8.

Lange, A., & P. Jakubowski. 1976—*Responsible Assertive Behavior.* Champaign Ill.: Research Press.

Larkin, Edward J. 1979—Controlled Drinking—Disease Concept Controversy: Suggestions for Synthesis. *Psychological Reports* 44(2):511-516.

Larsen, J. & Hepworth, D.H. 1978—Skill development through competency-based education. *Journal of Education for Social Work* 14:73-81.

Lazarus, Arnold A. 1968—Behavior Therapy in Groups. In *Basic Approaches to Group Psychotherapy and Group Counseling,* G.M. Gazda, (Ed.) Springfield, Ill.: Charles C. Thomas.

Lebow, Michael D. 1977—Can Lighter Become Thinner? *Addictive Behaviors* 2(1):87-93.

Lebowitz, M. D., & Burrows, B. 1976—Respiratory Symptoms Related to Smoking Habits of Family Adults. *Chest* 69(1):48-50.

Le Shan, E., & Le Shan, L. 1968—A Home is not a Lab. *New York Times Magazine,* April 7,

Levin, J. R., Marascuilo, L. A., & Hubert, L. J. 1978—N = Nonparametic Randomization Tests. In *Single Subject Research: Strategies for Evaluating Change.* T. Kratochwill, (Ed.), New York: Academic Press.

Lewinsohn, Peter M. 1975—Engagement in Pleasant Activities and Depression Level. *Journal of Abnormal Psychology* 84(6):729-931.

Libb, J. W., House, C., & Green, M. 1973—Charting and Contingency Management Procedures in a Children's Home. *Child Care Quarterly* 2(3):113-123.

Lichtenstein, Edward. 1977—Social Learning. In *Research on Smoking Behavior* (NIDA Research Monograph 17), Murray E. Jarvik, Joseph W. Cullen, Ellen R. Gritz, Thomas M. Vogt, and Louis Jolyon West, (Eds.), Washington, D.C.: U.S. Government Printing Office.

Lichtenstein, E., Harris, D. E., Birchler, G. R., Wahl, J. M., & Schmahl, D. P. 1973—Comparison of Rapid Smoking, Warm, Smoky Air, and Attention Placebo in the Modification of Smoking Behavior. *Journal of Consulting and Clinical Psychology* 40(1):92-98.

Licona, T. (Ed.) *Moral development and behavior.* New York: Holt, Rinehart & Winston, 1976.

Lindner, R., & Gurvitz, M. Restandardization of the revised beta examination to yield the wechsler type of IQ. *Journal of Applied Psychology,* 1946, *30,* 649-658.

Lindsley, O. R. Geriatric behavioral prosthetics. In R. Kastenbaum (Ed.), *New thoughts in old age.* New York: Springer, 1964.

Linehan, Marsha M. 1977—Issues in Behavioral Interviewing. *Behavioral Assessment: New Directions in Clinical Psychology,* J.E. Cone and R.P. Hawkins, (Eds.), New York: Brunner/Mazel.

Linsk, N., Howe, M. W., & Pinkston, E. M. Behavioral group work in a home for the aged. *Social Work,* 1975, *20*(60), 454-463.

Lipinski, D. P., Black, J. L., Nelson, R. O., & Ciminero, A. R. Influence of motivational variables on the reactivity and reliability of self-recording. *Journal of Consulting and Clinical Psychology,* 1975, *43,* 637-646.

Lipinski, D. P., & Nelson, R. 1974—The Reactivity and Unreliability of Self-recording. *Journal of Consulting and Clinical Psychology* 42(1):118-123.

Lobitz, W. C., & LoPiccolo, J. New methods in the behavioral treatment of sexual dysfunction. *Journal of Behavior Therapy and Experimental Psychiatry,* 1972, *3,* 265-271.

Locke, H. J., & Wallace, K. M. Short marital adjustment and prediction tests: Their reliability and validity. *Marriage and Family Living.* 1959, *21,* 251-255.

London, Perry 1964—The Modes and Morals of Psychotherapy. New York:

Holt, Rinehart and Winston.

LoPiccolo, J., & LoPiccolo, L., (Eds.). *Handbook of sex therapy.* New York: Plenum, 1978.

LoPiccolo, J., & Steger, J. C. The sexual interaction inventory: A new instrument for assessment of sexual dysfunction. *Archives of Sexual Behavior,* 1974, *3,* 585-595.

Lovaas, I., Schaeffer, B., & Simmons, J. Building social behavior in autistic children by use of electric shock. *Journal of Experimental Research in Personality,* 1965, *1,* 99-109.

Lovibond, S. H. 1977—Behavioral Control of Excessive Drinking. In *Progress in Behavior Modification,* volume five, Michel Hersen, Richard M. Eisler, and Peter M. Miller, (Eds.), New York: Academic Press.

Lovibond, S. H. & Caddy, G. 1970—Discriminated Aversive Control in the Moderation of Alcoholics' Drinking Behavior. *Behavior Therapy* 1(4):437-444.

Lovitt, T. C. & Curtiss, K. A. 1969—Academic response rate as a function of teacher- and self-imposed contingencies. *Journal of Applied Behavior Analysis* 2:49-53.

Lowe, Terry O. 1973—The utilization of verbal reinforcement by cadet teachers in the treatment of underachieving fourth-grade boys. Dissertation Abstracts International 33:6093A-6094A.

Lubar, J., & Bahler, W. Behavioral management of epileptic seizures following EEG biofeedback training of the sensorimotor rhythm. *Biofeedback and Self Regulation,* 1976, *1,* 77-104.

Lundman, R. J., McFarlane, P. T. & Scarpitti, F. R. 1976—Delinquency-Prevention-Assessment of Reported Project. *Crime and Delinquency* 22(3):297-308.

Maas, H. S. 1969—Children in long-term foster care. *Child Welfare* 48(6):321-333.

Maas, H. & Engler, R. 1959—*Children in Need of Parents.* New York: Columbia University Press.

Maccoby, E. M., & Jacklin, C. N. 1974—*The Psychology of Sex Differences.* Stanford, Calif.: Stanford University Press.

MacDonald, M. 1974—A Behavioral Assessment Methodology as Applied to the Measurement of Assertion. Unpublished doctoral dissertation, University of Illinois, Urbana.

Madsen, C., Madsen, C., & Thompson, F. 1974—Increasing Rural Head Start Children's Consumption of Middle-Class Meals. *Journal of Applied Behavior Analysis* 7(2):257-262.

Mager, R. F. 1975—*Preparing Instructional Objectives* (second edition). Belmont, California: Fearon.

Mahoney, M. J. Research issues in self-management. *Behavior Therapy,* 1972, *3,* 45-63.

Mahoney, Michael J. 1974—*Cognition and Behavior Modification.* Cambridge, Mass.: Ballinger.

Mahoney, Michael J. 1977—Cognitive Therapy and Research: A Question of Questions. Cognitive Therapy and Research 1(1):5-16 (b).

Mahoney, M., & Arnkoff, D. B. 1978—Cognitive and Self-Control Therapies. In *Handbook of Psychotherapy and Behavior Change,* 2nd edition, Sol L. Garfield and Allen E. Bergin, Eds. New York: John Wiley and Sons.

Mahoney, M. J., & Thoresen, C. E., (Eds.). *Self-control: Power to the person.* Monterey, California: Brooks/Cole, 1974.

Malmo, R., Davis, J., & Barza, S. Total hysterical deafness: An experimental case study. *Journal of Personality,* 1952, *21,* 188-204.

Maloney, K. B., Braukmann, C. J., Maloney, D. M., Braukmann, P., Ayala, H., Fixsen, D., Phillips, E., & Wolf, M. M. 1975—The Identification, Measurement, and Modification of Adolescent Social Interaction Skills. Paper presented at the annual meeting of the American Psychological Society, Chicago.

Marlatt, G. Alan. 1975—The Drinking Profile: A Questionnaire for the Behavioral Assessment of Alcoholism. In *Behavior Therapy Assessment: Diagnosis and Evaluation,* E. J. Mash and L. G. Terdal, (Eds.), New York: Springer.

Marlatt, G. Alan. 1978—Behavioral Assessment of Social Drinking and Alcoholism. In *Behavioral Approaches to Alcoholism,* G. Alan Marlatt and Peter E. Nathan, (Eds.), New Brunswick, NJ: Rutgers Center of Alcohol Studies.

Marlatt, G. A. & Donovan, D. M. Alcoholism and drug dependence: Cognitive social learning factors in addictive behaviors. In W. E. Craighead, A. E. Kazdin, and M. J. Mahoney (Eds.), *Behavior modification: Principles, issues, and applications* (2nd ed.). Boston: Houghton Mifflin, in press

Marlatt, G. A., & Gordon, J. R. 1979—Determinants of Relapse: Implications for the Maintenance of Behavior Change. In *Behavioral Medicine: Changing Health Lifestyles,* P. Davidson, (Ed.), New York: Brunner/Mazel.

Marston, A. Personality variables related to self-reinforcement. *Journal of Psychology,* 1964, *58,* 169-175.

Martin, P. A. *A Marital Therapy Manual.* New York: Brunner/Mazel, 1976.

Martinson, W. D. & Zerface, J. P. 1970—Comparison of individual counseling and a social program with nondaters. *Journal of Counseling Psychology* 17:36-40.

Masters, S., Garfinkel, I., & Bishop, J. 1978—Benefit-cost analysis in program evaluation. *Journal of Social Service Research,* 2(1):79-93.

Masters, W. H., & Johnson, V. E. *Human sexual response.* Boston: Little, Brown, 1966.

Masters, W. H., & Johnson, V. E. *Human sexual inadequacy.* Boston: Little, Brown, 1970.

Masters, W. H., Johnson, V. E., & Kolodny, R. C. *Ethical issues in sex therapy and research.* Boston: Little, Brown, 1977.

Mastria, E. O., Mastria, M. A., & Harkins, J. C. 1979—Treatment of Child Abuse by Behavioral Intervention: A Case Report. *Child Welfare,* 58 (4):253-

261.

Mayer, Jean. 1968—*Overweight: Causes, Cost, and Control.* Englewood Cliffs, NJ: Prentice-Hall.

McAlister, Alfred L. 1979—Tobacco, Alcohol, and Drug Abuse: Onset and Prevention. In *Healthy People: The Surgeon General's Report on Health Promotion and Disease Prevention—Background Papers,* DHEW (PHS) Publication No. 79-55071A. Washington, D.C.: U.S. Government Printing Office.

McAlister, A. L., Perry, C., & Maccoby, N. 1979—Adolescent Smoking: Onset and Prevention. *Pediatrics,* 63(4):650-658.

McCarthy, B. W. Strategies and techniques for the reduction of sexual anxiety. *Journal of Sex and Marital Therapy,* 1977, *3,* 243-248.

McCord, J. A thirty-year follow-up of treatment effects. *American Psychologist,* 1978, *33,* 284-289.

McCrary, J. L. *Sexual Myths and Fallacies.* New York: VanNostrand-Reinhold, 1971.

McFall, Richard M. 1970—Effects of self-monitoring on normal smoking behavior. *Journal of Consulting and Clinical Psychology* 35:135-142.

McFall, R. M., & Lillesand, D. B. 1971—Behavior Rehearsal with Modeling and Coaching in Assertion Training. *Journal of Abnormal Psychology,* 77:313-323.

McFall, R. & Marston, A. R. 1970—An experimental investigation of behavioral rehearsal in assertion training. *Journal of Abnormal Psychology* 76:295-303.

McHugh, G. *Marriage Counselor's Manual and Teacher's Handbook.* Saluda, New York: Plenum Press, 1968.

McMillan, Merna. 1977—Assertiveness as an Aid to Weight Control. In *Assertiveness: Innovations, Applications, Issues,* Robert E. Alberti, (Ed.), San Luis Obispo, CA: Impact.

McNees, M. P., Egli, D. S., Marshall, R. S., Schnelle, J. F., & Risley, T. R. 1976—Shoplifting Prevention: Providing Information Through Signs. *Journal of Applied Behavior Analysis* 9(4):399-405.

Meichenbaum, D. A cognitive-behavior modification approach to assessment. In M. Hersen & A. S. Bellack (Eds.), *Behavior assessment: A practical handbook.* New York: Pergamon Press, 1976.

Meichenbaum, D. *Cognitive-behavior modification: An integrative approach.* New York: Plenum Press, 1977.

Meichenbaum, D., & Cameron, R. The clinical potential of modifying what clients say to themselves. In M. J. Mahoney & C. E. Thoresen (Eds.), *Self-control: power to the person.* Monterey, California: Brooks/Cole, 1974.

Meichenbaum, D. & Goodman, J. 1971—Training Impulsive Children to Talk to Themselves: A Means of Developing Self-Control. *Journal of Abnormal Psychology,* 77, 115-126.

Mendels, Joseph 1970—*Concepts of Depression.* New York: Wiley.

Meyer, R. G. & Smith, S. S. 1977—A Crisis in Group Therapy. *American*

Psychologist 32:638-643.

Meyer, V. & Crisp, A. H. 1964—Aversion Therapy in Two Cases of Obesity. *Behaviour Research and Therapy* 2(2):143-147.

Meyers, A. W., & Schleser, R. Behavioral Community Psychology. In Behavior Modification: Principles, Issues, and Applications (2nd. ed.), W. E. Craighead, A. E. Kazdin, & M. J. Mahoney, eds. Boston: Houghton Mifflin, in press.

Miller, D. D. 1978—Children's services and Title XX from a national perspective. *Child Welfare* 57(2):134-139.

Miller, L. K., & Feallock, R. 1975—A Behavioral System for Group Living. In *Behavior Analysis: Areas of Research and Application,* Eugene Ramp and George Semb, (Eds.), Englewood Cliffs, NJ: Prentice Hall.

Miller, Peter M. 1978—Alternative Skills Training in Alcoholism Treatment. In *Alcoholism: New Directions in Behavioral Research and Treatment,* Peter E. Nathan, G. Alan Marlatt, and Tor Loberg, (Eds.), New York: Plenum.

Miller, P. M., Becker, J. V., Foy, D. W., & Wooten, L. S. 1976—Instructional Control of the Components of Alcoholic Drinking Behavior. *Behavior Therapy* 7(4):472-480.

Miller, P. M., & Hersen, M. 1972—Quantitative Changes in Alcohol Consumption as a Function of Electrical Aversive Conditioning. *Journal of Clinical Psychology* 28(4):590-593.

Miller, P. M., Hersen, M. Eisler, R. M., & Hilsman, G. 1974—Effectives of Social Stress on Operant Drinking of Alcoholics and Social Drinkers. *Behaviour Research and Therapy* 12(2):67-72.

Miller, William R. 1977—Behavioral Self-Control Training in the Treatment of Problem Drinkers. In *Behavioral Self-Management: Strategies, Techniques, and Outcomes,* Richard B. Stuart, ed. New York: Brunner/Mazel.

Miller, W. R., & Joyce, M. A. 1979—Prediction of Abstinence, Controlled Drinking, and Heavy Drinking Outcomes Following Behavioral Self-Control Training. *Journal of Consulting and Clinical Psychology* 47(4):773-775.

Mills, C., & Walter, T. L. 1979—Reducing Juvenile Delinquency: A Behavioral-Equipment Intervention Program. In *Progress in Behavior Therapy with Delinquents,* Jerome S. Stumphauzer, (Ed.), Springfield, Ill.: Charles C Thomas, 1979.

Mindick, B., Oskamp, S., & Berger, D. E. 1978—Prediction of Adolescent Contraceptive Practice. Paper presented at the annual meeting of the American Psychological Association, Toronto, August.

Minkin, N., Braukmann, C. J., Minkin, B. L., Timbers, G. D., Timbers, B. J., Fixsen, D. L., Phillips, E. L., & Wolf, M. M. 1976—The Social Validation and Training of Conversational Skills. *Journal of Applied Behavior Analysis,* 9:127-139.

Mischel, W. *Personality and assessment.* New York: Wiley, 1968.

Mischel, Walter 1975—The Self as the Person: A Cognitive Social Learning View. In A. Wandersman (ed.), *Behavioristic and Humanistic Approaches to*

Personality Change. New York: Pergamon Press.

Moore, N. Behavior therapy in bronchial asthma: A controled study. *Journal of Psychosomatic Research,* 1965, *9,* 257-276.

Morganstern, Kenneth P. 1974—Cigarettes Smoke as a Noxious Stimulus in Self-Managed Aversion Therapy for Compulsive Eating: Technique and Case Illustration. *Behavior Therapy* 5(2):255-260.

Morrow, W. R., & Wilson, R. C. 1965—Family relations of bright high-achieving and under-achieving high school boys. In *Underachievment,* Milton Kornrich, ed. Springfield, Ill.: Charles C. Thomas.

Mostofsky, D. & Balaschak, B. Psychobiological control of seizures. *Psychological Bulletin,* 1977, *84,* 723-750.

Mowrer, O. H. & Mowrer, W. M. 1938—Enuresis—A Method for Its Study and Treatment. *Journal of Orthopsychiatry* 8:436-459.

Mueller, D. J., & Atlas, L. Resocialization of regressed elderly residents: A behavioral management approach. *Journal of Gerontology,* 1972, *27*(3), 390-392.

Nagi, Saad Z. 1975—Child Abuse and Neglect Programs: A National Overview. *Children Today,* 4(3):13-17.

Nagi, Saad Z. 1977—*Child Maltreatment in the United States.* New York: Human Science Press.

Nathan, Peter E. 1978—Studies in Blood Alcohol Level Discrimination. In *Alcoholism: New Directions in Behavioral Research and Treatment,* Peter E. Nathan, G. Alan Marlatt, and Tor Loberg, (Eds.), New York: Plenum Press.

Nathan, P. E. & Lansky, D. 1978—Common Methodological Problems in Research on the Addictions. *Journal of Consulting and Clinical Psychology* 46(4):713-726.

National Association Of Attorneys General 1976—*Legal Issues in Foster Care.* Committee on the Office of Attorney General, 3901 Barrett Dr., Raleigh, North Carolina 27609.

Neisworth, J., & Moore, F. Operant treatment of asthmatic responding with the parent as therapist. *Behavior Therapy* 1972, *3,* 95-99.

Newman, E. & Turem, J. 1974—The Crisis of Accountability. *Social Work,* 19(1):5-16.

Newman, I.M. 1970—Peer Pressure Hypothesis for Adolescent Cigarette Smoking. *School Health Review,* 1(2):15-23.

Noble, Ernest P. 1978—*Third Special Report to the U.S. Congress on Alcohol and Health.* Washington, D.C.: U.S. Government Printing Office.

O'Conner, R.D. 1969—Modification of Social Withdrawal Through Symbolic Modeling. *Journal of Applied Behavior Analysis,* 2:15-22.

O'Dell, S. 1974—Training Parents in Behavior Modification: A Review. *Psychological Bulletin* 81(7):418-433.

O'Leary, D. D., Poulos, R. W., & Devine, V. T. 1972—Tangible Reinforcers: Bonuses or Bribes. *Journal of Consulting and Clinical Psychology* 38(1):1-8

O'Leary, D. E., O'Leary, M. R., & Donovan, D. M. 1976—Social Skill Acquisition and Psychosocial Development of Alcoholics: A Review.

Addictive Behaviors 1(2):111-120.

O'Leary, K. D., O'Leary, S., & Becker, W. C. 1967—Modification of a Deviant Sibling Interaction Pattern in the Home. *Behavior Research and Therapy* 5(2):113-120.

O'Leary, K. D., & Drabman, R. S. 1971—Token Reinforcement Programs in the Classroom. *Psychological Bulletin,* 75(6), 379-398.

O'Leary, K. D., O'Leary, S., & Becker, W. C. 1967—Modification of a Deviant Sibling Interaction Pattern in the Home. *Behavior Research and Therapy* 5:113-120.

O'Leary, K. D., & Wilson, G. T. 1975—*Behavior Therapy Applications and Outcome.* New Jersey: Prentice-Hall.

Osborn, S. M., & Harris, G. G. 1975—*Group Assertive Training for Women.* Springfield, Ill.: Charles C. Thomas.

Panyan, M., Boozer, H., & Morris, N. 1970—Feedback to Attendants as a Reinforcer for Applying Operant Techniques *Journal of Applied Behavior Analysis* 3(1):1-4

Papell, C.P. 1972—Sensitivity training: Relevance for social work education. *Journal of Education for Social Work* 8:42-55.

Parry-Jones, W., Santer-Westgate, J., & Crawley, H. Behavior Therapy in a case of hysterical blindness. *Behaviour Research & Therapy,* 1970, *8,* 79-85

Parsonson, B. S., & Baer, D. M. 1978—The Analysis and Presentation of Graphic Data. In *Single Subject Research: Strategies for Evaluating Change,* T. Kratochwill, (Ed.), New York: Academic Press.

Patterson, C., & Mischel, W. 1976—Effects of Temptation-Inhibiting and Task Facilitating Plans on Self-control. *Journal of Personality and Social Psychology* 33(2):209-217.

Patterson, Gerald R. 1971—Behavioral Intervention Procedures in the Classroom and in the Home. In *Handbook of Psychotherapy and Behavioral Change: An Empirical Analysis,* Allen E. Bergin and Sol L. Garfield (Eds.), New York: Wiley.

Patterson, Gerald R. 1971—*Families: Applications of Social Learning to Family Life.* Champaign, Ill.: Research Press.

Patterson, Gerald R. 1974—Intervention for Boys with Conduct Problems: Multiple Settings, Treatments, and Criteria. *Journal of Consulting and Clinical Psychology* 42: 471-481.

Patterson, Gerald R. 1971—*Families: Applications of Social Learning to Family Life.* (revised). Champaign, Ill.: Research Press, 1975.

Patterson, Gerald R. 1976—*Living With Children.* Champaign, Ill.: Research Press.

Patterson, G. R., Ray, R. S., & Shaw, D. A. 1968—Direct Intervention in Families of Deviant Children. *Oregon Research Institute Research Bulletin* 8(9).

Patterson, G. R., Ray, R. S., Shaw D. A., & Cobb, J. A. 1969—*Manual for Coding of Family Interactions,* sixth revision (Document NO. 01234) New

York: ASIS/NAPS, Microfiche Publications.

Patterson, G. R., Reid, J. B., Jones, R. R. & Conger, R. 1975—*Social Learning Approach to Family Intervention: Families With Aggressive Children.* Eugene: Castilia Publishing Company.

Paulson, M. J., Afifi, A. A., Thomason, M. L. & Chaleff, A. 1974—The MMPI: A Descriptive Measure of Psychopathology in Abusive Parents. *Journal of Clinical Psychology,* 30(3):387-390.

Paulson, M. J., Schwemer, G. T., Afifi, A. A., & Bendel, R. B. 1977—Parent Attitude Research Instrument (PARI) Clinical vs. Statistical Inferences in Understanding Abusive Mothers. *Journal of Clinical Psychology,* 33(3)848-854.

Pavlov, Ian P. 1928—*Lecturers on Conditioned Reflexes* (Translated by W.H. Grantt). New York: International.

Pelton, Leroy H. 1978—Child Abuse and Neglect: The Myth of Classlessness. *American Journal of Orthopsychiatry,* 48(4):608-617.

Phelps, S., & Austin, N. 1975—*The Assertive Woman.* San Luis Obispo: Impact.

Phillips, B.S. A role theory approach to adjustment in old age. *American Sociological Review,* 1957, *22,* 212-217.

Phillips, Elery L. 1968—Achievement Place: Token Reinforcement Procedures in a Home-Style Rehabilitation Setting for "Pre-Delinquent" Boys. *Journal of Applied Behavior Analysis* 1(3):213-223.

Phillips, E. L. Phillips, E. A., Fixsen, D. L., & Wolf, M. M. 1971—Achievement Place: Modification of the Behaviors of Pre-Delinquent Boys Within a Token Economy. *Journal of Applied Behavior Analysis* 4(1):45-59.

Phillips, E., Phillips, E. A., Wolf, M. M. & Fixsen, D. L. 1973—Achievement place: Development of the elected manager system. *Journal of Applied Behavior Analysis* 6:541-561.

Piaget, Jean 1963—*The Language and Thought of the child.* New York: Basic Books.

Pierce, C., & Risley, T. 1974—Improving Job Performance of Neighborhood Youth Corps Aides in an Urban Recreation Program. *Journal of Applied Behavior Analysis* 7(2):207-215.

Piliavin, I., & Briar, S. 1964—Police Encounters with Juveniles. *American Journal of Sociology,* 70:206-214.

Platt, J., Spivak, G., Altman, N., Altman, D., & Peizer, S. B. 1974—Adolescent Problem-Solving Thinking. *Journal of Consulting and Clinical Psychology,* 42(6):787-793.

Plummer, S., Baer, D. & Leblanc, J. 1977—Functional Considerations in the Use of Procedural Time Out and an Effective Alternative. *Journal of Applied Behavioral Analysis.* 10(4)689-705.

Polakow, R. L. Peabody, D. L. 1975—Behavioral Treatment of Child Abuse. *International Journal of Offender Therapy and Comparative Criminology,* 19(1):100-103.

Polich, J. M., Armor, D. J., & Braker, H. B. *Patterns of alcoholism over four* years. *Journal of Studies on Alcohol,* 1980, *41* 397-416.

Pomerleau, O. Behavioral medicine the contribution of the experimental analysis of behavior to medical care. *American Psychologist,* 1979, *34,* 654-663.

Poser, E. Issues in behavioral prevention and empirical findings. *Advances in Behaviour Research and Therapy,* 1979, *2,* 1-25.

Pothier, P.E. Patient compliance in therapy-bibliography. *Literature Search 75-12.* National Library of Medicine, 1975.

Premack, D. Reinforcement theory. In *Nebraska Symposium on Motivation,* D. Levine, ed., Lincoln: University of Nebraska Press, 1965.

Public Services Administration 1973—*A Guide to Protective Services for Abused and Neglected Children and Their Families.* New York: Community Research Applications, Inc.

Pumphrey, M. W., Goodman, M., & Flax, N. 1969—Integrating Individuals with Impaired Adaptive Behavior in a Group Work Agency. In *Social Work Practice 1969.* New York: Columbia University Press.

Purcell, K., & Weiss, J. Asthma. In *Symptoms of Psychopathology.* C. Costello, ed., New York: Wiley, 1970.

Quigley, M. E., Sheehan, K. L. Wilkes, M. M., & Yen, S. S. C. 1979—Effects of Maternal Smoking on Circulating Catecholamine Levels and Fetal Heart Rates. *American Journal of Obstetrics and Gynecology* 133(6):685-690.

Radin, Norma 1975—A personal perspective on school social work. *Social Casework* 56-605-613.

Radzinowicz, L. & Wolfgang, M. E. eds. 1971—*The Criminal in Confinement.* New York: Basic Books.

Rankin, H., Hodgson, R., & Stockwell, T. 1980—The Behavioural Measurement of Dependence. *British Journal of Addiction* 75(1):43-47.

Raths, L .E., Harmin, M., & Simon, S. B. *Values and teaching.* Columbus, Ohio: Charles E. Merrill Books, 1966.

Ravenberg, Ronald L. 1978—*Problem Oriented Record System.* Unpublished manuscript. Comprehensive Mental Health Center, Tacoma, WA.

Raymond, M.J. 1956—Case of Fetishism Treated by Aversion Therapy with Apomorphine. *Behavior Research and Therapy* 1(4):287-291.

Reavely, William and Marie-Therese Gilbert 1976—The Behavioural Treatment Approach to Potential Child Abuse Two Illustrative Case Reports. *Social Work Today,* 7(6):166-168.

Reckless, J. A behavioral treatment of bronchial asthma in modified group therapy. *Psychosomatics,* 1971, *12,* 178-183.

Reese, D., & Woolfenden R. *Conceptual Application of Elementary Principles of Behavior.* Kalamazoo, Michigan: Behaviordelia, Inc. 1973.

Rehm, Lynn P. and Albert R. Marston 1968—Reduction of social anxiety through modification of self-reinforcement: An instigation therapy technique. *Journal of Consulting and Clinical Psychology* 32:565-574.

Reid, John B. 1978—*A Social Learning Approach to Family Intervention, Volume 2: Observation in Home Settings.* Eugene, Ore.: Castalia, 1978.

Reid, John B. and Paul S. Taplin 1978—A Social Interactional Approach to the Treatment of Abusive Families. Unpublished manuscript.

Reid, William J. and Laura Epstein (eds.) 1977—*Task Centered Practice.* New York: Columbia University Press.

Reiss, M., Piotorwski, W., & Bailey, J. Behavioral community psychology: Encouraging low-income parents to seek dental care for their children. *Journal of Applied Behavior Analysis,* 1976, *9,* 387-397.

Repp, Alan C. and Deitz, Diane E. 1979—Improving Administrative-Related Staff Behaviors at a State Institution. *Mental Retardation* 17(3):185-192.

Reppucci, N. Dickon 1977—Implementation Issues for the Behavior Modifier as Institutional Change Agent. *Behavior Therapy* 8(4):594-605.

Reppucci, N. Dickon and Saunders, J. Terry 1974—Social Psychology of Behavior Modification: Problems of Implementation in Natural Settings. *American Psychologist* 29(9):649-660.

Resick, Patricia A. and Jerry J. Sweet 1979—Child Maltreatment and Intervention: Directions and Issues. *Journal of Social Issues,* 35(2):140-160.

Richey, C.A. 1975—Utilizing Self-Reinforcement in Group Assertion Training for Women: A Follow-Up Report. Paper presented at the Ninth Annual Convention of the Association for Advancement of Behavior Therapy, San Francisco.

Richmond, Mary E. 1922—*What is Social Casework? An Introductory Description.* New York: Russell Sage Foundation.

Rimm, Alfred A. and White, Philip L. 1977—Obesity: Its Risks and Hazards. In *Obesity in American,* George A. Bray, ed. Washington D.C.: U.S. Government Printing Office.

Rinn, R.C. and A. Markle 1979—Modification of Social Skill Deficits in Children. In *Research and Practice in Social Skills Training.* Alan S. Bellack and Michel Hersen, Eds. New York: Plenum.

Rinn, R.C. and Vernon, J.C. 1975—Process Evaluation of Outpatient Treatment in a Community Mental Health Center. *Journal of Therapy and Experimental Psychiatry* 6(1):5-11.

Risley, Todd R. 1975—Certify Procedures not People. In *Issues in Evaluating Behavior Modification,* W. Scott Wood, ed. Champaign, Ill.: Research Press.

Ritler, E. and L. Thome 1954—The gifted aren't delivering. *California Journal of Secondary Educaton* 29:480-482.

Roberts, Alan H. 1969—Self-control procedures in modification of smoking behavior: Replication. *Psychological Reports* 24:675-676.

Roberts, Maria 1979—Reciprocal Nature of Parent-Child Interaction: Implications for Child Maltreatment. *Child Welfare,* 58(6):383-392.

Robin, Arthur L. in press—Parent-Adolescent Conflict: A Skill Training Approach. In *Developing Social Competence: Programs for Children and Adults,* Diana P. Rathgen and J.P. Rathgen, Eds. New York: Plenum.

Robinson, Francis P. 1949—*Effective Study.* New York: Harper.

Robinson, John P., & Phillip R. Shaver 1973—*Measures of Social Psychological Attitudes.* Ann Arbor, Michigan: Survey Research Center, Institute for

Social Research, University of Michigan.

Roff, M.B. Sell and M.M. Golden 1972—*Social Adjustment and Personality Development in Children.* Minneapolis: University of Minnesota Press.

Rogers, Carl 1961—*On Becoming a Person: A Therapist's View of Psychotherapy.* Boston: Houghton/Mifflin.

Rogers, Carl and Skinner, B.F. 1956—Some Issues Concerning the Control of Human Behavior. A Symposium. *Science,* November 30.

Romans, J.T. 1979—The economic evaluation of mental health problems. In H.C. Schulberg and F. Baker (Eds.), *Program Evaluation in the Health Fields* (Vol. II). New York: Human Sciences.

Rose, S.D. 1972—*Treating Children in Groups.* San Francisco: Jossey-Bass.

Rose, S.D., 1977—*Group Therapy: A Behavioral Approach.* Englewood Cliffs, N.J.: Prentice-Hall.

Rose, S.D., Cayner, J.J. and Edleson, J.L. 1977—Measuring interpersonal competence. *Social Work* 22:125-129.

Rose, S.D., & Schinke, S.P. Assertive training. In H.H. Grayson & C. Loew (Eds.), *Changing approaches to the psychotherapies.* New York: Spectrum, 1978.

Rosenberg, Abraham. 1977—An Investigation into the Effect on Cigarette Smoking of a New Anti-Smoking Chewing Gum. *Journal of International Medical Research* 5(1):68-70.

Rosenthal, Ted L. and Albert Bandura 1978—Psychological Modeling: Theory and Practice. In *Handbook of Psychotherapy and Behavior Change,* 2nd edition. New York: John Wiley and Sons.

Rotter, Julian B. 1978—Generalized Expectancies for Problem Solving and Psychotherapy. *Cognitive Therapy and Research* 2(1):1-10.

Rowe, A., & Rowe, A. *Bronchial Asthma Its Diagnosis and Treatment.* Springfield, Ill.: Charles C. Thomas, 1963.

Roy, T. and R. Shields 1979—Alcohol Education in School Social Work. *Social Work in Education.* 1:43-53.

Rush, Augustus J., Aaron T. Beck, Maria Kovacs, and Steven Hollon 1977—Comparative Efficacy of Cognitive Therapy and Pharmacotherapy in the Treatment of Depressed Outpatients. *Cognitive Therapy and Research* 1(1):17-38.

Russell, M.A.H. and Feyerabend, C. 1975—Blood and Urinary Nicotine in Non-Smokers. *Lancet* 1(7900):179-181.

Russel, M.A.H., Raw, M., Taylor, C., Feyerabend, C., and Saloojee, Y. 1978—Blood Nicotine and Carboxyhemoglobin Levels After Rapid-Smoking Aversion Therapy. *Journal of Consulting and Clinical Psychology* 46(6):1423-1431.

Sackett, D.L., Haynes, R.B., Gibson, E.S., Taylor, D.W., Roberts R.S., & Johnson, A.L. Hypertension control, compliance and science. *American Heart Journal,* 1977, *94,* 666-667.

Sajwaj, T., Libet, J., & Agras, S. Lemon juice therapy: The control of life threatening rumination in a six-month-old infant. *Journal of Applied*

Behavior Analysis, 1974, *7,* 557-563.

Saltmarsh, R., & Hubele, G. Basic interaction behaviors: A microcounseling approach for introductory courses. *Counselor Education and Supervision,* 1974, *13,* 246-249.

Sanford, Donald A. and Richard D. Tustin 1973—Behavioral Treatment of Parental Assault on a Child. *New Zealand Psychologist,* 2(2):76-82.

Sarason, I.G. Text anxiety and cognitive modeling. *Journal of Personality and Social Psychology,* 1973, *28,* 58-61.

Sarason, Irwin G. and V.J. Ganzer 1971—Modeling: An Approach to the Rehabilitation of Juvenile Offenders (Final report to the Social Rehabilitation Service, Grant 15-P-55303). Washington, D.C.: DHEW.

Sarason, Irwin G. and V. J. Ganzer 1973—Modeling and Group Discussion in the Rehabilitation of Juvenile Delinquents. *Journal of Counseling Psychology.* 20:442-449.

Sargent, H., & Yorkston, N. Verbal desensitization in the treatment of bronchial asthma. *Lancet,* 1969, *7634,* 13 31-13 23.

Saunders, D.G. Marital violence: dimensions of the problems and modes of intervention. *Journal of Marriage and Family Counseling,* 1977, *3,* 43-52.

Savage, David G. 1976—Street academics. *Education Digest* 62:24-25.

Sayner, R., & Durrell, D. Multiple behavior therapy techniques in the treatment of sexual dysfunction. *Counseling Psychologist,* 1975, *5,* 38-40.

Schachter, Stanley. 1971—Some Extraordinary Facts About Obese Humans and Rats. *American Psychologist* 26(2):129-144.

Schachter, S., & Gross, L. P. 1968—Manipulated Time and Eating Behavior. *Journal of Personality and Social Psychology* 10(2):98-106.

Schinke, S.P. Bridging the accountability gap. *Practice Digest,* 1979, *1*(4), 28-29. (a)
cited: Prof. Competence & Accountability -1
17-14

Schinke, S.P. Evaluating social work practice: A conceptual model and example. *Social Casework,* 1979, *60,* 195-200. (b)
cited: Prof. Competence & Accountability-1

Schinke, S.P. Ethics. In R.W. Grinnell, Jr. (Ed.), *Social work research and evaluation.* Itasca, Ill.: F.E. Peacock, in press. (a)

Schinke, S. P., Blythe, B. J., & Doueck, H. J. Reducing cigarette smoking: Evaluation of a multifaceted intervention program. *Behavioral Engineering,* 1978, *4,* 107-112.

Schinke, S. P., Blythe, B. J., & Doueck, H. J. A broad-spectrum behavioral group approach to smoking reduction. In D. Upper & S.M. Ross (Eds.), *Behavioral group therapy, 1979: An annual review.* Champaign, Ill.: Research Press, 1979.

Schinke, S. P., & Gilchrist, L. D. Adolescent pregnancy: An interpersonal skill training approach to prevention. *Social Work in Health Care,* 1977, 999-167.

Schinke, S. P., Gilchrist, L. D., & Blythe, B. J. Interpersonal-skills training with teenagers at risk for unwanted pregnancy. *Health and Social Work,* 1980.

Schinke, S. P., Gilchrist, L. D., & Small, R. W. Preventing unwanted adolescent pregnancy: A cognitive-behavioral approach. *American Journal of Orthopsychiatry,* 1979, *49,* 81-88.

Schinke, S. P., Gilchrist, L. D., Smith, T. E., & Wong, S. E. Improving teenage mothers' ability to compete for jobs. *Social Work Research and Abstracts,* 1978, *14*(3), 25-29.

Schinke, S. P., Gilchrist, L. D., Smith, T. E., & Wong, S. E. Evaluation of contingency education effectiveness. *Journal of Education for Social Work,* in press.

Schinke, S. P., Smith, T. E., Gilchrist, L. D., & Wong, S. E. Assessing continuing education effectiveness. *Journal of Education for Social Work,* inpress.

Schinke, S. P., Smith, T. E., Gilchrist, L. D., & Wong, S. E. Interviewing-skills training: An empirical evaluation. *Journal of Social Service Research,* 1978, 1, 391-401.

Schinke, S. P., Smith, T. E., Meyers, A. K., and Altman, D. C. 1979—Crisis intervention training with paraprofessionals. *Journal of Community Psychology* 7(4):343-347.

Schinke, S. P., & Wong, S. E. Coding group home behavior with a continuous real-time recording device. *Behavioral Engineering,* 1977, *4,* 5-9. (a)

Schinke, S. P., & Wong, S. E. Evaluation of staff training in group homes for retarded persons. *American Journal of Mental Deficiency,* 1977, *3,*,, 000-137. (b)

Schinke, S. P., & Wong, S. E. 1978—Teaching Child Care Workers: A Behavioral Approach. *Child Care Quarterly* 7(1):45-61.

Schmahl, D. P., Lichtenstein, E., & Harris, D. E. 1972—Successful Treatment of Habitual Smokers with Warm, Smoky Air and Rapid Smoking. *Journal of Consulting and Clinical Psychology* 38(1):105-111.

Schneider, C., Hoffmeister J., & Helfer, R. 1976—A Predictive Screening Questionnaire for Potential Problems in Mother-Child Interaction. In *Child Abuse and Neglect, the Family and the Community.* R.H. Helfer and C.H. Kempe, (Eds.), Cambridge: Balager.

Schnelle, J. F., Kirschner, R. E., Galbaugh, F., Domash, M., Carr, A., & Larson, L. 1979—Program. Evaluation Research: An Experimental Cost Effectiveness Analysis of an Armed Robbery Intervention Program.*Journal of Applied Behavior Analysis* 12(4):615-623.

Schumacher, S., & Lloyd, C. W. Assessment of sexual dysfunction. In M. Hersen & A. S. Bellack (Eds.), *Behavioral assessment: A practical handbook.* New York: Pergamon Press, 1976.

Schwartz, A., & Goldiamond, I. 1975—*Social Casework: A Behavioral Approach.* New York: Columbia University Press.

Schwartz, R., & Gottman, J. 1974—*A Task Analysis Approach to Clinical Problems: A Study of Assertive Behavior.* Unpublished manuscript, Indiana University.

Schwartz, S.H. Words, deeds and the perception of consequences and responsibility in action situations. *Journal of Personality and Social Psychology*, 1968, *10*, 232-242.

Schwitzgebel, R., & Kolb, D. 1964—Inducing Behavior Change in Adolescent Delinquents. *Behavior Research and Therapy* 1(4):297-304.

Seaberg, J. R., Gillespie, D. F., Long, J., & Conte, J. 1975—Survey of Measures Available for Evaluation of Child Abuse and Neglect Demonstration Projects. Unpublished manuscript.

Seabury, Brett A. 1976—The Contract: Uses, Abuses, and Limitations. *Social Work*, 21 (1):16-21.

Seligman, Martin E.P. 1975—*Helplessness: On Depression, Development, and Death.* San Francisco: W.H. Freeman.

Shaw, Brian F. 1977—Comparison of Cognitive Therapy and Behavior Therapy in Treatment of Depression. *Journal of Consulting and Clinical Psychology* 45(4):543-551.

Shepard, D. S., & Thompson, M. S. 1979—First Principles of Cost-Effectiveness Analysis. *Public Health Reports* 94(6):535-543.

Sherif, M., & Sherif, W. *Social psychology.* New York: Harper and Row, 1969.

Sherman, E. A., Neuman, R., & Shyne, A. W. 1974—*Children Adrift in Foster Care: A Study of Alternative Approaches.* New York: Child Welfare League of America.

Sherwood, J.J. 1962—*Self-identity and Self-actualization: A Theory and Research.* Unpublished doctoral dissertation, University of Michigan.

Shorkey, Clayton T. 1979—A Review of Methods Used in the Treatment of Child Abuse. *Social Casework*, 60 (6):360-366.

Shrader, Carl 1979—Behavioral Group Therapy with Adolescents: A Review and Pilot Program. In *Behavioral Group Therapy, 1979: An Annual Review*, Dennis Upper and Steven M. Ross, (Eds.), Champaign, Ill.: Research Press.

Shyne, Ann E. 1969—*The Need for Foster Care.* New York: Child Welfare League of America.

Silverstein, S. J., Nathan, P. E., & Taylor, H. A. 1974—Blood Alcohol Level Estimation and Controlled Drinking by Chronic Alcoholics. *Behavior Therapy* 5(1):1-15.

Sirota, A., & Mahoney, M. Relaxing on cue: the self regulation of asthma. *Journal of Behavior Therapy & Experimental Psychiatry*, 1974, *5*, 65-66.

Skinner, B.F. 1953-*Science and Human Behavior.* New York: Macmillan.

Slavin, R. E., & Wodarski, J. S. 1978—Peer Tutoring and Student Teams. Center for Social Organization of Schools. The Johns Hopkins University, forthcoming.

Sluzki, C. Marriage therapy from a system theory perspective. In *Marriage and Marital Therapy: Psychoanalytic, Behavioral and Systems Theory Perspectives.* T.J. Paolina, & B.S. McCrady, (Eds.), New York: Brunner/Mazel, 1978.

Small, R. W. & Schinke, S. P. 1979—Cognitive-Behavioral Training for Preadolescents in Residential Treatment. Paper presented at the Association for Advancement of Behavior Therapy, San Francisco.

Smart, R. G., Gray, G. & Bennett, C. 1978—Predictors of Drinking and Signs of Heavy Drinking Among High School Students. *The International Journal of the Addictions,* 13:1079-1094.

Sobell, L. C., Maisto, S. A., Sobell, M. B., & Cooper, A. M. 1979—Reliability of Alcohol Abusers' Self-Reports of Drinking Behavior. *Behaviour Research and Therapy* 17(2):157-160.

Sobell, M. B., & Sobell, L. C. 1975—A Brief Technical Report on the Mobat: An Inexpensive Portable Test for Determining Blood Alcohol Concentration. *Journal of Applied Behavior Analysis* 8(1):117-120.

Sobell, M. B., & Sobell, L. C. 1976—Assessment of Addictive Behavior. In *Behavioral Assessment: A Practical Handbook,* Michel Hersen and Alan S. Bellack, (Eds.), Oxford: Pergamon Press.

Sobell, M. B., & Sobell, L. C. 1978—*Behavioral Treatment of Alcohol Problems: Individualized Therapy and Controlled Drinking.* New York: Plenum Press.

Spitzer, R. L., & Endicott, J. 1975—*Schedule for Affective Disorders and Schizophrenia.* NIMH Clinical Research Branch Collaborative Program on the Psychobiology of Depression. Unpublished manuscript.

Spitzford, Marianne 1978—*Cognitive Behavior Therapy with Depressed Women.* Unpublished dissertation proposal, University of Washington, Seattle, Washington.

Spivack, G., Platt, J., & Shure, M. 1976—*The Problem Solving Approach to Adjustment.* San Francisco: Jossey-Bass.

Staats, A. W., & Butterfield, W. H. 1965—Treatment of Nonreading in a Culturally Deprived Juvenile Delinquent: An Application of Reinforcement Principles. *Child Development* 36(4):925-942.

Staddon, J. Operant behavior as adaptations to constraint. *Journal of Experimental Psychology,* 1979, *108,* 48-67.

Stanton, A. H., & Schwartz, M. S. *The mental hospital.* New York: Basic Books, 1954.

Stanulis, R., & Glaros, A. Preventing iatrogenic illness: A critique of Johnson & Meyer. *Journal of Behavior Therapy and Experimental Psychiatry,* 1976, *7,* 309.

Steele, B. F., & Pollock, C. B. 1974—A Psychiatric Study of Parents Who Abuse Infants and Small Children. In *The Battered Child.* Ray E. Helfer and C. Henry Kempe, (Eds.), Chicago: The University of Chicago Press.

Steffy, R. A., Meichenbaum, D., & Best, J. A. 1970—Aversive and Cognitive Factors in the Modification of Smoking Behaviour. *Behaviour Research and Therapy* 8(2):115-125.

Steine, T. J., Gambrell, E. D., & Wiltse, K. T. *Children in Foster Homes: Achieving Continuity in Care.* New York: Praeger in press.

Stevenson, Kay M. 1978—Obesity Treatment: Research and Application. *Social Work in Health Care* 4(2):165-178.

Stokes, T., & Baer, D. M. 1977—An Implicit Technology of Generalization.

Journal of Applied Behavior Analysis, 10:349-367.

Stollak, Gary E. 1967—Weight Loss Obtained Under Different Experimental Procedures. *Psychotherapy: Theory, Research and Practice* 4(2):61-64.

Strayhorn, Joseph M. Jr. 1977—*Talking It Out: A Guide to Effective Communication and Problem Solving.* Champaign, Ill.: Research Press.

Strupp, Hans H. 1978—Psychotherapy Research and Practice: An Overview. In *Handbook of Psychotherapy and Behavior Change: An Empirical Analysis,* Sol L. Garfield and Allen E. Bergin, (Eds.), New York: Wiley.

Strupp, Hans H. 1979—A Psychodynamicist Looks at Modern Behavior Therapy *Psychotherapy: Theory, Research and Practice* 16(2):124-131.

Stuart, R. B., & Davis, B. 1972—*Slim Chance in a Fat World: Behavioral Control of Obesity.* Champaign, Ill.: Research Press.

Stuart, R. B., & Stuart, F. *The Marital Pre-Counseling Inventory.* Champaign, Ill.: Research Press, 1972.

Stuart, Richard B. and Freida Stuart 1975—*Family Pre-Counseling Inventory Program.* Champaign, Ill.: Research Press.

Stumphauzer, J., (Ed.), 1973—*Behavior Therapy with Delinquents.* Springfield, Ill.: Charles C. Thomas.

Stumphauzer, J.S. 1976—Modifying Delinquent Behavior: Beginnings and Current Practices. *Adolescence,* 41:13-28.

Stunkard, Albert 1972—New therapies for the eating disorders: Behavior modification of obesity and anorexia nervosa. *Archives of General Psychiatry* 26:391-398.

Sutherland, A., Amit, Z., Golden, M., & Roseberger, Z., 1975— Comparison of Three Behavioral Techniques in the Modification of Smoking Behavior. *Journal of Consulting and Clinical Psychology* 43(4):443-447.

Taylor, C., Farquhar, J., Nelson, E., & Agras, D. Relaxation therapy and high blood pressure. *Archives of General Psychiatry,* 1977, *34,* 339-343.

Taylor, F. G., & Marshall, W. L. 1977—Experimental Analysis of a Cognitive-Behavioral Therapy for Depression. *Cognitive Therapy and Research* 1(1):59-72.

Tharp, R. G., & Wetzel, R. J. 1969—*Behavior Modification in the Natural Environment.* New York: Academic Press.

Thomas, E. Uses of research methods in interpersonal practice. In N. Polansky (Ed.), *Social Work Research.* Chicago: The University of Chicago Press, 1975.

Thomas, E. J. Mousetraps, developmental research and social work education. *Social Service Review,* 1978, *52,* 116-121.

Thomas, E. J., & Walter, C. L. 1973—Guidelines for Behavioral Practice in the Open Community Agency: Procedure and Evaluation. *Behaviour Research and Therapy* 11(2):193-205.

Thomas, Lewis 1977—On the Science and Technology of Medicine. In *Doing Better and Feeling Worse: Health in the United States,* John H. Knowles, (Ed.), New York: W.W. Norton.

Thomas, William V. 1977—Obesity and Health. In *Editorial Research Reports on National Health Issues,* Hoyt Gimlin, (Ed.), Washington, D.C.: Congressional

Quarterly, Inc.

Thoresen, Carl E. in press—*Let's Get Intensive: Studying Change Over Time.* Englewood Cliffs: Prentice-Hall.

Thoresen, C. E., & Mahoney, M. L. *Behavioral self-control.* New York: Holt, Rinehart and Winston, 1974.

Timberlake, W., & Allison, J. Deprivation: An empirical approach to instrumental performance. *Psychological Review,* 1974, *81,* 146-164.

Tobias, J. Vocational adjustment of young retarded adults. *Mental Retardation,* 1970, *8,* 13-16.

Tompkins, Silvan A. 1968—A Modified Model of Smoking Behavior. In *Smoking, Health and Behavior,* Edgar F. Borgatta and Robert R. Evans, (Eds.), Chicago: Aldine.

Tori, C., & Worell, L. Reduction of human avoidant behavior: A comparison of counter conditioning, expectance and cognitive information approaches. *Journal of Consulting and Clinical Psychology,* 1973, *41,* 269-278.

Tracy, J. J., & Clark, E. H. 1974—Treatment of Child Abusers. *Social Work.* 19(3):338-342.

Truax, Charles B. 1966—Reinforcement and Non-Reinforcement in Rogerian Psychotherapy. *Journal of Abnormal and Social Psychology* 71(1):1-9.

Truax, C. B., & Carkuff, R. R. 1967—*Toward Effective Counseling and Psychotherapy: Training and Practice.* Chicago: Aldine.

Truax, C. B., & Mitchell, K. M. 1971—Research on certain therapist interpersonnal skills in relation to process and outcome. In *Handbook of Psychotherapy and Behavior Change: An Empirical Analysis,* A.R. Bergin and S.L. Garfield, (Eds.), New York: John Wiley and Sons.

Trupin, E. W., Gilchrist, L., Mairuo, R. D., & Fay, G. 1979—Social Skills Training for Learning Disabled Children. In *Behavioral Systems for the Developmentally Disabled: II. Institutional Clinic, and Community Environments.* New York: Brunner/Mazel.

Turkat, I. D., & Fuerstein, M. 1978—Behavior Modification and the Public Misconception. *American Psychologist* 33(2):194.

U.S. News and World Report 1976—2.4 million children who aren't in school, *U.S. News and World Report* 80:43-44.

Van Hasselt, V., Hersen, M., Whitehill, M.B., & Bellack, A. S. 1979—Social Skill Assessment and Training for Children: An Evaluative Review. *Behavior Research and Therapy,* 17:413-437.

Voegtlin, Walter L. 1940—The Treatment of Alcoholism by Establishing a Conditioned Reflex. *American Journal of the Medical Sciences* 199(6):802-810.

Vogler, R. E., Weissbach, T. A., Compton, J. V., & Martin, G. T. 1977—Integrated Behavior Change Techniques for Problem Drinkers in the Community. *Journal of Consulting and Clinical Psychology* 45(2):267-279.

Wahler, R. G., Winkler, G. H., Peterson, R. F., & Morrison, D. C. 1965—Mothers as Behavior Therapists for Their Own Children. *Behaviour Research and Therapy* 3:133-124.

Walen, S., Hausesrman, N., & Lavin, P. *Clinical Guide to Behavior Therapy.* Baltimore: Williams & Wilkins, 1977.

Walker, R.A. 1969—"Pounce": Learning Responsibility for One's Own Employment Problems. In *Behavioral Counseling: Cases and Techniques,* John D. Krumboltz and Carl E. Thoresen, (Eds.), New York: Holt, Rinehart and Winston.

Walsh, B. R., & Steggs, E. N. 1972—Group counseling for underachievers. *Clearing House* 46:496.

Ward, J. H., Jr., & Jennings, E. *Introducing to linear models.* Englewood Cliffs, New Jersey: Prentice-Hall, 1973.

Warren, M.Q. Correctional Treatment in Community Settings: A Report of Current Research. Paper presented at Sixth International Congress on Criminology, September 1970, Madrid, Spain.

Watson, D., & Friend, R. 1969—Measurement of Social-Evaluative Anxiety. *Journal of Consulting and Clinical Psychology* 33(4):448-457.

Wayne, Julianne L. 1979—A Group Work Model to Reach Isolated Mothers: Preventing Child Abuse. *Social Work With Groups,* 2 (1):7-18.

Weed, Lawrence L. 1971—*Medical Records, Medical Education, and Patient Care.* Cleveland: Case Western Reserve University Press.

Weiss, R. L., Hops, H., & Patterson, G. R. A framework for conceptualizing marital conflict: A technology for altering it. In *Behavior Change: Methodology, Concepts and Practice.* L.A. Hamerlynck, L.C. Handy, & E.J. Mash, (Eds.). Champaign, Illinois: Research Press, 1973.

Weiss, T., & Engel, B. Operant conditioning of heart rate in patients with premature ventricular contractions. *Psychosomatic Medicine,* 1971, *33,* 301-321.

Weissman, M. M., & Paykel, E. S. 1974—*The Depressed Woman: A Study of Social Relationships.* Chicago: University of Chicago Press.

Welch, G.B. Increasing compliance with structured sexual exercises: An experimental study. Paper presented at the 4th World Congress of Sexology, December 16-21, 1979, Mexico City, Mexico.

Wellington, C. B., & Wellington, J. 1968—*The Underachiever: Challenge and Guidelines.* Chicago: Rand McNally.

Wells, R.A. 1975—Training in facilitative skills. *Social Work* 20:242-243.

Welner, Z., Welner, A., & Robbins, E. 1977—Child Abuse: A Case for a Different Approach. *Comprehensive Psychiatry.* 18 (4):363-368.

Werner, J. S., Phillips, E. L., Minkin, N., Minkin, B. L., Fixsen, D. L., & Wolf, M. M. 1975—Intervention Package: An Analysis to Prepare Juvenile Delinquents for Encounters with Police Officers. *Criminal Justice and Behavior,* 2(1):55-84.

West, D. W., Graham, S., Swanson, M., & Wilkinson, G. 1977—Five Year Follow-Up of a Smoking Withdrawal Clinic Population. *American Journal of Public Health* 67(6):536-544.

Whaley, D., & Mallott, R. *Elementary Principles of Behavior.* New York: Appleton Century Crofts, 1973.

Whittaker, James K. 1970—Training Child Care Staff: Pitfalls and Promises. *Mental Hygiene* 54(4):516-519.

Whittaker, James K. 1974—*Social Treatment: An Approach to Interpersonal Helping.* Chicago: Aldine.

Whittaker, James K. 1975—The Ecology of Child Treatment: A Developmental/Educational Approach to the Therapeutic Milieu. *Journal of Autism and Childhood Schizophrenia* 5(3):223-237.

Whittaker, James K. 1979—*Caring for Troubled Children: Residential Treatment in a Community Context.* San Francisco: Jossey-Bass.

Williams, Carl D. 1959—The Elimination of Tantrum Behavior by Extinction Procedures. *Journal of Abnormal and Social Psychology* 59:269.

Willner, A. G., Braukmann, C. J., Kirigin, K. A., Fixsen, D. L., Phillips, E. L., & Wolf, M. M. 1977—The Training and Validation of Youth-Preferred Social Behaviors of Child-Care Personnel. *Journal of Applied Behavior Analysis* 10(2):219-230.

Wilson, G. Terence. 1978—Alcoholism and Aversion Therapy: Issues, Ethics, and Evidence. In *Behavioral Approaches to Alcoholism,* G. Alan Marlatt and Peter E. Nathan, (Eds.), New Brunswick, NJ: Rutgers Center of Alcohol Studies.

Wilson, G. T., & Davidson, G. C. 1969—Aversion Techniques in Behavior Therapy: Some Theoretical and Metatheoretical Considerations. *Journal of Consulting and Clinical Psychology* 33(3):327-329.

Wilson, R. C., & Morrow, W. R. 1965—School and career adjustment of bright high-achieving and under-achieving high school boys. In *Underachievement,* Milton Kornrich, (Ed.), Springfield, Ill.: Charles C. Thomas.

Winett, R. A. & Nietzel, M. T. 1975—Behavioral Ecology: Contingency Management of Consumer Energy Use. *American Journal of Community Psychology* 3(2):123-133.

Witkin, S. L., & Caynor, J. Communication and problem-solving skills training for couples: A case study. *In A Case Book in Group Therapy.* S.D. Rose (Ed.). Englewood Cliffs: Prentice-Hall, 1980.

Witkin, S. L., Shapiro, C. H., & McCall, M. In-service training in public welfare: Evaluation issues. *Public Welfare* (in press).

Wodarski, John S. 1976—Procedural Steps in the Implementation of Behavior Modification Programs in Open Settings. *Journal of Behavior Therapy and Experimental Psychiatry* 7(2):133-136.

Wodarski, J.S. 1978—The Prediction of Anti-Social Behavior: An Application of Regression Analysis. In *Corrective and Social Psychiatry,* in press.

Wodarski, J.S., & Feldman, R. A. 1975—Practical Aspects of Field Research. *Clinical Social Work Journal* 2(3): 182-193.

Wodarski, J. S., Feldman, R. A., & Pedi, S. J. 1976—Reduction of Anti-Social Behavior in an Open Community Setting Through the Use of Behavior Modification in Groups. *Child Care Quarterly* 5(3):198-210.

Wolf, Montrose, E. 1978—Social Validity: The Case for Subjective Measurement or How Applied Behavior Analysis is Finding its Hart. *Journal of Applied Behavior Analysis* 11(2):203-214.

Wolf, M., Birnbrauer, J., Williams, T., & Lawler, J. A note on apparent extinction of vomiting behavior of a retarded child. In *Case Studies in Behavior Modification.* L. Ullman & L. Krasner, (Eds.), New York: Holt, Rinehart & Winston, 1965.

Wolf, M. M., Phillips, E. L., Fixsen, D. L., Braukmann, C. J., Kirigin, K. A., Willner, A. G., & Schumaker, J. 1976—Achievement Place: The Teaching-Family Model. *Child Care Quarterly* 5(2):92-103.

Wolpe, J. *The Practice of Behavior Therapy.* New York: Pergamon Press, 1973.

Wood, D. D., Callahan, E. J., Alevizos P. N., & Teigen, J. R. 1977—A Behaviorally Based Logbook. *Journal of Applied Behavior Analysis,* 10 (4):706.

Author Index

Subject Index

www.ingramcontent.com/pod-product-compliance
Lightning Source LLC
LaVergne TN
LVHW102225300926
849160LV00005B/32
9780202362144